SOTHIS PRESS

Sothis Press aims to completely reimagine the public domain book with an emphasis on universal access to captivatingly designed print editions. We believe that technology will enable every single book ever published to be perpetually accessible in beautiful print form. Sothis is beauty in ubiquity.

www.sothis.press
1 Waterhouse Square, London, ECIN 2ST

An English Translation of the Sushruta Samhita

With a Full and Comprehensive Introduction, Additional Text, Different Readings, Notes, Comparative Views, Index, Glossary and Plates, Vol. 3 of 3

Kaviraj Kunja Lal Bhishagratna

SOTHIS PRESS

ISBN 978-1-83548-215-5

This edition is published by Sothis Press © 2023. The company is registered in England and Wales. The Company Number is 14900389.

AN ENGLISH TRANSLATION

OF

THE SUSHRUTA SAMHITA

Vol. III.

UTTARA-TANTRA

AN ENGLISH TRANSLATION

OF

THE SUSHRUTA SAMHITA

WITH

A FULL AND COMPREHENSIVE INTRODUCTION, ADDITIONAL TEXTS, DIFFERENT READINGS, NOTES, COMPARATIVE VIEWS, INDEX, GLOSSARY AND PLATES

(IN THREE VOLUMES)

EDITED BY

KAVIRAJ KUNJA LAL BHISHAGRATNA,
M. R. A. S. (LOND.)

Vol. III.

UTTARA-TANTRA

———:-:———

PUBLISHED BY

S. L. BHADURI, B. L

10, KASHI GHOSE'S LANE, CALCUTTA

1916

PRINTED AT THE BHARAT MIHIR PRESS BY M. BHATTACHARYYA OF
Messrs. SANYAL & Co.,
25, ROY BAGAN STREET, CALCUTTA.

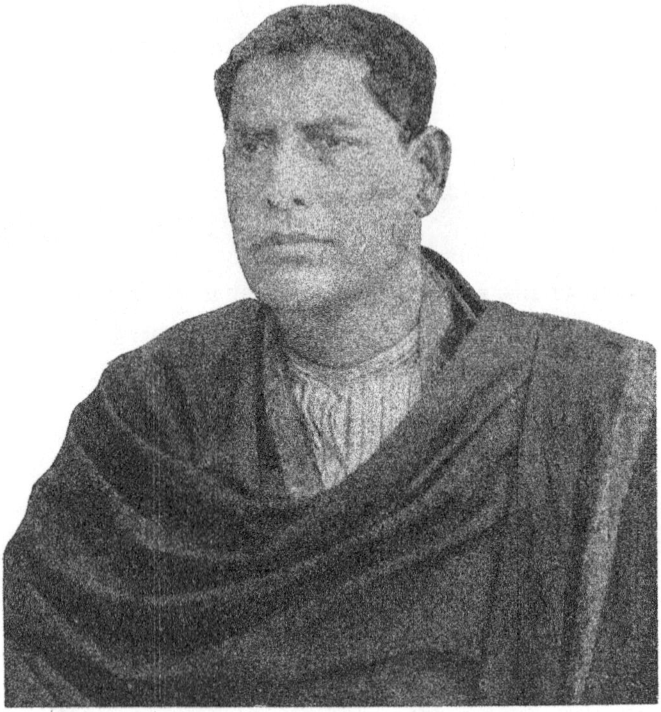

Kaviraj Kunja Lall Bhishgratna, M.R.A.S. (Lond.)

PREFACE.

It was some years ago that we took upon ourselves the rather ambitious task of bringing out the Sushruta Samhitá in English. And we may mention that the appreciation the first instalment of our undertaking met with at the hands of scholars at home and abroad considerably encouraged us in completing this huge undertaking.

We desire to record here our deepest feelings of gratitude towards His Highness the Maharaja Sir Sawai Jai Singh Bahadoor, K. C. S. I., of Alwar (Rajputana), who has, by his princely donation, enabled us to bring this highly important work to a completion. It is known throughout India that the illustrious Ruler of Alwar is a great patron of letters and a lover of Ayurvedic Science, and many noble undertakings in our country have depended largely upon his liberal support. No words of mine can adequately express my admiration for the good he is doing to our country.

Now that the whole work is before the public, its worth and importance will be duly judged Our translation does not claim to have any literary excellence, as our sole aim has been to render as faithfully as we could the original into one of the European languages. The technical terms occurring in the Sushruta Samhitá cannot be accurately translated into English, as there are no corresponding words in that language which would convey the exact meaning of the original. We have therefore retained the Sanskrit terms, and have in some cases put within brackets such English words as may approximately render the meaning of the original.

No apology is needed for placing before the learned world of the West a scientific treatise of ancient India. We may only mention that the Hindu system of medicine is not a thing of mere antiquarian interest. It is a living system, and even to-day millions of people in India are being treated according to this system. A system which has stood the test of centuries, and which still holds its own against rival systems of the day, cannot be lightly brushed aside as wholly unscientific. It has been said that a system which recognises prayer as one of the means of curing human ailments, can lay no claim to any scientific character. All that we need say in answer to this criticism is that humanity has not yet risen above prayer in any country in the world, and faith in the efficacy of prayer in curing diseases is, instead of dying out, gaining ground in the modern scientific world. Whatever that may be, in actual practice, Hindu medical men, like their brethren of Europe, rely chiefly upon medicine and surgery, but occasionally prescribe prayer also as an efficient form of remedy. While recognising the influence of mind on body, and the efficacy of faith in certain forms of disease, they treat it as a special method, falling more properly within the province of priests.

A few words, however, seem necessary to show what abiding interest there is for all time in such a work as the Sushruta Samhitá. We do not wish to enter into any historical criticism to prove that the different systems of medicine in other countries, new or old, have received more than a mere stimulus from the Indian System, and that many foreign discoveries may be traced to the work we are now presenting to the world. The opinions of some modern men of science, who cannot be accused of having any bias in favour of our system, will demonstrate its abiding value.

Surgeon General Sir Pardey Lukis, M. D., I. M. S., K. C. S. I., Director-General of Indian Medical Service, was pleased to remark in the course of his speech in the Imperial Legislative Council :—" Many of the so-called discoveries of recent years are merely *re-discoveries* of the facts known centuries ago to the ancients (Indians)." In noticing the first volume of this very work, the British Medical Journal observed in its issue of November, 1912 :—"It is certain that in this ancient medical book there are traces of knowledge which is comparatively recent in the West."

We do not know what reception will be accorded to this work by the public, but we may fairly hope that now that the ancient Indian Medical System and the Indigenous Drugs of this country are being investigated by scientific experts under the direction of the Government of India, this ancient system of Medicine and Surgery will attract the attention of those who have hitherto neglected it as unworthy of notice.

The encouragement which we have received from the Governments of Bengal and Nepal and from the States of Baroda and Mysore, has helped us a great deal and we take this opportunity of expressing our gratitude towards them. The active help extended to us in the preparation of this work by Vaidyaratna Kaviraj Jogindra Nath Sen, Vidyabhusan, M. A., Kaviraj Madhav Chandra Tarkatirtha, Kaviraj Jnanendranath Sen, Kaviratna, B. A., Prof. Satyendranath Sen, Vidyávágis'a, M. A., and Babu Sachindralal Bhaduri, B. A., B. L., we also specially and thankfully acknowledge. We offer our sincerest thanks also to Dr. U. D. Banerjee, L. R. C. P., M. R. C. S. Dr. Y. M. Bose, M. D. (Chicago), and Kaviraj Surendranath Goswami, Vidyavinode, B. A., L. M. S. who have never failed to give us their valuable suggestions whenever we have sought their advice.

10, KASHI GHOSE'S LANE,
CALCUTTA,
May 25, 1916.

KUNJA LAL BHISHAGRATNA.

CONTENTS.

(UTTARA-TANTRA.)

CHAPTER I.

CHAPTER II.

CHAPTER III.

CHAPTER IV.

CHAPTER V.

CHAPTER VI.

CHAPTER VII.

CHAPTER VIII.

CHAPTER IX.

CHAPTER X.

CHAPTER XI.

CHAPTER XII.

CHAPTER XIII.

CHAPTER XIV.

CHAPTER XV.

CHAPTER XVI.

CHAPTER XVII.

CHAPTER XVIII.

CHAPTER XIX.

CHAPTER XX.

CHAPTER XXI.

CHAPTER XXII.

CHAPTER XXIII.

CHAPTER XXIV.

CHAPTER XXV.

CHAPTER XXVI.

Here ends the Śálákya-Tantra.

CHAPTER XXVII.

CHAPTER XXVIII.

CHAPTER XXIX.

CHAPTER XXX.

CONTENTS.

CHAPTER XXXIX.

CHAPTER XL.

CHAPTER XLI.

CHAPTER XLII.

CHAPTER XLIII.

CHAPTER XLIV.

CHAPTER XLV.

CHAPTER XLVI.

CHAPTER XLVII.

CHAPTER XLVIII.

CHAPTER XLIX.

CHAPTER L.

CHAPTER LI.

CHAPTER LII.

CHAPTER LIII.

CHAPTER LIV.

CHAPTER LV.

CHAPTER LVI.

CHAPTER LVII.

CHAPTER LVIII.

CHAPTER LIX.

Here ends the Káya-chikitsá.

CHAPTER LX.

CHAPTER LXI.

CHAPTER LXII.

Here ends the Bhuta-Vidyá-Tantra.

CHAPTER LXIII.

CHAPTER LXIV.

CHAPTER LXV.

CHAPTER LXVI.

End of the Contents of the Uttara-Tantra.

—:o:—

ओं

THE

SUSHRUTA SAMHITÁ.

UTTARA-TANTARAM.

(SUPPLEMENTARY PART OF THE TREATISE).

—:o:—

CHAPTER I.

Now we shall discourse on the chapter which deals with the diseases, viz., of the eye, etc. **(Aupadravikam adhyayam).** 1.

Here commences that portion of the Sus'ruta Samhitá which is known as the Uttara Tantra (the supplementary part) to which references have been often made in the preceding one hundred and twenty chapters, as the fit place wherein to revert in detail to the topics cursorily mentioned therein. This part comprises within it the specific descriptions of a large and a varied number of diseases, viz., those which form the subject matter of the **S'ála'kya-Tantra** (Diseases of the eye, ear, nose and throat) as narrated by the king of Videha; the ætiology and symptomatology, etc. of diseases peculiar to infants and women (**Kaumára-bhritya**), the pathology, etc., of those diseases mentioned in the six books of the Practice of Medicine par excellence (**Ka'ya-chikitsa'**) compiled by the holy sages of old and diseases known as Upasarga (*e.g.* Bhutopasarga

—Demonology) as well as diseases of traumatic origin are also included in this supplementary text*. Herein are also mentioned the sixty-three combinations of the six different Rasas (tasces) as well as the laws of health and hygiene with their rationale (rules, interpretation and reasonings) and the classifications of different Doshas and organic principles of the body and various accessories and remedial agents required for their successful treatment and cure. 2.

I shall now begin with the description of the numbers, the pathology and the curability or incurability of those specific ailments of the body which are peculiar to the region of the head out of a myriad of other distempers reserved for treatment in this portion of the work (Uttara-tantra) which may be compared to the unfathomable deep in respect of the vastness of its depth and magnitude. 3.

Diseases of the eye and its appendages :—The eye-ball (Nayana-Budbuda) is two fingers (about an inch) in transverse diameter, about the breadth of one's own thumb in depth (Sagittal diameter), and two fingers and a half all round (in circumference). The eye-ball is almost round in shape and resembles the teat of a cow. It is made up of all the (five) elements of which the universe is built up. The element of the 'solid' earth (Bhu) contributes to the formation of its muscles, the element of 'heat' (Agni or Tejas) is in the blood (that courses in its veins and arteries), 'the gaseous element' (Vãyu) contributes to the formation of the black part (Iris, etc.) in which the pupil is situated, the fluid element (Jala) preponderates in the lucid

(1) The text has A'gantuka (traumatic diseases). Gayadãsa explains it to mean Apasmára, Unmáda, etc. (Hysteria, insanity, etc.).

(white) part (Vitreous body) and the void (ethereal) Space (Âkâs'a) is there to form lachrymal or the other ducts or sacs (As'rumârga) through which the secretions are discharged. 4.

I shall now proceed to describe the Drishti (the central part of Retina—'Macula Lutea') as set forth by expert ophthalmic physicians. The black portion of the eye (Krishna-mandala—Choroid) forms one third part of its whole extent while the Drishti, according to them, occupies only one-seventh part of the Krishna-mandala. The Mandalas or sub-divisions or circles of the eye-ball, the Sandhis or Joints (parts where these sub-divisions meet with one another) and the Patalas (layers or coats) of the eye are respectively five, six and six in number. 5-6.

Mandala and Sandhi :—The **Mandalas** of the eye are the following, viz., (1) the Pakshma-mandala (the circle of the eye-lashes), (2) the Vartma-mandala (the eye-lid) (3) the Śveta-mandala (the Sclerotic and Cornea), the Krishna-mandala (the choroid) and (4) the Drishti-mandala (the pupil). These circles are so arranged that the one preceding lies within the next in the list.* The **Sandhis** (which serve as lines of demarcation of the circles) already pointed out are six in number, the first binding the eye-lashes (Paksha-mandala) with the eye-lids (Vartma-mandala), the second the eye-lids and the Sclerotic coat (Śveta-mandala), the third binding the latter with the Krishna-mandala (choroid), the fourth situated between the latter and the Drishti-mandala, the fifth lying in the interior corner (Kaninakas) and the last (sixth) in the exterior (posterior) corner (Apángas) of the eye. 7-8.

* Evidently some line or lines are missing here as the line cannot give a complete sense by itself. Ed.

The Patalas :—Of the Patalas, two are in the eye-lid (Vartma-mandala) and four in the eye proper, wherein occurs the dreadful disease known as the Timira (loss of vision). Of these four the first or anterior coat (Patala) supports the humour Jala and light (Tejas), * the second coat or Patala (choroid) is supported by muscles ; the third coat or Patala (Sceroim and Cornea) consists of Medas (lit. fat) and there is the fourth which is a fifth part of the whole and is known as the Drishti. There are, however, divisions and sub-divisions of these coats. 9.

The different parts of the eye-ball are held together by the blood-vessels, the muscles, the Vitreous body and the choroid.† Beyond the choroid, the eye-ball is held (in the orbit) by a mass of Śleshmá (viscid substance—capsule of Tenon) supported by a number of vessels. The deranged Doshas which pass upward to the region of the eyes through the channels of the up-coursing veins and nerves give rise to a good many dreadful diseases in that region. 10.

Purva-rupa, etc. :—Cloudiness of vision, slight inflammation, lachrymation, mucous accumulation, heaviness, burning sensation, sucking pain (D. R.-aching pain) and redness in the eyes are indistinctly manifest (in the incubatory stage) in such cases. In cases of an inflammation of the Vartmas (eye-lids) the eye seems as if studded with the bristles of worms (Śuka) and attended with pain (as if pricked into with thorns) and a sensible impairment of the faculty of the eyes in detecting

* By "Jala" is meant here the serum (Rasa) in the skin, and by "Tejas" the blood in the veins (Sirá) carrying the (Tejas) known as the A'lochaka.

† D. R. vessels, muscles and aqueous humour (Medas) are most important for the maintenance of Krishna-mandala.

colours and in closing and opening the eye-lids freely. An intelligent physician will conclude from these symptoms that the eyes have been affected by the (deranged) Doshas, with a due consideration whereof the remedies should be (carefully) administered, otherwise the eye-diseases might become too serious. The simple maxim or principle to be followed in the treatment of a disease is simply to forego the primary pathological causes of that disease. The special remedial measures that would pacify the different Doshas, Vâyu, etc. have been described in detail. 12-13.

Causes of Eye-disease :—The local Doshas deranged and aggravated by such causes as diving in water immediately after an exposure to the heat and the glare of the sun, (constant) gazing at distant objects, sleep in the day time and keeping up late hours in the night, fixed and steady gaze, excessive weeping or over-indulgence in grief, worry and fatigue, a blow or a hurt, sexual excesses, the partaking (in inordinate quantities) of Śukta, Áranála (fermented rice-water), acid gruel, Másha pulse, and Kulattha pulse, voluntary repression of any call of nature, exposure (of the eyes) to smoke or dust, trickling down of the drops of sweat (into the eyes), excessive or impeded vomiting, repression of tears, constant contraction of the eyes to adjust the sight to extremely small objects, etc., beget disorders of the organs of vision. 14.

Classification of the Eye-diseases :—Seventy-six different kinds of eye-diseases have been come across in practice ; of these ten are originated by the deranged **Váyu**, ten by **Pitta** and thirteen by **Kapha**. Sixteen are produced by vitiated **blood**, and twenty-five by the concerted action of the deranged Doshas (**Tri-Doshaja**), and lastly, two are produced by external causes i. e., they are **traumatic** in their origin. 15.

Prognosis of the Vátaja Type :—Of the diseases of the eyes which are due to the action of the deranged Váyu, those known as Hatádhimantha, Nimisha, Gambhiriká affecting the vision, and Váta-hata-vartma (Váyu-afflicted Sclerotic coat) is said to be incurable. A temporary cure (Yápya) is all that can be effected in a case of Kácha (cataract) due to the action of the deranged bodily Váyu ; while the affection of the eyes known as the Anyato-Vàta, Adhi-mantha (ophthalmia), Śushkàkshi-páka, Abhishyanda and Maruta-Paryaya are curable. 16.

Prognosis of the Pittaja Type :—Of the diseases due to the deranged action of the Pitta known as Hrasva-jádya and Jala-srâva should be deemed incurable ; and palliative measures are the only remedies in cases of Kàcha, Parimlàyi and Nila, while Abhishynda, Adhi-mantha Amládhyushita, Sùktiká, Pitta-Vidagdha-Drishti, Pothaki and Lagana are curable. 17.

Prognosis of Kaphaja Type :—Of the diseases due to the aggravation of Kapha, the one known as the Sràva-roga is incurable and (Kaphaja) Kácha (cataract) admits of only palliative treatment, while a cure may be be effected in the following cases, viz,, Abhishyanda (conjunctivitis), Adhi-mantha, Balása-Grathita, Śleshma-Vidagdha-Drishti, Pothaki, Lagana, Krimi-granthi, Pariklinna-Vartma, Śuklárma, Pishtaka, Śleshmo-panáha. 18.

Prognosis of the Raktaja Type :—Of the diseases of the eyes due to the vitiated condition of the blood, those known as Raktasráva, Ajakájâta, Avalambita (pendent), Śonitárśas and Śukra-roga should be regarded as incurable, and the type of Kácha (cataract) due to the same cause admits of only palliative measures, while the diseases known as Adhi-mantha, Abhishyanda, Klishta-vartma, Sirâ-harsha and Sirotpàta, Anjana, Sirâ-jàla, Parvani, Avrana (non-ulcerated), Śukra-roga, Śonitárma and Arjuna may be included within the group of curables. 19.

Prognosis of the Tridoshaja Type, etc. :—Of the eye-diseases due to the concerted action of the three aggravated Doshas, those known as Puya-sráva, Nakulándhya, Akshipákátyaya and Alaji are incurable and palliative measures are only possible in cases of Kâcha (cataract) or Pakshma-kopa ; while those known as Vartmávabandha, Sıràja-pidakâ, Prastár-yarma, Adhi-mánsárma, Snayvarma, Utsangini, Puyà-lasa, Arvuda, Śyáva-vartma, Kardama-vartma, Arśo-vartma, Śukrárśas, Śarkará-vartma, the two forms of inflammation with or without local swelling known as) Saśopha-páka and Aśopha-páka, Bahala-vartma, Kumbhiká and Visa-vartma yeild to the curative efficacy of appropriate remedial agents. Both the forms of eye-disease due to the **external** causes* should be considered as incurable. 20—21.

Their Localities :—Thus we have finished enumerating the seventy-six types of eye-diseases, of which nine are confined to the **Sandhis** (binding unions), twenty-one to the **Vartma** (eye-lids), eleven to the **Śukla-bhága** (the Vitreous body), four to the **Krishna-bhága** (the region of the Choroid), seventeen to the **entire region** (eye-ball) and twelve to the region of the **Drishti** (pupil or the crystalline lens, etc.). The

*The one due to any external blow or hurt (**Sa-nimitta**) and the other originating from the sudden sight of any celestial being of extreme brilliancy (**A-nimitta**).

two cases due to the extraneous cause (are chiefly located in the **Drishti** though affecting the whole of the eye-ball and) are very painful and incurable. The characteristic symptoms of all these will be hereafter described in detail. 22—23.

Thus ends the first chapter of the Uttra-tantra in the Sus'ruta Samhitá which deals with the diseases, viz. of the eye, etc.

CHAPTER II.

Now we shall discourse on the chapter which deals with the pathology of diseases which are peculiar to the joints or binding membranes of the eye (**Sandhi-gata-Roga-Vijnaniya**).

The names of those diseases :—Diseases peculiar to the joining (Sandhi) of the eye are nine in number and are named Puyálasa, Upanáha, (the four kinds of) Sráva (viz. Puya-sráva, Sʹleshma-sráva, Rakta-sráva, Pitta-sráva), Parvani, Alaji and Krimi-granthi. 2.

Symptoms of Puyálasa and Upanáha :—A suppurated swelling occurring at any of these joining and exuding a sort of fetid and dense * pus is called **Puyálasa**. A painless cyst (Granthi) of considerable size occurring at the union of the pupil (with the Krishna-mandala) and attended with an itching sensation and a little suppuration is called **Upangha**. 3. A.

Symptoms of Sráva :—The (deranged) Doshas † of the locality passing through the lachrymal ducts into the binding tissues of the four different Sandhis (joinings) set up a painless ‡ secretion (Sráva) from the localities characterised by the specific symptoms of the different Doshas involved. These are known as **Srávas**, which according to some, are also called

* According to Mádhava's reading, the swelling should be painful (सतोद:). There is no mention whether the pus should be dense (सान्द्र) or otherwise.

† The term "Dosha" here means S'leshmá, Pitta, Rakta (blood) and the concerted action of the above three Doshas. It should be noted that Vâyu is excluded from the list as it does not produce any secretion.

‡ Mâdhava does not mention this (painlessness) to be a symptom.

Netra-nádi and are classified into four different groups, the different symptoms of which will be described presently. A suppuration (D. R. swelling) in any of the unions (Sandhi) of the eye marked by a discharge of pus is called **Puyá-sráva.** This is due to the concerted action of the Doshas (Kapha, Pitta and blood). The secretion of slimy, white and thick muco-purulent discharges marked by the absence of pain * is called **Śleshmá-sráva.** The flow of thin, warm† and blood-streaked copious discharge due to a contaminated state of the local blood is called **Raktá-sráva.** A warm, water-like and yellowish blue (D. R. reddish yellow) discharge from the middle part of the union (owing to the deranged condition of the Pitta) is called **Pittá-sráva.** 3.

Symptoms of Parvani, etc. :—A small, round and copper-coloured swelling occurring at the joining of the Krishna-mandala and Śukla-mandala, due to the vitiated state of the local blood and attended with a burning sensation and aching pain, is called **Parvani.** A swelling possessed of the preceding features and occurring at the very same joining is called **Alaji** (Keratitis) ‡. A cyst or swelling (Granthi) characterised by an itching sensation appearing on the joining of the eye-lids and eye-lashes owing to the germination of parasites (Krimi) in those localities, is called **Krimi-granthi.** Parasites of different forms in such a case are found to infest the regions where the inner lining of the Vartma-

* According to Mâdhava's reading, the absence of pain is not a necessary concomitant in this case.

† According to Mâdhava's reading thinness and warmness are not essential.

‡ The difference between a case of **Parvani** and that of **Alaji** is that the swelling in a case of Parvani is smaller, and that in the Alaji is larger.

mandala (eye-lid) is connected with the Śukla-mandala (Sclerotic coat) of the eye and to invade and vitiate the substance of the eye-ball. 4—5.

Thus ends the second chapter of the Uttara-Tantra in the Sus'ruta Samhitâ which deals with the pathology of the diseases peculiar to the Sandhi (unions) of the eye.

CHAPTER III.

Now we shall discourse on the chapter which deals with the pathology of diseases peculiar to the region of the eye-lids (**Vartmagata-Roga-Vijnániya**). 1.

Causes and Names :—The Doshas of the body jointly or severally expanding through the nerves and veins, (Sirâ) of the eye-lids (Vartma) bringing about an augmentation of the quantity of the blood and the growth of the flesh in the localities (determination of blood toward formation of fleshy growth in the affected parts) give rise to a host of local diseases which are known as Utsangini, Kumbhikâ, Pothaki, Vartma-Śarkará. Arśo-vartma, Śushkârśas, Anjana, Bahala-vartma, Vartmâvabandha, Klishta-vartma, Kardama-vartma, Śyáva-vartma, Praklinna-vartma, Pariklinna-vartma, Vâtáhata-vartma, Arvuda, Nimisha, Śonitarsas, Lagana, Visha-vartma and Pakshma-kopa. These twenty-one diseases are restricted to the eye-lids (Vartma). 2.

The Specific symptoms of the diseases of the eye-lids :—The names of these have been enumerated ; now hear me describe their specific symptoms. A (rolled up and indented) boil or eruption (Pidakâ) appearing along the lower eye-lid on its exterior side with its mouth or head directed inward is called **Utsangini**. A number of boils or pustules (Pidakâ) to the size of a Kumbhikâ seed appearing on the joint of the eye-lids and the eye-lashes and becoming inflamed after being burst is called **Kumbhiká** *. 3—4.

* This disease (Kumbhiká) is due to the concerted action of the three Doshas.

A number of red and heavy (hard) boils or pustules (Pidaká) resembling red mustard seeds attended with pain, itching and exudation is called **Pothaki.** A rough and large pustule (Pidaká) surrounded by other very small and thick erythematous pustules (covering the entire length of the eye-lid) is called **Vartma-śarkará.** 5—6.

Vegetations of small (D. R. soft) and rough papilæ (Pidakâs) on the eye-lid resembling *Ervâruka* seeds and attended with very little pain are called **Arśo-vartma.** Long, rough, hard, and numbed papilæ (Amkura) on the eye-lid (2) are called **Śushkárśas.** 7—8.

A small, soft, copper-coloured pustule (Pidakâ) appearing on the eye-lid and attended with burning, pricking sensation and a slight pain is called an **Anjana.** Vegetations of pustules (Pidaká) of equal size (D. R.—attended with hardness) occurring all along the eye-lid and resembling it (or each other) in colour are called **Bahala-vartma.** 9-10.

Such swelling of the eye-lid attended with an itching sensation and a slight pain as impedes or interferes with its being evenly opened is called **Vartma-bandha.** A mild and copper-coloured inflammatory swelling of both the eye-lids simultaneously attended with a slight pain and changing suddenly into redness (D. R.—suddenly discharging blood therefrom) is called **Klishta-vartma.** 11-12.

A case of Klishta-vartma in which the Pitta has deranged and affected the blood and much dirty matter (mucus) is discharged as a consequence is called a case of **Vartma-kardama.** A dark brown colour of the eye-lids both internally and externally marked by a

(2) According to Mâdhava, the papilæ in such cases occur in the inner side of the eye-lid.

swelling (D. R.—pain) and attended with a discharge of pus and with burning and itching sensations is called **Syáva-vartma.** 13-14.

An external swelling of the eye-lid with a deposit of mucous matter in its inner surface accompanied with a little pain as well as a discharge, itching and pricking sensation, is called a **Praklinna-Vartma.** A sticking together of the eye-lids even in the absence of any suppuration and in spite of the eyes being constantly washed (with water) * is called **Pariklinna-vartma.** 15—16.

The drooping down (lit.—inactivity) of the eye-lids, whether attended with any pain or not, (so as to obstruct the opening of the eye-lashes) where the eye-lids seem to be out of joint is called **Vátáhata-vartma.** A red and knotty swelling (Granthi) of an uneven size or shape, growing hastily on the interior side of the eye-lid and attended with a little pain is called an **Arvuda** or tumour. 17—18.

Constant wrinklings of the eye-lids owing to the incarceration of the (deranged) Vâyu within the nerves or veins (Sirâ) controlling their wrinkings (closing and opening) are known as **Nimesha.** Soft and fleshy growths (Amkura) on the eye-lid which reappear even after being removed with a knife, and are attended with pain, itching and burning sensation are called **Sonitársas** and should be ascribed to the vitiated condition of the blood. 19-20.

A thick, slimy, hard and painless nodular swelling (Granthi) on the eye-lid resembling a **Kola** fruit in size and marked by an itching sensation and absence of suppuration is called **Lagana** †. An inflammatory swelling

* A different reading reads 'whether washed or not.' This, however, not a good reading.

† Certain editions read **Nagana.**

of the eye-lid dotted with minute punctures like the pores in the stem of a water-soaked lotus plant is called **Visa-vartma**. 21-22.

An accumulation of the deranged Doshas about the eye-lashes makes them rough and sharp-pointed, which give pain to the eye and give relief when drawn off. The disease is known as **Pakshma-kopa** in which the eye cannot bear the least wind or heat or the glare of fire. 23.

Thus ends the third chapter of the Uttara-Tantra in the Sus'ruta Samhitá which deals with the pathology of the diseases of the eye-lids.

CHAPTER IV.

Now we shall discourse on the chapter which deals with the pathology of diseases of the Sclerotic coat (white coat) of the eye (**Śuklagata-Roga-Vijnáníya**). 1.

Names :—The eleven different forms of diseases which are peculiar to the Sclerotic coat (white) of the eye, are Prastâryarma, Śuklârma, Kshatajàrma (Raktâ-rma), Adhimânsârma, Snáyvarma, Śuktikâ, Arjuna, Pishtaka, Sirâ-jâla, Sirâ-pidakâ, and Balâsa-grathita. 2.

Symptoms :—A thin and extended glandular swelling (Granthi) coloured reddish blue and apearing on the Sclerotic coat (Śukla) is called **Prastáryarma.** A crop of soft and whitish growths slowly extending over the entire length of the Sclerotic coat is called **Śuklárma**. The fleshy growth on the white coat of the eye resembling a (red) lotus flower in colour is called **Lohitárma**. The soft, extended, thick and dark-brown and liver-coloured growth of flesh on the white coat is called **Adhi-mánsárma**. The rough, yellowish (D. R. white) growth of flesh on the white coat, and gaining (slowly) in size, is called **Snáyvarma**. 3-7.

The appearance of dark brown specks resembling flesh in colour or of those having the colour of an oyster-shell on the white coat (Śukla) of the eye is called **Śuktiká**. The appearance of a single dot or speck on the Sclerotic coat (Śukla), coloured like a (drop of the) hare's blood, is called **Arjuna**. A raised and circular dot or speck appearing on the white coat and coloured white like pasted rice and (as transparent as) water is called **Pishtaka**. Red and extensive patches of hardened veins spreading over the white coat and looking like a net-work is called **Sirá-jála**. The crop of white pustular growths (Pidakâ) on the Sclerotic coat (Śukla), near the limit of the black coat (Iris) and covered over with shreds of veins are called the **Sirá-Pidaká**. The disease in which a speck coloured like the Indian bell-metal (Kàmsya) and covered over with a vein (Sirá) appears on the region of the Scleratic coat is called the **Balása***. 8-13.

Thus ends the fourth chapter of the Uttara-Tantra in the Sus'ruta Samhitá which treats of the pathology of the diseases of the Sceloretic region of the eye.

* The reading in Mâdhava's Nidâna is quite different here, and Dallana seems to support that. It is defined as the disease in which a hard speck appears like a drop of water on the white coat and looks like bell-metal in colour.

CHAPTER V.

Now we shall discourse on the chapter which deals with the pathology of the diseases of the black part of the eye—Choroid including the Iris (**Krishna-gata-Roga-Vijnániya**). 1.

The diseases which are found to invade the region of the Choroid including the Iris (Krishna-mandala) have been briefly said to be four in number. Their names are Sa-vrana-Śukra, A-vrana-Śukra, Pâkâtyaya and Ajakâ. 2.

Symptoms :—A puncture-like dip in the region of the (Krishna-mandala) with a sensation there as if the part has been pricked with a needle and attended with an excruciating pain and a hot exudation is called **Sa-vrana-Śukra**. If the seat of this disease considerably remote from the pupil—entire part of the Drishti (Retina) be marked by the absence of pain and discharge and be not deep-seated and if there be not double spots, it offers very little chance of remedy. 3-4.

Symptoms and Prognosis of A-vrana-Śukra :—A whitish film appearing on the region of the Choroid including the Iris (Krishna) like a speck of transparent cloud in the sky, and attended with lachrymation and slight pain due to the eye-disease known as Abhishyanda (Ophthalmia—lit. secretion) is called the **A-vrana-Śukra**. This is easily curable. A case of Avrana-Śukra (non-ulcerated film) which is thickened, deep-seated and long-standing, may be cured only with the greatest difficulty, while an long-standing case of this disease, if it is mobile, covered with shreds of flesh, vein-ridden, stretching down to the second layer of skin (in the eye) and obstructing the vision, severed in the middle and marked with a reddish tint in the extremities, should be deemed as incurable. Several authorities aver that the appearance of *Mudga*-like specks or films on the region of the Iris, attended with growths of pustules and hot lachrymations, should be like-wise regarded as incurable. The fact of its (speck) assuming the colour of the feather of a *Tittira* bird is an additional indication of the incurable nature of this disease. 5.

The appearance of a whitish milky film over the black part of the eye slowly shrouding it entirly with its mass and attended with acute pain is known as the **Akshi-Pákátyaya**. This is invariably found to result from an attack of Akshi-kopa* and is due to the concerted action of all the Doshas. A painful reddish growth, like the head of a goat, found to shoot forth from beneath the surface of the black part and attended with reddish slimy secretion is called an **Ajaká**. 6–7.

Thus ends the fifth chapter of the Uttara-Tantra in the Sus'ruta Samhitâ which treats of the pathology of the diseases of the black part of the eye.

* According to Mâdhava's reading in his Nidâna, this disease need not necessarily result from an attack of Akshi-kopa, and there need not be an acute pain, and it would be incurable.

CHAPTER VI.

Now we shall discourse on the chapter which deals with the (symptoms and) pathology of the diseases affecting the eye as a whole **(Sarva-gata-Roga-Vijnániya)**. 1.

Names and causes :—The fcur types of Abhishyandha (Ophthalmatis), the four types of Adhimantha, the two forms of Akshi-páka (suppuration of the eye) attended with or without swelling, these ten, as well as Hatádhimantha, Anila-Parjáya, Śuskákshipáka, Anyato-váta, Amládhyushita, Drishti, Śirotpáta and Śirá-Harsha are the names of the (seventeen kinds of) diseases which affect the eye as a whole. Nearly all these forms of eye-diseases may result from the Abhishyanda (Ophthalmitis). Hence a wise physician shall try speedily to remedy a case of Abhishyanda (Ophthalmitis) as soon as it is found out. 2.

Specific symptoms of Abhishyanda :—The symptoms which mark a case of **Abhishyanda** due to the action of the deranged **Váyu** are pricking pain (in the eyes), numbness, horripilation and irritation in the eyes, roughness and parchedness of the organ, cold lachrymations and headache. A case of **Pittaja-Abhishyanda** exhibits the following features, *viz.*, burning and inflammatory suppuration of the eyes, longing for coldness (in the eyes), excessive hot lachrymations, cloudy vision and a yellowness of the eye. In the **Kaphaja** type of the disease, the affected organ longs for the contact of warm articles and is attended with a heaviness, itching sensation, swelling, excessive whiteness and a constant deposit and discharge of slimy mucus. The special type of this disease which has its origin in the vitiated condition of the blood, *i. e.*, the **Raktaja type** is marked by redness of the eyes, flow of copper-coloured tears, as well as the symptoms of the Pittaja type of the disease and the presence of deep red stripes all along. 3-6.

Causes of Adhimantha :—All the (four) forms of chronic Abhishyanda, if not properly attended to and remedied at the outset, may run into as many cases of **Adhimantha** which is attended (invariably) with an excruciating pain in the eye, which seems as if being torn out, the pain extending upward to and crushing, as it were, the half the region of the head. The characteristic symptoms of the Doshas involved in each case are also seen to supervene. 7.

Symptoms of Vátaja Adhimantha :—In the **Vátaja** type of Adhimantha the eye becomes cloudy and seems as if being torn out and churned as with an Arani (fire-producing wooden stick) attended with an irritating, piercing and cutting pain, as well as with a swelling of the local flesh, and a half of the head (on the side of the affected eye) is afflicted with a twisting and cracking sensation as well as with local swelling, shivering and pain. 8.

Symptoms of Pittaja Adhimantha :—The symptoms which mark the **Pittaja** type of Adhimantha are the blood-streaked eye attended with secretion and a sensation therein of being burnt with fire, as well as swelling, perspiration and suppuration in the affected organs, yellowish vision, fainting fits and a burning sensation in the head. The eyes in this case become liver-coloured and seem as if ulcerated or rubbed with an alkali. 9.

Symptoms of Kaphaja Adhimantha :—In the **Kaphaja** type of Adhimantha the eye is swollen with a slight congestion (inflammation). Discharges with a sensation of itching, coldness and heaviness in the localities set in, and there is horripilation. The eye becomes slimy with deposit of mucous matter. The sight becomes cloudy, the nostrils are dilated, the head aches and all objects seem to be full of dust. 10.

Symptoms of Raktaja Adhimantha: —A pricking pain in and a blood-streaked secretion from the affected organ which looks (bright red) like a *Bandhujiva* flower, are the symptoms which mark the type of **Raktaja** Adhimantha (due to the vitiated blood). The eye becomes painful and incapable of bearing the least touch or contact, and the objects of vision seem as if enveloped in flames. The extremities of the eye become red and the whole origin of the cornea (black coat of the eye) looks like an *Arishta* fruit submerged in blood. 11.

The prognosis :—A course of injudicious diet, conduct or medical treatment may usher in the blindness of vision in seven days from an attack of the Kaphaja type of Adhimantha (Ophthalmia) and in five days from that of the blood-origined (Raktaja) type, in six days in a case of the Vátaja Adhimantha and instantaneously within three days of the attack) in the Pittaja type of (*i. e.*, Adhimantha. 12.

Symptoms of Sa-ŝopha and A-ŝopha Akshi-páka :—A case of **Sa-śopha-Netra-páka** exhibits the following symptoms, *viz.*, itching sensation, deposit of mucous matter (in the eye), lachrymation and a redness of the eye like the colour of a ripe *Udumbara* fruit. There is a burning sensation in the eye-ball which becomes copper-coloured, heavy, and attended with a pricking pain and horripilation. The eye becomes swollen and constantly secretes either cold or hot slimy discharges, and ultimately suppurates. All these symptoms except swelling mark the (non-swollen) **A-śopha-Netra-páka** type of the disease. 13.

The deranged Váyu getting incarcerated in the optic nerve (Sirá) impairs the faculty of sight, and gives rise to an incurable disease which is called **Hatádhimantha** (blinding Ophthalmia). A shifting pain experienced sometimes in the region of the eye-lashes* or of the eye-brows and sometimes in the region of the eye, owing to the coursing of the deranged and incarcerated Váyu in those localities, is called **Váta-Paryáya**. 14–15.

The disease in which the eye-lids become dry and hard and remain always closed, the vision becomes cloudy and hazy, and it becomes very painful to open the eye-lids, is called the **Śushkákshi-páka**.† The excessive pain in the eyes or in the eye-brows due to the action of the deranged Váyu incarcerated in the region of the head, the ears, the cheek-bones, the back of the neck (Avatu), the Manyá (a particular nerve on either side of the neck), or in any other (adjacent) place, is called the **Anyato-váta**. 16–17.

The swelling of the eye attended with a bluish red tint all about, owing to the partakings of meals composed of an unduly large proportion of acid articles, or of such food as is followed by a digestionary acid reaction, is called the **Amládhyushita-Drishti**. The disease in which the veins all over the eye become copper-coloured and are frequently discoloured, whether attended with pain or not, is called the **Sirotpáta**. 18–19.

* Mádhava in the Nidána does not mention the eye-lashes.

† Mádhava in the Nidána reads "दन्दह्यते" which means that a highly burning sensation is produced in the affected eye, in place of "विलोकने"—a word which seems redundant.

A case of Sirotpáta, if not attended to and remedied in time through ignorance, gives rise to transparent and copper-coloured discharges in copious quantities from the eyes and produce a complete blindness of vision. This is known as the **Sirá-harsha**. 20.

Thus ends the sixth chapter of the Uttara-Tantra in the Sus'ruta Samhitá which treats of the diseases affecting the eye as a whole.

CHAPTER VII.

Now we shall discourse on the chapter which deals with the pathology of the diseases which are peculiar to the Drishti (pupil) of the eye (**Drishti-gata-Roga-Vijnániya**). 1.

Experts well-versed in the anatomy of the eye aver that the **Drishti** (pupil) of the eye is the quintessence of the five material elements with that of the eternal light predominating therein—this principle of light neither increasing nor decreasing in this case. It is naturally accustomed to cold from the very nature of its temperament and is covered by the outer coating (Patala) of the organ proper. It looks like a hole and is equal in dimension to that of a *Masúra* seed or pulse*. The pupil of the eye resembles in its action the phosphorescent flash of a glow-worm or that of a minute particle of fire (in not burning the things coming in contact with it). Now we shall describe the pathology of the twelve kinds of disease peculiar to the region of the **Drishti** (pupil), as well as of the one which is known as Timira (loss of vision) affecting the **Patala** (coating over the pupil). 2.

All external objects appear dim and hazy to the sight when the deranged Doshas of the locality passing through the veins (Sirá) of the eye, get into and are incarcerated within the **first Patala** (innermost coat) of the pupil (Drishti). 3.

Symptoms—when second Patala attacked:—False images of gnats, flies, hairs, nets or cob-webs, rings (circular patches), flags, ear-rings appear

* According to Nimi, quoted in Mádhava's commentary by S'rikantha, the dimension of the **Drishti** is equal to only a half of that of a *Masura-pulse*.

4

to the sight, and the external objects seem to be enveloped in mist or haze or as if laid under a sheet of water or as viewed in rain and on cloudy days, and meteors of different colours seem to be falling constantly in all directions in the event of the deranged Doshas being similarly confined in the **second Patala** (coat) of the Drishti. In such cases the near appearance of an actually remote object and the contrary (*Miopia* and *Biopia*) also should be ascribed to some deficiency in the range of vision (error of refraction in the crystalline lens) which incapacitates the patient from looking through the eye and hence from threading a needle. 4.

Symptoms—when third Patala attacked :—Objects situate high above are seen and those placed below remain unobserved when the deranged Dosha are infiltrated into the **Third Patala** (coat) of the Drishti. The Doshas affecting the Drishti (crystalline lens), if highly enraged, impart their specific colours to the objects of vision. Even large objects seem to be covered with a piece of cloth. The images of objects and persons with ears and eyes, etc., seem to be otherwise *i.e.*, bereft of those organs. The deranged Doshas situated at and obstructing the lower, upper and lateral parts of the Drishti (crystalline lens) respectively shut out the view of near, distant and laterally-situate objects. A dim and confused view of the external world is all that can be had when the deranged Doshas spread over and affect the whole of the Drishti (crystalline lens). A thing appears to the sight as if cut into two (bifurcated) when the deranged Doshas affect the middle part of the lens, and as triply divided and severed when the Doshas are scattered in two parts ; while a multifarious image of the same object is the result of the manifold distributions of movability of the Doshas over the Drishti. 5.

Symptoms—when fourth Patala attacked :—Loss of vision (**Timira**) results from the fact of the deranged bodily Doshas being confined within the **fourth Patala** (choroid) of the organ. When the vision is completely obstructed by the aforesaid cause, it is called a case of **Linga-nása** (blindness). Only a faint perception of the images of the sun, the moon and the stars, the heaven, a flash of lightning or any other such highly brilliant objects is possible in a case of superficial (not deep-seated) Linga-nása. The Linga-nása (blindness) is also called Nfliká and Kácha. 6.

Specific traits of Timira :—All external objects are viewed as cloudy, moving, crooked and red-coloured in the **Vátaja** type (of Timira), while in the **Pittaja** type they appear to be invested with the different colours of the spectrum or of the rain-bow, of the glow-worm, of the flash of lightning, or of the feathers of the pea-cock, or with a dark blue tint bordering on black ; while in a case of **Kaphaja** Timira, a thick white coat like that of a pack of white clouds or a deep white chowri (Chámara) seems to intervene in everything which look white and oily and dull and appear hazy and cloudy in a fine day, or as if laid under a sheet of water. In a case of the **Raktaja** type of Timira, all objects appear red or envoloped in gloom, and they assume a greyish, blackish or variegated colour. In a case of **Sánnipátika** Timira, the outer world looks vareigated and confused, appears as doubled or trebled to the vision (of the patient), and stars and planets, either defective or supplied with additional limbs, seem to float about in the vision. 7-11.

Parimláyi :—The quarters of the heaven look yellow and appear to the sight as if resplendent with the light of the rising sun, and trees seem as if sparkling with the tangles of fire-flies in a case of **Parimláyi**, which should be ascribed to the action of the deranged **Pitta** in concert with the vitiated **blood.** 12.

The different colours of the pupil in cases of Linga-nása :—Now we shall describe the colours of the pupil in the six different types of Linga-nása. The pupil assumes a reddish (Aruna) colour in the **Vátaja** type of the disease ; looks blue or bluish yellow in the **Pittaja**, white in the **Kaphaja** and blood-red in the **blood-origined** one, while it assumes a variegated hue in the **Sánnipátika** type of Linga-nása. A circular patch (Mandala) tinged with a shade of bluish or bluish yellow colour and looking like fire or a piece of thick grass, is formed on the pupil owing to the diseased and aggravated condition of the **blood** (with **pitta**) in a case of **Parimláyi**. In this case the patient is sometimes permitted to catch faint glimpses of the external objects owing to the spontaneous and occasional filtering away of the deranged Doshas obstructing the vision. 13–15.

Specific Traits of Linga-násâ :—The circular patch (over the pupil) in a case of **Vátaja** Linga-nása is red-coloured, and is moving and rough to the touch, while that in a case of **Pittaja** Linga-nása is bluish or yellow or coloured like bell-metal. The circular patch in a case of **Kaphaja** Linga-nása is thick, oily and as white as a conch-shell, a *Kunda* flower or the moon—resembling a white drop of water on the moving lotus leaf and moving away to and fro when the eye is rubbed. The circular patch over the pupil in a case of **Raktaja** (blood-origined) Linga-nása is red-coloured like a coral or a (red) lotus-petal. A **Sánuipátika** type of the disease is marked by a variegated colour of the Drishti (pupil) and by the specific symptoms of the different Doshas. 16.

The total number of diseases peculiar to the Drishti

is twelve. The six types of Linga-náśa (Drishti) have been described above. The six other forms of the disease, peculiar to the Drishti (pupil) are named as Pitta-vidagdha-Drishti, Śleshma--vidagdha-Drishti, Dhûma-darśin, Hrasva-Jâtya, Nakulândhyatá and Gambhîriká. 17.

The disease in which the region of the Drishti (pupil) assumes a yellowish colour, and all external objects appear yellow to the sight owing to the presence of the vitaited (and augmented) Pitta in the region of the Drishti is called **Pitta-Vidagdha-Drishti**. It is due to an accumulation of the deranged Dosha (Pitta) in the **third Patala** (coat) of the eye, and the patient cannot see anything in the day, but can see only in the night. 18.

The external objects appear white to the sight when it is affected by the accumulation of the deranged Kapha. The deranged Dosha (Kapha), in this case, is simultaneously divided over all the three Patalas (coats) of the eye. In consequence of this the patient is attacked with nocturnal blindness, being able to see only in the daytime owing to the (melting and) decrease of the deranged Kapha through the heat of the sun. This is known as **Śleshma-vidagdha-Drishti**. 19.

The external objects appear dusky or smoke-coloured when the sight is affected through grief, (high and protracted) fever, over-straining or excessive physical exercise, or injury to the head, etc. The affection of vision thus engendered is called **Dhuma-Drishti** (smoky sight). 20.

The disease in which small things can be viewed only with the greatest difficulty (even) in the daytime, but can be viewed (easily and clearly) in the night owing to the subsidence of the deranged **pitta** through the coldness of the atmosphere (and a general cooling of the Earth's surface)* is called **Hrasva-játya**†. 21.

The form of occular affection in which the colour of Drishti (pupil) of a man affected by the Doshas resembles (and is found to emit (luminous) flashes like) that of a mungoose in consequence of which the external objects appear multi-coloured in the day time,‡ is called **Nakulándhya**. The form of occular affection due to the action of the deranged **Váyu**, and in which the Drishti (pupil) is contracted and deformed and sinks into the socket, attended with an extreme pain in the affected parts, is called **Gambhiriká**. 22–23.

Besides the above, there are two more forms of **Linga-násá** of traumatic origin, *viz.*, Sa-nimitta (of ascertainable origin) and A-nimitta (without any manifest or ascertainable cause). Under the first group may be arranged those which are produced by such causes as an over-heated § condition of the head (brain, etc.), and marked by the specific symptoms of (blood-origined) Abhishyanda, while the second comprises those in which the loss of one's vision is due to causes, such as the witnessing of divine halo or effulgence emanating from the ethereal person of a god, or a Gandharva (demi-god), a holy saint, a celestial serpent, or such other

* The latter part of the text here seems to be incongruous. Mádhava does not read the last line in his Nidána, nor does Dallana include it in his commentary. Dallana, on the other hand, says that some read this line, but holds, on the authorityof Videha, that the reading is incongruous, in as much as "Hrasva-játya" is said to cause one of the four types of night-blindness.

† Some read Hrasva-jádya in place of Hrasva-játya.

‡ This shows that a man affected with this form of disease cannot see anything in the night.

§ The head is liable to be over-heated by the smelling of poison or poisonous objects or any other strong-scented flower, etc.

highly bright object. In this case the eye is not outwardly affected and the pupil (Drishti) looks as bright and clear as a Vaidûrya gem, while in the former case (of ascertainable origin) the eye is characterised by a sunken or pierced or impaired aspect of the pupil. 24.

We have thus finished describing separately the diagnostic traits of the seventy-six forms of disease which affect the organ of vision. We shall hereafter separately deal with the nature of the medical treatment to be pursued in each case. 25.

Thus ends the seventh chapter of the Uttara-Tantra in the Sus'ruta Samhitá which treats of the pathology of the diseases peculiar to the pupil of the eye.

CHAPTER VIII.

Now we shall discourse on the chapter which deals with the classification of occular affection according to the different modes of treatment **(Netra-Roga-Chikitsá-Vibhága-Vijnániya).** 1.

Classification :—We have already described the names and symptoms of the seventy-six kinds of eye disease. We shall now briefly and severally deal with the nature of treatment to be pursued in them. Of these seventy-six kinds eleven should be treated with incision operations (**Chhedya**), nine with scarification (**Lekhya**), five with excision (**Bhedya**), fifteen with venesection (**Vyádhya**) ; twelve cases should not be operated upon and seven admit only of palliative measures (**Yápya**), while fifteen should be given up by an experienced physician (Ophthalmic surgeon) as incurable. The two kinds of eye-disease of traumatic origin should be likewise held as incurable or admitting only of palliative measures at the best. 2.

Names of the Chhedya and Lekhya eye-diseases :—Diseases which should be treated with **incision** are Ars'o-vartma, Śushkárs'as, Arvuda, Sirá-Pidaká, Sirá-jâla, the five types of Arman*, and Parvaniká (thus numbering eleven in all). Diseases in which **scarification** should be resorted to (numbering seven in all) are Utsanginî, Bahala-vartma, Kardama-vartma, Śyáva-vartma, Vaddha-vartma, Klishta-vartma, Pothaki, Kumbhîkinî, and Śarkará-vartma. 3-4.

Names of Bhedya and Vyádhya eye-diseases :—Optical diseases in which the affected

* See Chapter IV, para 2, Uttara-Tantara.

localities should be treated with **excisions**, are Śleshmo-panáha, Lagana, Visa-vartma, Krimi-granthi and Anjana—thus numbering five in all. The two kinds of eye-disease beginning with Sirá *viz.*, Sirotpáta and Sirá-harsha, the two kinds of Akshi-páka attended or un-attended with swelling, *viz.*, Saśothâkshi-páka and Aśothákshi-páka, and Anyatováta, Puyálasa, Váta-viparyaya and the four types of Abhishyanda and the four types of Adhimantha should be treated with **Venesection** (Sirá-vyadhana). 5–6.

Eye-diseases—not to be operated :— Operations should not be resorted to in cases of Śushká-kshi-páka, Kapha-Vidagdha-Drishti, Pitta-Vidagdha-Drishti, Amládhyushita-Drishti, Śukra-roga, Arjuna, Pishtaka, Aklinna-vartma, Dhuma-darśin, Śuktiká, Prak-linna-vartma and Valása—thus making twelve in all. In the traumatic forms also of eye-disease surgical operations are not advised by experts. 7.

Names of curable and incurable eye-disease :—Palliative or temporary relief is all that can be offered in any of the six types of Kâcha described before, as well as in the affection known as Pakshma-kopa, if the patient retains the faculty of sight. Four of the Vâyu-origined, two of the Pittaja, one of the Kaphaja, four of the blood-origined and four of the types caused by the concerted action of the three Doshas, as well as the two traumatic forms of optical affections should be regarded as beyond all cure. 8–9.

Thus ends the eighth chapter of the Uttara-Tantra in the Sus'ruta Samhitá which deals with the classification of eye-diseases according to the different modes of treatment.

CHAPTER IX.

Now we shall discourse on the remedial measures of Abhishyanda (Ophthalmia) due to the action of the deranged Vâyu **(Vátábhishyanda-Pratishedha)*** 1.

The patient should be treated with old and matured clarified butter, both in a case of (Vátaja) Abhishyanda (Ophthalmia) and (Vátaja) Adhimantha (Conjunctivites). The diseased organ should be then duly* fomented and local venesection resorted to. Then after having effected full purging with the help of a Sneha-vasti (oleaginous enema), such measures as Tarpana, Puta-pâka, fumigation, sprinklings (Ás'chyotana) †, snuffing (Nasya), oily washings, S'iro-vasti (errhines) or washing the organ with Kânjika (Amla) or with any decoction prepared with the drugs of the Váyu-subduing group or with that of the flesh of any aquatic (Jalaja) animal, or of one frequenting the marshy places (Ánupa), should be resorted to. A compound consisting of clarified butter, curd, fat and marrow should be applied luke-warm to the affected organ, which should also be

* It should be noted that the part of the forehead adjoining the eye and not the eye itself—should be fomented, since fomentation should not be applied directly over the eye.

† Ás'CHYOTANA (EYE-DROP)—Consists in dropping into the eye with the two fingers, honey, A'sava, drug-decoction or any oleaginous substance. Its doses are eight drops for scarifying purposes, ten drops for lubricating the part with any oleaginous substance (Snehana), twelve drops for the healing of any local ulcer (Ropana). They should be dropped luke-warm in winter and cold in summer into the eyes. In diseases of Vátaja origin they should be of a bitter taste ; oleaginous in diseases due to the Pitta ; and bitter,—warm and parching in diseases due to Kapha. —VAIDYAKA NIGHANTU as quoted in the Vaidyaka-S'abda-Sindhu. Cf. also Chapter XVIII, Uttara-Tantra.

covered with a compress or linen soaked with the preceding lardacious compound. Milk, Veśavára, Śâlvana Poultice, Porridges (Páyasa), etc., should be used by a physician in poulticing the affected organ. A portion of clarified butter cooked with the decoction of *Triphalá*, or simply old and matured clarified butter, or milk duly cooked with the drugs of the Vâyu-subduing group, or of the first group (viz., *Vidári-Gandhádi Gana*) should be taken after the meal. 2. A.

The application of any lardacious substance other than oil cooked with the admixture of the Váyu-subduing drugs will prove beneficial for **Tarpana** purposes in such cases. The use of medicated *Sneha* in the shape of **Putapáka, Dhuma** (fumigation) and **Nasya** (snuffs) is likewise recommended. Oil (duly) cooked with *Sthirá*, milk and the drugs of the *Madhura* group should be employed as a snuff (in such cases). The milk of a she-goat duly cooked with the admixture of the leaves, roots or barks of *Eranda* plants, or with the roots of *Kantakári*, should be employed lukewarm in **washing** (Sechana) the affected organ. A liquid compound containing half milk and half water, and boiled together with *Saindhava*, *Válá*, *Yashti-madhu* and *Pippali*, should be used in washing the eye as well as an **Aśchyotana** (eye-drop). A liquid compound consisting of the milk of a she-goat diluted with the addition of water, boiled with the admixture of *Hrivera*, *Chakra* (Tagara), *Manjishthá*, and *Udumbara*-barks is considered to be the best **eye-drop** in cases of there being any pain (Śula) in the eye. 2. B.

A thin plaster compound of *Yasthi-madhu*, *Rajani*, *Pathyá* and *Devadáru*, pasted together with the milk of a she-goat should be used as an **Anjana** (collyrium) in a case of acute Ophthalmia (Abhishyanda), and it proves very effective. *Gairika*-earth, *Saindhava*, *Krishná*, (Pippali) and *S'unthi*—the quantity of each subsequent one being double of that of the one preceding it in the order of enumeration, should be pasted together with water, made into Gutiká (a large pill) and be likewise applied (to the eye) in the manner of the application of an **Anjana**. The use of Snaihika (lardacious) Anjana (Collyrium) is beneficial in such cases. These will be duly dealt with later on. 2.

Physicians should likewise adopt this method in treating cases of **Anyato-váta** and **Váta-paryaya**. Draughts of (medicated) clarified butter and of milk before the meal, are highly efficacious. Clarified butter duly cooked with (two parts of) *Vrikshádani*, *Kapittha* and major *Pancha-mula*, (one part of) the expressed juice (or decoction) of *Karkata* and (one part of) milk should be taken in such cases*. In the alternative, Ghrita duly cooked with (the decoction of) *Pattura*, *Agnika* (Ajamodá) and *Ártagala* and with milk, or clarified butter duly cooked with milk and (the decoction of) *Mesha-s'ringi*, or of *Viratara* should be similarly taken. 3.

Treatment of Śushkákshi-páka :— *Saindhava*, *Devadáru* and *S'unthi* and the expressed juice of *Mátulunga*, water, breast-milk and clarified butter mixed together and duly prepared (in the manner of Rasa-kriyá) should be prescribed as an Anjana in cases of **Śushkákshi-páka**. The taking of clarified

* According to Dallana and Gayadása, this Ghrita should be prepared without any Kalka. S'rikanta holds that the drugs *Vrikshadáni*, *Kapittha* and the *Pancha-mula* should be taken as Kalka and the Ghrita prepared with three parts of milk. S'ivadása also seems to support this view.

butter cooked with the drugs of the *Jivaniya* group and the filling of the cavity of the eye with the same, as well as snuffing with the *Anu-taila** are also efficacious in such cases. Washes composed of cold milk with the admixture of Saindhava salt or of milk cooked with *Rajani* and. *Deva-dáru* and mixed with (a little quantity of) Saindhava are efficacious. *Mahaushadha* (S'unthi) rubbed over a stone-slab with clarified butter and breast-milk is also recommended as an **Anjana** (eye-salve)†. The Vasá (essence of the flesh) of aquatic animals or of those which frequent swampy grounds, mixed with a little quantity of powdered *S'unthi* and *Sanidhava* salt (and rubbed on stone-slab) should be applied to the eyes as an Anjana (collyrium) in a case of S'ushkâkshipâka (Non-secreting type of conjunctivites). Let the intelligent physician treat the sight-destroying Vátaja affections of the eye of what-soever kind in accordance with the principle herein inculcated. 4-5.

Thus ends the ninth Chapter of the Uttara-Tantra in the Sus'ruta Samhitá which deals with the medical treatment of Vátaja Abhishyanda.

* According to Dallana, this Anu-taila is not the one described in Chapter V of the Chikitsita Sthána ; but the one described in the S'álákya-Tantra.

† This couplet may also be translated as follows :—Anjana (black-antimony) rubbed over a stone-slab with clarified butter and breast-milk is also recommended as a best remedy in such cases.

CHAPTER X.

Now we shall discourse on the curative treatment of Abhishyanda (Ophthalmia) due to the action of deranged Pitta (**Pittá-bhishyanda-Pratishedha**). 1.

General Treatment :—Blood-letting and purgatives, eye-washes and plasters round the eyes, medicinal snuffs and Anjana (collyrium), as well as the remedial measures for Pittaja-Visarpa (Erysipelas) should be employed in a case of Pittaja Abhishyanda (Ophthalmia) and Pittaja Adhimantha (Conjunctivites). 2.

Clarified butter or goat's milk duly cooked with *Gundrá*, *S'áli* (paddy), *S'aivála*, *S'aila-bheda*, *Dáru-haridrá*, *Elá*, *Utpala*, two parts of *Lodhra*, *Abhra* (Mustaka), *Padma*-leaves, sugar, *Durvá*, *Ikshu*, *Tála*, *Vetasa*, *Padmaka*, *Drákshá*, honey, (red) *Chandana*, *Yashti-madhu*, breast-milk, *Haridrá* and *Ananta-mula*, should be employed as a **Tarpana** measure* or as a **wash** or **snuff** in the present case. As an alternative, all the preceding drugs or as many of them as would be available should be daily used in the manner of any of the four forms of Nasya†. 3.

Anjanas :—All the Pitta-subduing measures, may be employed in such cases. Application of medicinal snuffs (as well as eye-drops, etc.) with *Kshira-Sarpih* (clarified butter churned from milk) at the interval of three days, as well as that of Anjana (collyrium) with the expressed juice of *Palás'a* or of *S'allaki*, mixed with honey and sugar, should be likewise resorted

* See Chapter XVIII, ibid.

† The four forms of Nasya are (1) Pratimarsha.* (2) Avapida (3) Nasya (snuff) and (4) S'iro-virechana.

to. The thick liquid extract (Rasa-Kriyá)* of *Pálindi* or *Yashti-madhu* mixed with honey and sugar, should be likewise employed. As an alternative, a compound consisting of *Musta, Samudra-phena, Utpala, Vidanga, Elá, Dhátri* and *Vijaka* and prepared in the manner of Rasa-kriyá should be employed (as an **Anjana**). 4.

Acompound of *Tálisa* (D. R.—Kás'is'a), *Elá, Gairika, Us'ira* and *S'amkha* (conch-shell) pasted with breast-milk should be applied to the affected organ in the manner of an **Anjana** (eye-salve). As an alternative, the powder or the Rasa-kriyá of *Dhátaki* and *Syandana* (D. R.—Chandana) mixed with breast-milk should be used as an Anjana. Gold-leaf rubbed with breast-milk, or the flowers of *Kims'uka* rubbed with honey, or of a compound of *Rodhra, Drákshá,* sugar, *Utpala, Vacha* and *Yashti-madhu* rubbed with breast-milk should be used as an **Anjana**. Barks of *Varnaka*† pasted in cow's milk, or (red) *Chandana* wood, *Udumbara* and *Toya* (Válá) pasted in the same, or *Samudra-phena* rubbed either in honey or breast-milk should be likewise applied to the eyes in the manner of an **Anjana**. 5.

Áŝchyotana :—*Rodhra, Yashti-madhu, Drákshá,* sugar and *Utpala* should be soaked in breast-milk. It should then be folded inside a piece of silk (*Kshauma*) and employed as an **Ás'chyotana** (eye-drop). A compound of *Yashti-madhu* and *Rodhra* rubbed in clarified butter should be similarly used. A compound of *Kás'mari* (Gámbhári) *Dhátri, Pathyá* (Haritaki) and *Toya* (Vâlà),

* For preparation of Rasa-kriyá see Chapter XVIII, ibid.

† According to Dallana, '*Varnaka*' means '*Rochanika*'. It may also mean '*Karnika'ra*' which is not accepted either by Gay or by Dallana. It may also mean '*Chandana*' which is most probably the meaning here.

as well as that of *Katphala* and *Ambu* (Vâlâ) should be similarly* prepared and applied. 6.

All the above remedial measures with the exception of blood-letting should be resorted to in a case of Amlá-dhyushita-Drishti and Śukti-pâka. The medicated Ghritas known as the **Traiphala Ghrita** or the **Tilvaka Ghrita**† should be prescribed, or simply old and matured clarified butter should be given in such cases. 7.

In a case of **Śukti-páka** an Anjana with cooling drugs should be speedily employed in the event of the Doshas being located in the lower part of the eye. Fine powder of Vaidurya gem, *Sphatika* (crystal), *Vidruma* (coral) and *Muktá* (pearl), *Samkha* (conch-shell), silver and gold mixed with sugar and honey and used as an anjana would prove a speedy remedy in a case of Śukti-pâka. 8.

Clarified butter should be administered in a case of **Dhuma-darśin** and the procedure and the remedial measures laid down in connection with Rakta-pitta and Pitta-origined Visarpa (Erysipelas) as well as the Pitta-sub-duing remedies ‡ should be likewise employed therein. 9.

Thus ends the tenth chapter in the Uttra-Tantra of the Sus'ruta Samhitá which deals with of the curative treatment of Pittábhishyanda.

* In the first two compounds, some take 'Toya' and '*Ambu*' for water. But Dallana having explained '*Toya*' as '*Valaka*' in a preceding compound we adopt that meaning of the word here also.

† Traiphala-Ghrita is prepared by duly cooking clarified butter with the Kalka and decoction of *Triphala'*. For Tilvaka-Ghrita see chapter III. Chikistsita-Sthána.

‡ By Pitta-subduing remedies Dallana means the remedial measures laid down in connection with the treatment of Pitta-Vidagdha- Drishti.

CHAPTER XI.

Now we shall discourse on the chapter which deals with the curative treatment of Abhishyanda due to the deranged action of Śleshmá (**Śleshmábhishyanda-Pratishedha**). 1.

General Treatment :—An attack of Śleshmaja Abhishyanda or Adhimantha during the stage of acute aggravation should be treated by opening a local vein* or by the employment of fomentation, Avapida-Nasya, Anjana, fumigation, washes, plasters, gargles or non-fatty (Ruksha) eye-drops (Áśchyotana) and Puta-páka. The patient should be made to fast on each fourth day and to take a potion of Tikta-Ghrita† in the morning, and his diet should consist of such articles as do not lead to the aggravation of the bodily Kapha. 2-3.

Tender twigs or leaves of *Kutannata*, *Áshpotá*, *Phanijjhaka*, *Vilva*, *Pattura*, *Pilu*, *Arka* and *Kapittha*‡ should be employed in (mildly) **fomenting** the affected eye. A thin plaster composed of *Válaka*, *S'unthi*, *Devadáru* and *Kushtha*, should be likewise applied to the affected eye. 4.

Hingu, (Asafœtida), *Triphalá*, *Yashti-madhu*, *Saindhava*, *Prapaundaika*, *Anjana* (black Antimony), *Tuttha* (Sulphate of copper), and copper pasted together with

* The word 'Atha' (अथ) in the text means says Dallana, that the local vein should be opened as the best resource, when fomentation, etc. would fail to effect a cure.

† See Chikitsita-sthána, chapter IX.

‡ In place of "*Kutannata*" and "*Arka*" both Vrinda and Chakrapáni read "*Surasa*" and "*Arja*". S'rikantha the commentator of Vrinda however is of opinion that Arka should be better reading in place of that of "*Arja*".

water and made into a stick (Varti) should be applied as an **Anjana** to the affected eye. As an alternative, sticks (Varti) composed of *Pathyá*, *Haridrá*, *Yashti-madhu* and *Anjana* should be similarly applied. Compounds made of the equal parts of *Pippali*, *Maricha*, *S'unthi*, *Haritaki*, *Ámalaki*, *Vibhitaka*, *Haridrá* and *Vidanga*-seeds, or of *Válaka*, *Kushtha*, *Deva-dáru*, (burnt) conch-shell, *Páthá* (Ákanidhi), *Anala* (Chitraka roots), *Pippali*, *Maricha*, *S'unthi* and *Manah-s'ilá* (Realgar) and the flowers of *Játi*, *Karanja* and *S'obhánjana** pasted together with water should be applied to the eye. The seeds† of *Prakiryá* (Karanja), or of *S'igru* with the seeds and flowers of the two kinds of *Vrihati* mixed with *Rasánjana*, *Chandana*, *Saindhava*-salt, *Manah-s'ilá*, *Haritaki*, and garlic taken in equal parts and pasted together with water should be made into sticks (Varti) and used as an **Anjana** in all forms of Kaphaja eye-diseases. 5.

The following medicinal compounds should be prescribed by experts as an **Anjana** (eye-salve) in a case of **Valása-Grathita** after the system of the patient had been properly cleansed by means of blood-letting. A quantity of blue barley with the horns should be soaked (for a week or two) in milk and dried (after the manner of Bhávaná saturation). It should then be burnt into ashes. These ashes should then be mixed with an equal part of burnt ashes of *Arjaka*, *Áshphotaka*, *Kapittha*, *Vilva*, *Nirgundi* and *Játi* flowers and an alka-

* Dallana quotes the reading of "*Panjika'ka'ra*" (another commentator of Sus'ruta) according to whom *Murva'* and the flowers of *Ja'ti* only should be taken instead of the flowers of *Jati*, *Karanja* and *S'obha'njana*. This reading seems to be the correct one inasmuch as this makes the number of the drugs in the list twelve in all, as given by Dallana himself.

† According to some commentators both the seeds and flowers of *Prakiryá* and of *S'igru* should be taken.

line solution should be duly prepared therewith. *Saindhava*, *Tuttha* (Sulphate of copper) and *Rochaná* should now be added to the above alkaline solution and duly boiled. The compound thus prepared should be applied as an **Anjana** with an iron pipe (Nâdi). This is prescribed in a case of Valâsa-Grathita. Alkaline preparations may be similarly prepared with (the flowers, etc. of) *Phanijjhaka* etc., and may be employed in a similar manner. 6.

A (thin) plaster composed of *S'unthi*, *Pippali*, *Musta*, *Saindhava* and white *Maricha** pasted with the expressed juice of *Mátulunga* and applied to the eye as an Anjana, would bring about a speedy cure of the eye-disease known as **Pishtaka**. 7.

Vrihati fruits should be gathered when ripe and a paste compound of (the equal parts of) *Pippali* and *Srotánjana* should be kept inside those seedless fruits for seven nights. The (preserved) paste should then be taken out and applied to the eye as an Anjana. It proves beneficial in a case of **Pishtaka**. Paste may similarly be preserved inside a *Vártáku* (brinjal), *S'igru*, *Indra-Váruni*, *Patola*, *Kiráta-tikta* and *Ámalaki* and used for the same. 8.

Kâsîs'a (Sulphate of iron), *Samudra*†, *Rasánjana* and buds of *Játi*-flowers pasted together and rubbed in honey, is advised to be prescribed as an **Anjana** in a case of **Praklinna-Vartma**. 9.

A single application as an Anjana of the compound composed of excellent *Nádeya* (Saindhava) ‡ salt,

* Dallana explains white *Maricha* as *S'igru* seeds.

† *Samudra* may either mean *Samudra-phena* or Samudra salt, i. e. *Karakacha* salt. The commentators are silent on this point.

‡ Dallana explains Nádeya as meaning Saindhava, but it generally eans Srotanjana (black antimony).

white *pipper** and *Nepála-játa* (Realgar-lit., that which is produced in Nepála) taken in equal parts and pasted together with the expressed juice of *Mátulanga*, would alleviate the itching sensation (Kandu) in the eyes. Similarly a compound of *S'ringa-vera, Deva-dáru, Musta, Saindhavá* salt and buds of *Játi* flowers pasted together with wine and used as an **Anjana** would prove efficacious in a case of swelling (Śopha) and itching sensation of the eyes. The above eye-diseases should be judiciously treated in accordance with the principles laid down in the treatment of the cases of Abhi-shyanda and Adhi-mantha. 10.

Thus ends the eleventh chapter of the Uttara-Tantra in the Sus'ruta Samhitá which treats of the curative treatment of S'leshmâbhishyanda.

* Dallana explains "S'veta-Maricha" as "S'igru-seeds", but there is a particular kind of Maricha which is white in colour and this is also supported by some commentator.

CHAPTER XII.

Now we shall discourse on the curative treatment of the type of Abhishyanda (Ophthalmia) which has its origin in the vitiated condition of the blood **(Raktábhishyanda-Pratishedha).** 1.

General Treatment :—A wise physician shall pursue the same course of medical treatment in those four diseases known as Adhimantha, Abhishyanda, Śirotpâta and Śirá-harsha due to the vitiated condition of the blood. Persons suffering from any of the aforesaid four complaints should be first anointed and lubricated with old and matured clarified butter technically known as *Kaumbha* Ghrita*, or with a copious quantity of clarified butter. **Venesection** should then be resorted to. The patient, having been made thus to bleed as much as required, should be treated with clarified butter duly cooked with Śiro-virechana drugs and mixed with sugar, as an errhine for cleansing the head. Plasters, washes, snuffs (Nasya), inhalations (Dhuma) of medicated smokes, eye-drops (Áśchyotana), Abhyanjana†, Tarpana (soothing measures), Sneha-karma (emulsive measures) and Puta-pâka should then be prescribed according to the nature of the deranged Dosha involved in each case. 2-5.

A plaster (**Pralepa**) composed of *Nilotpala*, *Us'ira*, *Dâru-haridrá*, *Kâliya*, *Yashti-madhu*, *Musta*, *Lodhra* and *Padma-Kâshtha* (taken in equal parts and) mixed with Ghrita—duly washed, should be applied round the region

* See Chapter XLV, Sutra-Sthána.

† Dallana explains "Abhyanjana" as collyrium, but he also says that some commentators take it in its usual sense of anointment with clarified butter washed hundred times in water, or such other Sneha.

of the affected eye. Mild fomentations (Sveda), or leeches should be applied to the region around the eye in the event of there being intolerable pain (due to any defect in bleeding) in the affected organ. Large draughts of clarified butter tend to alleviate the pain. Remedial measures and agents mentioned in connection with Pittâbhishyanda, should be as well employed. 6-7.

Rain-water with powdered *Kas'eru* and *Yashti-madhu* added thereto may be squeezed with benefit through a piece of linen into the affected organ* as an **Áschyotana**. Flowers of *Pâtalá*, *Arjuna*, *S'riparni*, *Dhâtaki*, *Dhátri*, *Vilva*, the two kinds of *Vrihati*, and of *Vimbi-lota* and *Manjishthâ* taken in equal parts and pasted together with honey or expressed juice of sugar-cane and applied to the affected organ as an **Anjana** (Collyrium) is said to be a curative in cases of Raktábhishyanda. 8-9.

A similar compound consisting of *Chandana*, *Kumuda*, *Patra*, *S'ilá-jatu*, *Kumkuma*, powders of dead iron and dead copper, *Tuttha* (Sulphate of copper), lead, bell-metal, *Rasânjana* and the resinous exudation of a *Nimba* tree taken in equal parts should be pasted with honey and made into large **Vartis** (sticks). These are always recommended to be applied to the affected eye as an **Anjana**. 10.

Treatment of Śirotpáta :—A compound consisting of honey and clarified butter and applied as an Anjana should be regarded as a patent cure in cases of **Śirotpáta** eye-disease. A compound composed of *Saindhava* (salt), *Kás'is'a* (Sulphate of iron) and pasted together with breast-milk should be similarly used. The

* Both Dallana and S'ivadàsa say that pure transparent water may be used in preparing the compound if rain-water is not available. Dallana says further that the affected eye should also be washed with the liquid compound thus prepared. S'ivadása, however, supports this latter view.

application as an Anjana of *S'amkha* (conch-shell), *Manah-s'ilá*, *Tuttha*, *Dáru-haridrá*, and *Saindhava* pasted with honey, or of (white) *Maricha* pasted with the juice of *S'irisha* flowers, honey and wine, or of *Svarna-Garika* pasted with honey would be attended with beneficial results in cases of **Sirotpáta**. 11.

Sirá-harsha :—A compound consisting of *Phánita* (treacle boiled down to a sticky consistency) and honey should be applied to the affected organ as an **Anjana** in a case of **Sirá-harsha**. Similar applications of compounds composed of *Rasánjana* (Antimony) pasted with honey, or of *Saindhava* and *Kás'is'a* (Sulphate of iron) pasted with honey, or of *Vetrámla** and *Saindhava* pasted with *Phánita* and breast-milk would likewise prove highly efficacious. 12.

Treatment of Arjuna :—All the measures and remedies for Pittábhishyanda should be employed in cases of **Arjuná** eye-disease. The expressed juice of sugar-cane, honey, sugar, breast-milk, *Dáru-haridra*, *Yashti-madhu* and *Saindhava* should be used in combination as a wash (**Seka**), or as an **Anjana**. *Amla* (Kánjika, &c.) should also be used as an **Áschyotana** (eye-drop) in such cases. The following drugs, *viz.*, sugar, *Yashti-madhu*, *Katvanga*, *Mastu*, *Amla*, honey, *Saindháva*, *Vija-puraka*, *Kola* and *Dádimba* of acid taste and other acid fruits either singly or in combination of two or three should be judiciously used (as an **Áschyotana** with a due consideration of the vitiated Dosha in each case). 13–14.

These two following compounds viz., of *Sphatika*

* Dallana explains "*Vetrámla*" as "*Amla vetasa*". Some, however, divide it into two words *viz.*, "Vetra" and "Amla" meaning thereby sprouts of *Vetra* (cane) and *Amla-vetasa* respectively.

(crystal), *Vidruma* (coral), *S'amkha* (conch-shell), and *Yashti-madhu*, pasted with honey, as well as of *S'amkha*, sugar, and *Samudra-phena* pasted with honey, if used as an **Anjana** would prove curative in a case of **Arjuna** eye-disease. *Saindhava* and *Kataka* pasted with honey, or *Rasánjana* pasted with honey, or *Kás'isa* (Sulphate of iron) pasted with honey, should constantly be applied as an Anjana to the affected organ. 15.

Scarifying-Anjana :—All kinds of powdered (dead) metals (Gold, Silver, Iron, Copper, etc.) and metallic substances (*Manah-s'ilá, Gairika*, etc.), (the five officinal kinds of) salt, all kinds of gems (*Vaidurya*, coral etc.), the teeth (of cows, horses, etc.), the horns (of cows, etc.), the drugs of the sedative (Avasádana) * group, pulverised shells of hen's eggs, *Las'una* (garlic), *Trikatu*, *Karanja* seeds and *Elá* (cardamom) mixed together and used as an Anjana, should be regarded as **Scarifying** (Lekhya) in their action. 16.

Treatment of Śukra :—In a case of non-ulcerated (A-vrana) **Śukra** (milky film or white fleshy growth in the eye) a skilful physician shall (first) adopt all the preceding measures prescribed in the treatment of (Blood-origined) Abhishyanda,† beginning with Rakta-visrávana (Venesection) and ending with Puta-pâka (and these failing, the Lekhyánjana—collyrium for scarifying) should be adopted. A case of ulcerated (Sa-vrana) **Śukra** whether superficial or deep-seated ‡ or rough should be treated in the same manner. 17-18.

* The group beginning with Kás'is'a—See Chapter XXXVI, Sutra-Sthana, page 334, Vol. I.

† See paras 3 and 4 of this Chapter.

‡ "Superficial" (Uttâna) is here used in the sense of "seated in the first layer" and "deep seated" (Avagádha) 'seated in the second layer'.

. In a case of **S'ukra** the affected part should be rubbed (scarified) with a compound consisting of *S'irisha*-seeds, *Maricha*, *Pippali* and *Saindhava* pounded together, or with *Saindhava* alone. A compound composed of powdered copper, *Manah-s'ilá*, *Maricha* and *Saindhava* each preceding drug being taken in a quantity double the one immediately succeeding it in the order of enumeration*, should be pounded together and made into a thin paste. Applied as an **Anjana** to the seat of the disease, it will cure a case of **S'ukra**. As alternatives, the two compounds composed of *S'amkha*, stones of *Kolas*, *Kataka*, *Drákshá*, *Yashti-madhu*, *Mákshika* (honey), or of teeth (of cows, etc.), *Samudra-phena* and *S'irisha* flower and honey should be applied to the affected locality inthe manner of applying an Anjana. The **Kshá-ránjana** (alkaline collyrium) mentioned in connection with the medical treatment of Valása-grathita,† may as well be profitably employed as an Anjana (eye-salve) in the present disorder. Eye-salves made of fried huskless *Mudga* pulse, (burnt) *S'amkha* and sugar mixed with honey, or of the pith of *Madhuka* pasted with honey, or of the inner pulps of the stones of *Vibhitaka* pasted with honey should be constantly used as an Anjana, in cases of the eye-disease known as **S'ukra**. A compound consisting of conch-shell, oyster-shell, *Drákshá*, *Yashti-madhu*, *Kataka* and honey may be used and soothing application (**Tarpana**) antidotal to the deranged bodily Váyu, should be resorted to in cases of S'ukra, if the second layer (Patala) of the eye is attended with pain (S'ula). 19-21.

* One part of *Saindhava*, two parts of *Maricha*, four of *Manah-s'ilá*, eight of *S'amkha* and sixteen parts of copper should be taken in the preparation of the compound.

† See Chapter XI, para 6.

Young bamboo-sprouts, *Arushkara*, *Tála* (palm) and *Nárikela* (cocoanut)* should be burnt to ashes and alkaline water should be duly prepared therewith. The burnt ashes of elephant's bones should be soaked several (seven) times with the above alkaline preparation in the manner of Bhávaná saturation. The application of this preparation in the manner of an Anjana tends to remove the discolouring nature (whiteness) of a case of S'ukra †. 22.

Treatment of Ajaká :—The thin watery matter accumulated in the eye in a case of **Ajaká** should be drained by making a puncture on either side (of the cornea) with a needle after which the incidental ulcer should be filled with powdered beef mixed with clarified butter. Scarification should be many times made in the event of the ulcer becoming raised. 23.

Treatment of Akshi-páka :—Applications of Sneha and of Sveda (fomentation) to the affected locality should be made in cases of the two kinds of eye-disease known as Sa-s'opha and A-s'opha **Akshi-páka** (inflammation of the eye-lid whether attended with any local swelling or otherwise). Venesection should then be resorted to. Eye-washes, eye-drops (Ás'chyotana), errhines (Nasya) and Puta-páka measures should also be employed. 24.

After having cleansed the system of the patient both internally and externally the following compounds should be used as an Anjana (in cases of the two kinds

* The spathe (Jatá) of the palm tree and the shell of the cocoanut fruit should be taken in preparing the compound —S'ivadása.

† The prepared powder of elephant's bone should be mixed with honey and rubbed over the affected part (S'ukra) with the tip of the finger or with a S'aláká (rod). The eye should then be washed with the infusion of *Triphalá*.—Dallana.

of **Akshi-páka**). *Saindhava* and clarified butter pasted together in a copper vessel with flesh or *Maireya* or curd or with curd-cream should be used as an **Anjana**. As an alternative, the rust of bell-metal pasted with clarified butter, or *Saindhava* pasted with breast-milk, or equal parts of the pith of *Madhuka* tree and *Gairika* pasted with honey, or *Saindhava* and copper pasted with breast-milk and clarified butter should be used as **Anjanas**. The compounds of *Dádimba*, *Araveta*, *As'-manta*, *Kola*, and *Saindhava* pasted with any acid juice* should be applied to the affected organ in the manner of a **Rasa-kriyá** measure for the cure of (the two kinds of) Akshi-páka. 25-26.

Animal flesh and *Saindhava* salt soaked in clarified butter and mixed with *S'unthi* and breast-milk should be applied to the affected organ in the manner of an **Ás'chyotana** or as an **Anjana**. A compound consisting of *Játi* flower, *Saindhava*, *S'unthi*, *Pippali* and huskless *Vidanga* pasted together with honey, may as well be used as an **Anjana** with advantage in a case of **Akshi-páka**. 27-28.

Treatment of Puyálasa :—Blood-letting (after the application of Sneha and Sveda) and poulticing (Upanáha) of the affected locality are efficacious in the affection of the eye, known as **Puyálasa**. The measures and remedies which prove curative in cases of Akshi-páka should as well be employed with discretion in this case by a physician. An **Anjana** (eye-salve) composed of *Árdraka*, *Saindhava* and *Kás'isa* (Sulphate of iron), or *Kás'isa Saindhava*, *Árdraka*, iron and copper dust pasted together with honey, should be applied to the affected eye in the manner of an Anjana (in a case of Puyálasa). 29-30.

* Some add honey in the list.

Treatment of Praklinna-vartma :— The deranged Doshas of the system should be duly* removed (corrected) and the patient should be duly soothed in a case of **Praklinna-vartma**, after which washes, eye-salves, eye-drops (Ás'chyotana), snuffs (Nasya) and fumigation (Dhumá) should be resorted to according to the Dosha involved in each case. A compound composed of *Musta*, *Haridrá*, *Yashti-madhu*, *Priyangu*, *Siddhártha*, *Rodhra*, *Utpala-sárivá* † pasted together ‡ should be employed in the manner of an **Ás'chyotana** measure. As an alternative, the compound consisting of *Rásánjana* and honey should be used as an **Anjana**. 31-32.

The decoction of the leaves and fruits of *Ámalaka* should be duly prepared (in the manner of Rasa-kriyá) and used as an **Anjana**. **Rasa-kriyá** preparations prepared with (the expressed juice of) the roots of bamboo, or **Vartis** prepared with the same by (condensing it by) cooking it (again) in a copper vessel, should be used for the above purpose. Rasa-kriyá preparations prepared with *Triphalá*, flowers of *Palása*, or *Khara-manjari*, should be similarly applied to the affected organ. Eye-salves made of powdered *Káms'ya-mala* and cotton fibres (Tantu) burnt together and pasted with the milk of a she-goat and mixed with (white) *Maricha* and powdered copper should be used as a *Pratyanjana* to the eye (already weakened by the use of Anjana.) 33-34.

* Dallana says that the deranged Doshas of the system should be cleansed with the application of Sneha, Venesection, purgative, errhines and A'sthápana.

† In place of 'रोध्रोत्पलसारिवाभिः' some read 'लोध्रासितसारिवाभिः', meaning in this case 'Syâma-latâ' by the term 'Asita-sárivâ'. Others again mean 'Rasánjana' by the term 'Asita'.—Dallana.

‡ Dallana recommends 'rain water' as the liquid for the preparation.

An eye-salve or an Anjana made of *Samudra-phena*, *Saindhava*, conch-shell, *Mudga* and white *Maricha* mixed together (in the shape of a powder) should be prescribed in a case of **Aklinna-vartma** as it would promptly alleviate the local itching. The foregoing measures and remedies should be likewise employed in a case of **Praklinna-vartma** according to the nature of the deranged Doshas involved therein. An Anjana prepared with the admixture of *Kajjala* and *Tuthhaka* (Sulphate of copper) rubbed in clarified butter on the surface of a copper vessel, would be similarly used (in such cases). 35-36.

Thus ends the twelfth chapter of the Uttara-Tantra in the Sus'ruta Samhitá which treats of the curative treatment of Raktábhishyanda.

CHAPTER XIII.

Now we shall discourse on the curative treatment of eye-diseases in which Scarification should be resorted to (**Lekhya-Roga-Pratishedha**). 1.

The general course of treatment to be adopted in the nine kinds of eye diseases which are amenable to Scarifying (Lekhana) operations is as follows :—The patient should be laid in a chamber not exposed to the sun and the gales of wind, after having been treated with proper emulsive measures (Sneha-karma)* and subjected to a course of emetics and purgatives. The eye-lid should be over-turned with the thumb and the index finger and should be very carefully fomented with a piece of linen soaked in lukewarm water and squeezed. The eye-lid should be covered with a piece of linen and over-turned with the thumb and the index finger at the time to guard against its movement and enclosing. The (part of the) eye-lid to be scraped, should be wiped with a linen and marked with a surgical instrument and the scraping should be effected therein with a scraping knife or any (rough) leaf according to the exigencies of the case. After the subsidence of the bleeding, the part should be fomented and then gently rubbed (Pratisárana) with a medicinal compound consisting of *Manahs'ilá* (Realgar), *Kás'isa* (Sulphate of iron), *Trikatu*, *Anjana* (black antimony), *Saindhava* salt and *Mákshika* finely pounded together. After this the part should be washed with lukewarm water and lubricated with clarified butter. The subsequent treatment thereof should be

* It should be noted that the patient should also be fomented (Sveda) after being treated with the emulsive measures.

like that of an ulcer (Vrana).* Fomentations, Avapida, etc., should also be employed after three days. Thus I have described to you the general measures to be observed in scraping an affected locality in the eye. 2.

Satisfactory and deficient scarification :—Stoppage of bleeding, subsidence of the swelling and itching, a smooth level aspect of the part like the surface of a finger nail are the features, which mark a **proper** and **satisfactory** scarification. Redness of the eyes, swelling and discharge of blood from the operated locality, occurrence of Timira (blindness or darkness of vision), non-ameliorations of the disease under treatment, brownness, heaviness, numbness, itching, horripilation and coating (as if with foreign matter) of the eye-lids and a consequent high inflammation of the eye if not attended to in time, are the symptoms which attend an **incomplete** and **unsatisfactory** scarification, and this should be remedied by anointing† and scarifying the affected part again. 3-4.

Excessive Scarification :—Excessive discharge and pain in the locality together with an upturning of the eye-lids and spontaneous uprooting of the eye-lashes should be ascribed to **excessive** scraping. Fomentation, application of Sneha and employment of Váyu-subduing measures should be resorted to in such cases. 5.

In the following diseases of the eye, *viz.*, Vartmávabandha, Klishta-vartma, Bahala-vartma and Pothaki, the affected part should first be gently scraped and then

* For the first seven days the treatment should be like that of an incidental ulcer (Sadyo-vrana) after which period, the case should be treated, if necessary, as a case of S'árira-Vrana.

† Dallana says that some read 'स्वेदयित्वा' (fomenting) in place of 'स्नेहयित्वा' (anointing).

scarified. In Śyâva-vartma and Kardama-vartma, the intelligent physician will gently scarify the affected part neither deeply nor superficially. In cases of Utsangini, Śarkará and Kumbhikini, the seat of the disease should be first cut (with a knife) and then carefully scarified. An incision should be followed by a scarification in the case of small, very hard, supperated, copper-coloured, Pidakás (pustules) occurring on (the inner membrane of) the eye-lid. Small and slightly swelling Pidakás (pustules) occurring on the exterior surface of the eye-lid should be remedied with fomentations, plasters and the general corrective remedies. 6.

Thus ends the thirteenth chapter of the Uttara-Tantra in the Sus'ruta Samhitá which treats of the curative treatment of (eye-) diseases amenable to scarification.

CHAPTER XIV.

Now we shall discourse on the curative treatment of eye-diseases which require surgical incisions (**Bhedya-Roga-Pratishedha**). 1.

Treatment of Visa-granthi:—In a case of suppurating **Visa-granthi**, it should be first fomented, and its puncture-like holes should be completely incised (so as to remove any swelling in the affected part). It should then be dusted with *Saindhava*, *Kás'is'a*, *Mágadhi*, *Pushpánjana*, *Manah-s'ilá* and *Elá* pounded together*. Honey and clarified butter should then be applied (over the dusted part), and it should be duly (loosely) bandaged (for the complete union of the parts). 2.

Lagana:—An incision should be made into the affected part in a case of **Lagana**, and any of the following drugs, *viz.*, *Rochaná*, *Yava-kshára*, *Tuttha*, *Pippali* and honey should be applied to the incised part; while in serious (lit.—big) cases cauterization with alkali or with fire will be the remedy. 3.

Anjana:—In a case of **Anjana**, the affected part should be duly fomented and if it spontaneously bursts open, it should be well pressed and rubbed (Pratisárana) with a plaster-compound of *Manah-s'ilá*, *Elá*, *Tagara-páduká* and *Saindhava*, pasted together with honey. If, however, the surgeon wants to open it, it should be rubbed with honey and *Rasánjana* mixed together and

* Both Vrinda and Chakradatta read only the first two lines of the text and hold that the incision should be dusted with *Saindhava* only. Their commentators, however, accept the reading there to be Sus'ruta's. They supply the next two lines of Sus'ruta, and notice the consequent alteration in the sense.

then coated with a warm collyrium made with the lamp-black collected from a burning lamp flame. 4.

Krimi-granthi :—In a case of **Krimi-granthi**, the affected part should be duly fomented after it has been incised and it should then be treated with the Rasa-kriyá solution prepared with (the decoction of) *Triphalá* (with the addition of) *Tuttha**, *Ká-sisa* and *Saindhava*. In a case of **Upanáha** (in the eye) due to the action of the deranged Kapha, the affected part should be opened and rubbed with powdered *Pippali* and *Saindhava* mixed with honey. It should then be scraped with a Mandalágra instrument. The surrounding parts should also be gently scratched all around. 5.

In the foregoing five cases of incisable eye-disease, until the setting in of suppuration therein, the affected eye should first be treated with Sneha and then with light fomentation with (the help of) tender leaves (as a cover over the eye). In all the remedies to be adopted in the treatment of these (incisable eye) diseases, the application of a Sneha should be first adopted. In cases, however, where suppuration had already set in, the remedies for the healing up of the ulcer, should be carefully adopted. 6.

Thus ends the fourteenth chapter of the Uttara-Tantra of the Sus'ruta Samhitá which deals with the curative treatment of (eye-) diseases requiring incisions.

* Both Vrinda and Chakrapáni read '*Mutra*' (cow's urine) in place of '*Tuttha*'. Both of them also recommend the addition of *Rasánjana* in the compound.

CHAPTER XV.

Now we shall discourse on the curative treatment of eye-diseases, which should be cured with excisions **(Chhedya-Roga-Pratishedha).** 1.

Treatment of Armas :—The patient should be first treated with a Sneha-predominating food before being surgically operated upon in a case of **Arman** marked by the manifest vegetation or polypus (on the affected eye). The patient should then be made carefully to sit at ease and the affected eye should then be irritated by casting powdered *Saindhava*-salt into its cavity after which the eye-ball, without any loss of time, should be duly fomented and rubbed with the hand. The intelligent physician will then ask the patient to look at his Apánga (the interior corner of his own affected eye) and the cyst or the polypus (thus turned up), should be carefully secured with a hook (Vadiśa) and held with a Muchundi instrument or with a thread-needle. It is dangerous to suddenly uplift the eye-lid under the circumstances. The two eye-lids should be firmly drawn asunder so as to guard against their being anywise hurt during the operation. The polypus, thus made flabby and pendent with the means of the three aforesaid accessories, should be fully got rid of by scraping it with a sharp Mandalágra instrument. The root of the polypus should be pushed asunder from the Krishna-mandala (Sclerotic region) and the Śukla-mandala (region of the cornea), to the extremity of the Kaninaka (pupil) and then removed. The Kaninaka (pupil) should be duly guarded so as not to be hurt. A quarter layer of the flesh (of the polypus) should be left back and then the operation would not in any way hurt or injure the eye. An operation at a point beyond the aforesaid limit of the Kaninaka (might hurt the pupil and) would set up a hœmorrhage and beget a sinus (as well as pain) in the locality. The vegetation or polypus is sure to grow up again to its former size if it is cut off insufficiently. 2.

A shreddy or netted Arman in the form of a membranous growth (Jála) in the eye should be made pendent by rubbing it (with *Saindhava*-salt) and then cut with a bent Vadiśa instrument at the junction of the Śukla-mandala (cornea) and the Vartma-mandala (conjunctiva or eye-lid). The affected part should then be rubbed with a compound consisting of *Yava-kshára*, *Trikatu* and *Saindhava*-salt (pounded together) and then (duly) fomented and bandaged up by the skilful physician. Lardaceous or oily (Sneha) application should thereafter be prescribed with due regard to the nature of the place*, the season, the time (day or night) and the strength of the patient, and the incidental wound should be treated as an ulcer. The bandage should be removed after three days and the affected part should be (mildly) fomented with the application of heated palms of the hands and treated with corrective or purifying remedies. 3.

Milk duly cooked with *Karanja* seed, *Ámalaka* and *Yashti-madhu* and mixed with honey (when cold), should be dropped twice a day (morning and evening) into the affected eye in the event of there being any pain in it. A cold plaster composed of *Yashti-madhu*, polens of lotus (*Utpala*) and *Durvá*-grass pasted together with milk and mixed with clarified butter is recommended in such cases to be applied to the scalp. 4.

* In place of 'देश'—the particular part and nature of the country, some read 'दोष'—the particular Dosha involved in each case.

Any residue of the **Arman**, left after the excision, should be removed with the application of Lekhya* (scraping) Anjana or eye-salve. An Arman (Cyst-like papilla or protruberance) which is as white as curdled milk (Dadhi), or which looks blood-red or blue or grey, should be treated like a case of Śukrárman (Opacity of the cornea or a flimy and fleshy growth in the eye). An Arman which is very thick and looks like a piece of skin and covered over with fibres of flesh and nerves †, as well as one occurring on the Krishna-mandala (region of the iris) should be excisioned. The eye assumes its former and natural colour and function, and becomes free from pain and other complications by the proper excision of an Arman. 5-8.

Treatment of Sirá-Jála and Sirá-pidaká :—In a case of **Sirá-Jála**, the hardened veins (Sirá) should be hung down with a hook (Vadiśa) and scraped with a Mandalágra (round-topped) instrument. Cysts or pimples (Pidakás) appearing on the diseased veins in a case of the aforesaid Sirá-Jála and not proving amenable to the application of medicines, should be excisioned as in a case of Arma with a Mandalâgra instrument. Pratisárana (rubbing) as in a case of Arma and Lekhana (scraping) with due regard to the nature of the deranged Doshas involved in each case, are also recommendad in both the diseases (Sirá-Jála and Sirá-Pidaká) under discussion. 9.

Treatment of Parvaniká :—In a case of **Parvaniká** the place of junction ‡ (of the lachrymal

* For Lekhya Anjana see Chapter XII, para 16 of this Uttara Tantra.

† Some here read 'सिरा' (veins) in place of 'घन' ।

‡ The 'junction' is the junction of the Krishna-mandala and the S'ukla-mandala of the eye.—Dallana.

sac and the cornea) should be duly fomented. A quarter part only of the protuberance or growth should be kept apart, while the remaining upper three quarters should be secured with a hook and cut with a knife. Half of the aforesaid quarter part should then be cut away (very carefully), as lachrymal sinus (and consequent lachrymation) would otherwise set in. The seat of operation should be subsequently rubbed (Pratisárana) with a compound of honey and *Saindhava*-salt. Scarifying (Lekhana) powders should then be applied to the affected part for the complete recovery of the disease (any complaint still remaining). 10.

Churna-Anjana :—Powders of *S'amkha* (conch-shell), *Samudra-phena*, marine oyster-shell, crystal, ruby, coral, *As'mantaka*, *Vaidurya* (Lapis lazuli), pearl, iron, copper and *Srotonjana* (antimony) taken in equal parts and mixed together, should be stuffed in a ram's horn* and then let the intelligent one apply this **Churna-anjana** (powder) to the affected locality, morning and evening everyday, as such applications are extremely efficacious in all types of Armans, Pidakás, Sirá-jála, Arsás, Śushkárśas and Arvuda, etc., in the eye. 11.

Treatment of inner part of the eye-lids :—The mode of treatment in a case of any affection in the inner lining of the Vartma (eye-lid) is given below. The affected part should be first fomented and then the eye-lid should be over-turned (held at an angle), and the diseased growth or swelling should be carefully lifted up with a needle, when an experienced physician should cut it at its root or base with the help of a sharp Mandalágra instrument. After that the affected part should be rubbed with a pulverised compound consist-

* Dallana explains '*Mesha-s'ringa*' as a kind of *Ingudi* tree.

ing of *Saindhava*, *Kásisa* (Sulphate of iron) and *Pippali*. The affected eye-lid should then be carefully cauterised with a (red-hot) rod after a (complete) cessation of the bleeding. The residue of its root or base, if any, should be scarified with a scarifying alkaline (caustic) preparation. Decoctions of strong emetic and purgative drugs* should be (internally) administered for the elimination of the Doshas (from the Vrana—ulcer). The measures and remedies mentioned in connection with Abhishyanda (Ophthalmia) should also be prescribed with regard to the nature of the bodily Doshas involved in the case. The patient shall observe strict regimen of diet and conduct for a month after the surgical operation. 12.

Thus ends the fifteenth chapter in the Uttara-Tantra of the Sus'ruta Samhitá which treats of the remedies of eye-diseases requiring excisions or surgical operation.

* Some commentators say that emetics and purgatives should be internally administered, but Dallana and the Panjiká-kára oppose this view.

CHAPTER XVI.

Now we shall discourse on the curative measures for the remedy of diseases occurring on the eye-lashes and hence on the eye-lid **(Pakshma-kopa Pratishedha).** 1.

Surgical Treatment :—In a case of **Pakshma-kopa** which is an affection of the eye-lid and which has been described before as admitting only of palliative treatment, the patient should be first treated with a Sneha and made to take his seat (in a proper position). A cut in the shape and size of a barley corn should be made in the eye-lid horizontally parallel to (the part of the eye-ball lying between) the Kaninaka (pupil) and the Apánga (exterior corner of the eye) leaving two parts below the eye-brow and one part above the eye-lashes. The surgeon should then diligently suture up the two edges of the incisions with (horse's) hair. After the application of honey and clarified butter to the operated part, it should be treated in the manner of an (incidental) ulcer. A piece of linen should be tied round the forehead and the horse's hair sewing up the operated part should be attached thereto. The stitching hair should be carefully removed after the complete adhesion* of the two edges of the incidental ulcer. 2.

Cauterisation :—In case of the failure of the preceding measure, the eye-lid should be carefully examined and lifted up in an inverted posture and the diseased cyst (Bali) should be very carefully **cauterised** with fire or alkali. As an alternative, the Pakshma-

* According to Vágbhata, the stitching hair should be removed on the fifth day.

málá (eye-lashes) should be all removed and the affected eye-lid having been carefully secured with three hooks (Vadis'a) should be rubbed with pasted *Haritaki* and *Tuvaraka* (Lodhra). The four aforesaid measures* as well as purgatives, eye-drops (Ás'chyotana), medicinal snuffs, inhalations (fumigations), Plasters, Collyrium, Sneha and Rasa-kriyá, should be likewise held as beneficial† in cases of Pakshma-kopa. 3-5.

Thus ends the sixteenth chapter of the Uttara-Tantra in the Sus'ruta Samhitá which treats of the remedies of Pakshma-kopa.

* The four measures are (*a*) operation, (*b*) cauterisation with fire, (*c*) cauterisation with alkali, and (*d*) application of medicinal drugs.

† It should be noted that this disease cannot be radically cured, but is amenable only to palliative treatments (याप्य).

CHAPTER XVII.

Now we shall discourse on the curative treatment of the diseases of the pupil and the Crystalline lens (**Drishti-gata-Roga-Pratishedha**). 1.

Of the diseases included within the present group, three are curable, three are incurable, while the remaining six admit only of palliative treatment. The curative remedies of the disease known as **Dhuma-dars'i** (smoky or dusky vision) has been already described (in connection with the medical treatment of Pittaja Ophthalmia) *. All the remedies applicable in cases of deranged Pitta and Kapha as well as application of Nasya (snuff), Seka (sprinkling), Anjana (Collyrium), A'lepa (plaster), Puta-páka and Tarpana (soothing) remedies with the exception of surgical operation should be respectively administered in cases of Pitta-affected (Pitta-vidagdha) and Kapha-affected (S'leshma-vidagdha) vision. Traiphala-Ghrita should be prescribed in a case of **Pitta-vidagdha-Drishti** and Traivrita-Ghrita in a case of **S'leshma-vidagdha-Drishti**. Potions of old and matured clarified butter as well as of Tailvaka-Ghrita are equally efficacious in both cases †. Collyriums (Anjanas) should be prepared with *Gairika*, *Saindhava*, *Pippali*, and the charred remains (Masi) of cow's teeth, or with beef, *Maricha*, *S'irisha*-seeds and *Manah-s'ilá*, or with the stalk of a *Kapittha* fruit together with honey, or with *Átmaguptá* pasted with honey ; these four

* See Chapter X, 9, Uttara-Tantra.

† Traiphala-Ghrita, Traivrita-Ghrita and Tailvaka-Ghritá should be prepared with both the decoction and Kalka of Triphalá, Trivrita and of Tilvaka respectively.

Anjanas may be used with advantage in both the types under discussion. 2-3.

Pushpa'njana :—Powders of the flowers of *Kubjaka, As'oka, S ála, Ámra, Priyangu, Nalini* and of *Utpala*, as well as powdered *Renuká, Pippali, Haritaki* and *Ámlaki* mixed with honey and clarified butter, should be kept inside a hollow bamboo and applied to the eye in the manner of a collyrium (Anjana) in cases of Pitta-vidagdha and Śleshmá-vidagdha eye-diseases. 4.

Dravánjana and Gudikánjana :—As an alternative, *Renuká* pasted with the expressed juice of the flowers of *Ámra* (mangoe) and *Jambu* (black-berry) and mixed with honey and clarified butter, should be used in both the above cases as an Anjana. Pollens of *Nalini* (red lotus) and of *Utpala* (blue lotus) as well as *Gairika* * pasted together with the Rasa (watery secretions) of cow-dung † and made into large pills (Gudiká) may be profitably applied to the eye as an Anjana alike in cases of day-blindness and night-blindness. This Anjana is called the Gudikánjana. 5.

Treatment of Day-blindness :—*Rasánjana, Rasa* (Juice) ‡, honey, *Tális'a-patra* and *Svarna-gairika* should be pasted together with the Rasa of cow-dung and applied (in the manner of an Anjana) in cases of Pitta-affected vision *i.e.* **day-blindness**. *S'ita*

* Chakradatta does not read 'Gairika' in the list.

† In place of "गोशकृत्" some read "गोयकृत्" *i.e.*, the liver of a "गो" which may mean a cow or any animal, such as goat, sheep, etc.

‡ According to Dallana, Rasa (lit :—Juice) means the juice of *A'malaka*. According to others, however, it means the juice of the leaves of *Játi* flower. Chakradatta, however, reads "घृत" (clarified butter) in place of "रस".

(Rasánjana, or according to some Camphor), and *Sauvira* should be soaked in Rasa (meat-juice) * and then pasted together. It should then be soaked again in the bile of a tortoise or of a *Rohita* fish and dried and reduced to powder. The present compound is called the **Churna-anjana** (powdered Collyrium) and may be used beneficially for the pacification of Pitta (in cases of Pitta-vidagdha-Drishti). *Kás'mari* flowers, *Yashti-madhu*, *Dárvi*, *Rodhra* and *Rasánjana*, should be pounded together and mixed with honey. Used as an Anjana it is always efficacious in the affections of the eye. 6-8.

Treatment of nocturnal blindness :—The application of a medicinal **Varti** (stick) composed of *Sauviránjana*, *Saindhava*, *Pippali* and *Renuká* pasted together with the urine of a she-goat would prove highly beneficial in cases of **nocturnal blindness**. Similarly the application of a medicinal **Varti** (stick) composed of *Kálánu-Sárivá*, *Pippali*, *S'unthi*, *Yashti-madhu*, *Tális'a-patra*, the two kinds of *Haridrá*, and *Musta*, pasted with the Rasa of cow-dung † and dried in the shade, proves beneficial in such cases. *Manah-s'ilá*, *Haritaki*, *Trikatu*, *Balá*, Kálánu-sárivá and (*S'amudra-*) *Phena* pasted together with the milk of a she-goat and similarly prepared in the shape of a **Varti** is also recommended. 9-11.

Rasa-Kriya'njana :—The urine, bile and dung of a cow ‡ together with wine, should be boiled (in the manner of Rasa-kriyánjana preparation) in the

* Rasa may also, from the context, mean the watery secretions of cow-dung.

† Dallana's reading is evidently 'गोयकृत्रस' which he explains as meaning the juice or serum of the liver of a goat, &c.

‡ The text has "गोमूत्रपित्त" । The term "गो" which literally means a cow, here stands for any female quadruped, such as a she-goat, etc.

expressed juice of *Dhátri*, or in the Rasa (serum) of the liver of an animal (e.g. a goat), or in the decoction of *Triphalá*. It is called the **Kshudránjana**, and should be applied to the affected organ in the manner of an Anjana (collyrium). An Anjana consisting of cow's urine, clarified butter, *Samudra-phena*, *Pippali*, *Katphala*, *Saindhava* and honey mixed together should be first kept inside a hollow bamboo and subsequently applied (in night-blindness) as a collyrium. The Medas (fat) and liver of a goat, together with a quantity of clarified butter skimmed out of the milk of a she-goat, mixed with *Pippali* and *Saindhava* should be boiled and cooked with the (expressed) juice of *Ámalaka* (in the manner of Rasa-kriyá preparations). It should then be mixed with honey and kept in a closed vessel made of *Khadira* (Catechu) wood. The use of this (compound), known as the Kshudrânjana, as an Anjana (collyrium) would be attended with good results. *Harenu*, *Pippali*-seeds (without pericarps), *Elâ* and the liver (of a goat, etc.) should be pasted with the Rasa of cow-dung. Used as an Anjana, it would prove efficacious in a case of Kapha-affected vision (Śleshma-Vidagdha-Drishti). 12-14.

The liver of a Godhâ (a kind of wild lizard) should be partially opened and stuffed with *Pippali* and roasted in fire (having been coated with clay). The use of the compound * for only once † as an Anjana (with honey)

* According to Dallana the Pippali so roasted should be used with honey as an Anjana.

† Both Vrinda and Chakradatta read 'यकृत्' in place of 'सकृत्' and the commentators of both of them say that the sentence means—the liver should be taken internally and the Pippali should be used as an Anjana. The commentator of Vrinda further says that the practice is to use both of them together as an Anjana.

would be found to be highly beneficial in cases of *night-blindness*. Similarly a single application of an Anjana made of a goat's liver stuffed with Pippali * and roasted in fire as in the preceding case would speedily and certainly cure an attack of night-blindness. As an alternative, both the spleen and the liver (of a goat or of a lizard) would be cut into pieces, mixed with oil and clarified butter, and roasted on a spit. Used internally or used as an Anjana with mustard oil, it would speedily cure an attack of night-blindness. 15-17.

An Anjana or a pill composed of *Nadija* (Saindhava), *S'imbi* (D. R.—Śamkha—conch-shell), *Kataka*, *Anjana* (Rasánjana), *Manah-s'ilá*, the two kinds of *Nis'á*, pasted together with the juice of the liver † (of a cow) and mixed with red-sandal paste is recommended in a case of **day-blindness**. 18.

Treatment of palliative types:—Bleeding by opening the (local) veins should be resorted to in the six kinds of ocular affections in which the palliative treatment is all that is open to us. The patient should be as well kept constantly purged with draughts of matured clarified butter duly cooked with the admixture of suitable purgative drugs. In a Vátaja

* Both Vágbhata and Dallana plainly say that the roasted *Pippali* only should be used with honey as an Anjana in cases of night-blindness.

† There is a confusion in the reading of this couplet. In place of "यकृद्रसे" i.e. pasted with the juice of the liver (of a cow or any other animal), Chakradatta reads "गवां यकृत्" i.e. to say—the liver of a cow (and of no other animal) should be taken. Vrinda, however, reads and his commentator accepts the reading "अगवां यकृत्" (the liver of an animal other than a cow) ; but this reading is objectionable on the ground of a faulty construction. "शकृद्रसे" i. e. pasted in the watery secretions of cow-dung, is yet another variant noticed by both the commentators of Vrinda and of Chakradatta.

type (of any of these six affections) purging should be induced with castor oil taken through the vehicle of milk. Administration of **Traiphala-Ghrita** is also recommended for purgative purposes, especially in the Pittaja blood-origined types. Purging with (clarified butter duly cooked with) *Trivrit* should be induced in types having their origin in the deranged Kapha, while oil duly cooked with *Trivrit* should be administered (for the purpose) in cases of affections having their origin in the concerted action of all the three deranged Doshas. The use in any shape of old and matured clarified butter, kept in an iron vessel, proves beneficial in cases of **Timira** of any type. Clarified butter cooked with (the Kalka and decoction) of *Triphalá* or *Mesha-s'ringi* always proves efficacious in Timira of any type. The patient should be made to lick a compound of powdered *Triphalá* with a copious quantity of clarified butter in cases of Pittaja blindness, with oil in the Vataja type, and with a copious quantity of honey in the Kaphaja type, of this disease (Timira—loss or darkness of vision). 19-21.

The use as a Navana (errhine) of a medicated oil cooked and prepared with the decoction of cow-dung would be attended with beneficial results in all types of Timira. Clarified butter * alone is beneficial in the Pittaja type; similarly clarified butter prepared by churning the milk of a ewe or a she-goat and cooked with the admixture of the drugs of the *Madhura* (Kákolyádi) group would prove beneficial in the Pittaja type of Timira. Oil cooked with the drugs of the *Sthirádi* (Vidári-gandhádi) or the *Madhura*

* Some say that this clarified butter is to be prepared from the milk of a ewe or she-goat

group * as well as the Anu-taila (see Chapter V, Chikitsita Sthána), might be prescribed with the greatest advantage in the types of the disease due respectively to the action of the deranged Váyu and vitiated blood of the system. A medicated oil duly cooked with an admixture of *Sahá*, *As'va-gandhá*, *Ati-valá*, *S'atávari*, *Trivrit* and the three fatty substances, Ghrita, lard and marrow, mentioned before (in connection with the treatment of Mahá-Váta-Vyádhi, Chapter VI, Chikitsita Sthána) might be advantageously employed as an errhine in cases of Vátaja Timira. Butter churned out of the milk duly cooked with the flesh of any aquatic or marsh-frequenting fowl or beast should be employed as an errhine ; it would prove curative in cases of Vátaja Timira (loss of vision). 22-23.

The flesh of a vulture and of a deer of the Ena species, *Saindhava* salt, honey and clarified butter should be prepared and applied (to the affected eye) in the manner of **Puta-páka** (see next Chapter). The lard of vultures, snakes and cocks and *Yashti-madhu* should be pasted together (with honey) and applied (to the affected organ) in the manner of an Anjana (eye-salve)†. 24.

Antidotes :—*Srotonjana* should be successively soaked in meat-juice, ‡ milk and clarified butter in

* The part of the text within the two *s from 'Similarly' in the last page to 'group' in this page is not to be found in either Vrinda or Chakradatta. The commentator of Chakradatta, moreover, does clearly say that this part is an interpolation and cannot be found in some of the Mss. of Sus'ruta Samhitá.

† According to Dallana the lards of vultures, snakes and cocks may be jointly or separately used—taken either one, two or all the three at a time. But in all cases they should be mixed with honey and *Yashti-madhu.* It should be noted that the lard of a Krishna-Sarpa (venomous serpent) should be used.

‡ Flesh of those animals which give strength to the sight should be used in the preparation of meat-juice.

the manner of Bhávaná saturation and used as a **Pratyanjana** * (in cases of Vátaja Timira unattended with redness). In cases of Vátaja Timira attended with redness of the eye, however, the *Srotonjana* should be placed inside the blades of *Kus'a* grass and preserved for a month inside the mouth of a (dead) black cobra. Then it should be taken out and mixed with *Saindhava* salt and the burnt ashes of *Málati* (Játi) flowers. It should then be applied as an Anjana to the affected organ. As an alternative, *Srotonjana* should be soaked in milk for three successive days and applied to the seat of the disease in a case of (Vátaja) **Kácha** (cataract) which is said by experts to be remediable by this Anjana. 25.

Treatment of Pittaja-Kácha :—Clarified butter skimmed from milk (and not from curd) and duly cooked with the drugs of the *Madhura* (Kákolyâdi) group † should be employed as a snuff **(Nasya)**, or as a Tarpana in the **Pittaja** type of this disease. The flesh of Jángala animals (deer, etc.) and the drugs of the *Kákolyâdi* group should be used in the manner of **Puta-páka** in the Pittaja type of Kácha. A Kshudránjana composed of *Rasánjana*, sugar, honey *Manah-s'ilá*, and *Yashti-madhu* may likewise be applied. The use of an Anjana composed of *Rasánjana* and *Tutthaka* taken in equal parts and finely pounded, is also recommended by experts ‡ in such cases. Powdered *Tutthaka* soaked in the decoction of *Bhillota* and the drugs of

* Pratyanjana (secondary eye-salve) is an antidote for the over-use of an Anjana.

† According to some commentators the milk should be first cooked with the drugs of the *Madhura* group, and butter should then be churned out of that milk.

‡ A benumbed condition of the eye through the abuse of eye-salves calls for the use of this Anjana as an antidote.

the *Eládi-gana* would be used as a **Pratyanjana**, and would be found beneficial in such cases. The use (as an Anjana) of *Mesha-s'ringi* and *Srotonjana* taken in equal parts and two parts of conch-shell pounded together is efficacious in the Pittaja type of this disease (Kâcha).

The juice of *Paláś'a*, *Rohita* and *Madhuka* (flower) mixed with honey and the surface layer of wine (taken in equal parts) should be prepared (in the manner of Rasa-kriyá and applied as an eye-salve in this type). 26-27.

Treatment of Kaphaja Type :—The drugs known as *Us'ira*, *Rodhra*, *Triphalá* and *Priyangu* duly cooked together (with Tila oil) should be employed for the purposes of **snuffing** (Nasya) in the Kaphaja Type. **Fumigation** (Dhumana) with the vapours of *Vidanga*, *Páthá*, *Kinihi* and *Ingudi*-bark would also prove beneficial in the Kaphaja type of cataract (Timira). The affected part should be likewise lubricated with the medicated Ghrita duly cooked with the decoction of *Vanaspati* (the milk-exuding trees, e. g., those of the species of Indian holy fig) with pasted *Haridrá* and *Us'ira* (as Kalka). The essence of the meat of Jángala (forest) animals, mixed with *Pippali* and profusely saturated with *Saindhava* and honey, should be prepared in the manner of *Puta-páka* (and applied to the affected part). *Manah-s'ila*, *Trikatu*, *Saindhava*, *Mákshika* (honey), *S'amkha*, *Kásisa* and *Rasánjana* should be combinedly used for the purposes of *Rasa-kriyá* (in the type under discussion). *Kásisa*, *Rasánjana*, *Guda* (old and matured treacle) and *Nágara*, may be likewise used with benefit. 28.

Treatment of Tri-doshaja Ka'cha :— *Anjana* (Antimony) many times heated and (subsequently) soaked in the decoction of *Triphalá* prepared with (the eight kinds of) urine, should be put inside the hollow (marrowless) bone of a nocturnal bird (such as the vulture, etc.) and kept immersed for a month in unruffled (currentless) water. The Anjana thus prepared may be used with advantage, in combination with *Madhuka* (Yashti-madhu) and the flowers of *Mesha-s'ringi* in the **Tri-doshaja** types of **Kácha**. As an alternative, all the measures and remedies (e. g., Tarpana, Puta-páka, etc.) * applicable in all the three Doshas should be employed in such cases. 29.

Treatment of blood-origined Parimláyi :—Measures and remedies mentioned in connection with the Pittaja type of Timira should be employed in a case of blood-origined **Parimláyi**. In the alternative, the remedial agents prescribed for the treatment of the different kinds of Ophthalmia (Abhishyanda) should be as well prescribed according to the nature of the deranged Doshas involved in the case. In case the deranged Doshas are not thereby subdued, *Nasyas* of the proper drug, as well as the many other *Anjanas* (collyrium) mentioned in the (next) Chapter on Kriyá-kalpa should be employed. 30.

Diet :—A person carefully partaking of old and matured clarified butter, *Triphalá*, *S'atávari*, *Patola*, *Mudga*, *Ámalaka*, *Yava* (barley) as diet enjoys immunity from all attacks of the dreadful **Timira**. Simply the *Páyasa* † prepared with *S'atávari*, or with *Ámalaka* or a meal of barley corns cooked with the decoction

* According to some, the measures and remedies to be applied in such cases are the measures of Rasa-kriyá applicable in cases of Vátaja, Pittaja and Kaphaja Timira.

† The **Páyasa** of *S'ata'vari* and *A'malaki* should be prepared by duly cooking *S'ata'vari* or *A'malaki*, as the case may be, with milk and sugar. According to others, however, it means the gruel (Yavágu) prepared with the expressed juice of *S'ata'vari* or *A'malaki*.

of *Triphalá* and a copious quantity of clarified butter would remove (an attack of) Timira. The use of such edibles as *Jivanti, Sunishannaka, Tanduliyaka, Vástuka, Chilli, Mulaka* as well as meat of birds (such as Làva, etc.) and Jángala animals (e g. deer, etc.) should be considered as invigorating to eye-sight. The use of the leaves or fruit (as the case may be) of *Patola, Karkotaka, Káravella, Vártáku, Tarkári, Karira* (tender bamboo plants), *S'igru* or *Ártagala*, cooked with clarified butter, proves beneficial (invigoratiog) to the sight. 31.

Blood-letting (venesection) should never be resorted to in a case of **Timira**, marked by the redness of the affected eye in as much as it might bring about an aggravation of the deranged Doshas ending in blindness of the patient. 32.

Prognosis :—A case of **Timira** marked by the absence of any redness of the eye and in which the first Patala (coat) of the organ is the seat of the disease, is curable (**Sádhya**). The case in which the eye assumes a bright red hue and the second coat or Patala of the organ is the seat of the disease, may be regarded as a curable one though only with the greaterst difficulty (**Krichchhra-Sádhya**). The case in which the third coat or Patala of the organ is the seat of the disease (characterised by the redness of its outer coat) should be regarded as (an incurable affection) admitting only of palliative treatment (**Yápya**). Proper palliative measures and remedies mentioned before should be employed in cases of Timira marked by a redness (of the affected organ), and leeches may also be applied to the region of the affection (to relieve it of its exuberance of the Dosha in cases of emergency). 33.

Surgical treatment of Kaphaja Linga-nás'a :—Now we shall describe the (surgical) measures to be employed for curing a case of **Linga-nása** (obstruction or choking up at the pupil with a cataract) due to the action of the deranged Kapha. In cases where the deranged Dosha in the organ, *i.e.*, the affected part of the organ does not appear semi-circular or thin in the middle, nor, fixed, (hard) nor irregular (in shape), nor marked by a large number of lines or a variety of tints, or where it does not resemble a pearl or a drop of water in shape, or if it does not become painful and red coloured, the patient should be first treated with Sneha and Sveda at a season of the year which is neither too cold nor too hot for the purpose. Then the hands, etc., of the patient should be secured with proper fastenings and he should be made to sit, looking simultaneously (with his two eyes) at (the tip of) his nose. Then the intelligent surgeon leaving off two portions of the white part of the eye-ball from the end of the Apánga (the end of the eye) and having fully and carefully drawn apart the eye-lids with his thumb and the index and the middle fingers, should insert the Yava-vaktra (needle) instrument* through the sides of the natural apperture-like point near the external angles of the eye, neither above nor below, care being taken not to pierce the veins. The left eye should be pierced with the right hand, and the right with the left. The satisfactory nature of the operation (perforation) should be presumed from the characteristic report or sound and the emission of a drop of water † from the affected region, following upon the perforation. 34-35.

* Both S'rikantha Datta and S'ivadása, the commentators respectively of Vrinda and Chakradatta, read 'शलाकया ताम्रमय्या' meaning that the S'aláká (rod) should be made of copper.

† Blood would come out if the perforation be not satisfactorily done.

instantly with the perforation the affected organ should be sprinkled over with breast-milk. The Śaláká should be retained in its place and the diseased growth or appearance (cataract), whether fixed or mobile, should be duly fomented from the outside with the help of the tender leaves of Váyu-subduing efficacy, and the region of the Drishti-mandala should be subsequently scraped with the (pointed) end of a Saláká. The mucus or phlegm (Kapha) accumulated in the affected eye should be removed by asking the patient to snuff it off by closing the nostril on the other side of the operated eye-ball. The part should be regarded as properly scraped when it would assume the glossiness of a resplendent cloudless sun and would be free from pain. Then the Śaláká (rod) should be gently withdrawn as soon as it would be able to perceive vision, and then the (affected) eye should be sprinkled over with clarified butter and bandaged with a piece of linen. During this period * the patient should be laid on his back in a comfortable chamber (free from dust and smoke), and be warned against indulging in all those bodily functions such as eructation, coughing, yawning, spitting, sneezing, etc. The regimen of diet and conduct thereafter should be the same as observed by one internally treated with a Sneha (See Chapter XXXI, Chikitsita-stha'na). 36-A.

The bandage should be removed on every fourth day, and the organ should be washed with the decoction of the drugs of Váyu-subduing properties and bandaged again with a fresh one. The eye should be (mildly) fomented on every fourth day as before, so that the bodily Váyu might not be aggravated. This rule should be

† The period during which these rules should be followed is 'seven days' according to Vágbhata. But according to Dallana it is only the period during which the operation lasts.

followed for ten days, as it would impart a fresh vigour to the sight. After-measures (such as snuffs, errhines, Tarpanas, etc.) should then be employed and the Diet should consist of light articles of food and be given only in moderate quantities. 36.

Persons declared unfit for venesection (viz., infants, old men, etc.) in the chapter on venesection * should not be subjected to any surgical operation, in cases of **Niliká** except at the place mentioned before (viz. the natural aperture—Daiva-krita Chhidra). 37.

Symptoms and treatment of the disorders resulting from an injudicious operation :—If the incidental hæmorrhage (from a puncture in a wrong place) fill in the cavity of the eye, in that case the eye should be beneficially sprinkled over with clarified butter duly cooked with *Yashti-madhu* and breast-milk. An incision (puncture) close to the exterior corner (Apánga) of the eye would usher in swelling, pain, lachrymation and redness of the eye, which should be remedied by poulticing (Upanáha) the part between the arches of the eye-brows, and sprinkling (Sechana) the eye over with tepid clarified butter. In the event of the organ being punctured near the Krishna-mandala (region of the iris) and the Krishna-mandala being affected thereby, the affected part should be sprinkled over with clarified butter, purgative should be administered and blood-letting (by means of leeches) should be resorted to. A distressing pain ensues from the puncture being made on the upper part of the eye (Krishna-mandala) and this should be cured by sprinkling drops of lukewarm clarified butter on the seat of affection. Excessive lachrymation sets in

* S'árira-Sthána, Chapter VII.

with pain and redness of the eye in the event of the puncture being made on the lower part of the eye (Krishna-mandala) and such cases should be treated in the preceding manner. Emulsive (Sneha) application and fomentation (Sveda) of the parts as well as applications of Anuvâsana enema should be considered as remedies in cases of redness, lachrymation, pain, numbness and bristling (of the eye-lashes) in the eye, as the result of an excessive and improper handling of the instrument during the operation. 37-38.

If removed in its acute stage (in a case of Linga-nás'a) the Dosha is liable to have an upward course and produce relapse in the red-coloured specks or films (opacity) in the S'ukra (white part of the eye), and it tends to give rise to an excruciating pain in the locality and completely obstruct the vision. The remedy in such a case consists in sprinkling the eye with clarified butter duly cooked with the drugs of the *Madhura-gana*, and in the application of the same in the manner of S'iro-vasti (errhine). Meat diet should be prescribed for the patient in such cases. As a full-bodied cloud coming in contact with the wind meets its destruction, so the fully aggravated Dosha meets its doom, if operated upon with the surgeon's S'áláká (rod). 39-40.

Causes of Relapse :—A relapse of the deranged Dosha is caused by a blow on the head, physical exercise, sexual excesses, vomiting, epileptic fits, or by an act of piercing the Linga-nás'a (cataract) during its partially developed (D. R. immature) stage. 41.

Symptoms produced by the defects of the S'aláka' :—Care should be taken not to remove the cataract with a roughly shaped **S'aláká** (rod) as it might usher in an acute and aching pain in the affected organ. A rod with an unsmooth body might lead to an aggravation of the deranged Doshas. A thick-topped rod would necessarily create an extensive ulcer, whereas a sharp one begets the apprehension of hurting the eye in many ways. An excessive lachrymation sets in from using a rod with an unequal or irregular top or mouth, whereas its unsteadiness (in the course of the operation) makes the operation an abortive one. Hence a Śaláká (rod) should be constructed and used for the purpose in such a manner as to preclude the possibility of the foregoing defects and injuries. 42.

Description of the Śaláká :—The Śaláká (rod) should be made to measure eight fingers in length, its middle part being covered with strings of thread and resembling the upper section of the thumb in circumference and its ends terminating in the form of a bud. The rod (Śaláká) should be prepared of copper, iron or gold. 43.

Derangements due to defective operation :—Redness of the eye, local swelling, sucking pain, (appearance of) Arvuda or Vudvuda, hog-like eye (Śukarákshitá) * and ophthalmia &c. are due to the improper handling of the rod or to the use of improper regimen of diet and conduct. These should be remedied according to the nature of the deranged Dosha involved in each case. 44.

Their treatment :—Now again hear me discourse on the (specific) medicines to be employed in cases of pain or redness in the eyes. A medicinal plaster composed of *Gairika*, *S'árivá*, *Durvá*, and barley pasted with milk † and clarified butter, should be

* Both Virinda and Chakradatta reads "Kekarákshitá" *i. e.* a squinting look.

† Vrinda and Chakradatta following Vágbhata do not read "*Payas*" (milk) and they read the first line of this couplet in a different form.

applied lukewarm (about the eyes) for the subsidence of pain and redness. A plaster (Lepa) prepared of *Siddhárthaka* (white mustard seeds) and slightly fried sesamum seeds pasted with the expressed juice of *Mátulunga*, or one prepared of *Payasyá* (Kshira-kákoli), *Sárivá*, *Patra*, *Manjishthá* and *Yashti-madhu* pasted together with the milk of a she-goat, if applied lukewarm to the affected region, removes the pain and redness of the eyes. A plaster composed of *Dáru*, *Padmaka*, and *S'unthi*, prepared and used in the same way is likewise recommended for the purpose. A plaster of *Drákshá*, *Yashti-madhu*, *Kushtha* and *Saindhava* should be likewise used. Cow's milk cooked with *Saindhava* should also be used for the alleviation of pain and redness of the eye. Clarified butter duly cooked with the admixture of *S'atávari*, *Prithak-parni*, *Musta*, *Ámalaka*, *Padmaka* and the milk of a she-goat, should be applied (cold) to the affected organ (eye) for the alleviation of pain and burning sensation therein. Clarified butter duly cooked with the Kalka of the drugs of the *Kákolyádi* group with a quantity of milk four times the weight of the clarified butter, previously cooked with the drugs of the Váyu-subduing (*Bhadradárvádi*) group (in the manner of Kshira-páka) should be considered as efficacious in any form (internally or externally) in cases of ocular affections. The affected organ should be treated with Sneha emulsive (applications) and (Sveda), fomentation and opening of the veins (Sirá) or cauterisation (by honey, clarified butter, or treacle) as described before, should be resorted to in cases where the foregoing remedies would fail to produce any effect. 45-46.

Eye-sight-invigorating Anjana:— Now hear me describe two beneficial *recipes* of **Anjana**

which would invigorate the eye-sight and impart a clearness of vision. Flowers of *Mesha-S'ringi*, *S'irisha*, *Dhava* and of *Málati* together with pearl and *Vaidurya* (ruby) should be pounded and made into a paste with the addition of the milk of a she-goat. The compound thus prepared should be kept in a copper vessel for a week and then made into **Vartis** (sticks) of convenient lengths and applied to the eyes in the manner of an Anjana. A **Varti** (stick) should be similarly prepared with *Srotonjana*, coral, *Samudra-phena*, *Manah-s'ilá* and *Maricha* and used similarly as an Anjana (eye-salve). It imparts steadiness of vision. The many other Anjanas to be described in the next Chapter (Kriyá-kalpa) may also be beneficially applied for the purpose. 47-48.

Thus ends the seventeenth chapter in the Uttara-Tantra of the Sus'ruta-Samhitá which treats of the curative measures of the diseases of the Drishti (pupil).

CHAPTER XVIII.

Now we shall diseourse on the Chapter which treats of the preparations and uses of the medicinal measures (external applications) to be adopted or employed in treating ocular affections in general **(Kriyá-kalpa)**. 1.

Here follows a general exposition of the instructions which the sainted lord of Benares, the holy Dhanvantari of profound intellect imparted to his disciple the son of Viśvámitra (Suśruta) regarding the different medicinal measures (Kriyá) such as **Tarpana** (soothing), **Seka** (sprinkling), **A'schyotana** (eye-drops), **Puta-pákas Anjanas** (eye-salves), etc., mentioned before in different places to be employed in diseases of the eye. 2-3.

The Tarpana Measure :—The measure known as **Tarpana** should be employed in respect of an affected eye either in the fore-noon or in the after-noon under the auspices of propitious astral combinations, after having purged the head and bowels of the patient and subsequent to the digestion of any food previously taken. The patient should be laid on his back in a chamber not exposed to the rays of the sun, and the gust of the wind, and where the atmosphere is not charged with minute particles of floating dust. The region of his eye (i. e. eye-lids) should be thickly coated with powdered *Másha* pulse, pasted (with water) in the form of a circular wall which should be even, hard and compact. Then a quantity of the transparent upper layer of clarified butter should be stirred with the admixture of a quantity of lukewarm water and poured (Purana) into the cavities of the eye up to the eye-lashes and retained therein for as long a period as one would take to count five hundred, six hundred, eight hundred, and ten hundred syllabless respectively in cases of healthy persons and persons with Kapha-origined, Pitta-origined and Váyu-origined diseases of the eye. According to certain authorities, the periods of such retention (of clarified butter) should vary with the seat of the affection (in the eye-ball). The clarified butter mentioned above should, according to them, be retained in the cavities of the eye for as long a period as one would take to utter three hundred, five hundred, seven hundred, one thousand, or eight hundred syllables respectively in cases of the diseases confined to the region of the Sandhi, Vartman, Śukla, Krishna, the eye in general (Sarva-gata) and the Drishti of the eye*. The clarified butter should then be secreted through the interior corner of the affected organ which should be purified by applying poultices of pasted barley. The Kapha, deranged by the use of this Sneha-Purana should be then conquered by making the patient inhale some kind of Kapha-subduing Dhuma (smoke). This rule † should be observed for one, three or five days in succession. 4.

Symptoms of satisfactory, excessive and defective Tarpana:—Sleep at the first call, unembarrassed waking, cessation of secretion, clearness of vision, agreeable sensation, perceptible amelioration of the disease, and lightness of the organ

* Accordtng to some, the **'Purana'** should be retained in the eye for a period required to count one thousand syllables in cases of Sarva-gata and eighteen hundred words in cases of Drishti-gata eye-diseases.

† According to Gayadása, this rule should be observed for one, three, or five days in cases of the preponderance of Váyu, Pitta and Kapha respectively, and according to Jejjata, in cases of mild, moderate and severe attack respectively.

are the symptoms which result from a proper and **satisfactory** Tarpana of the eye. Cloudiness of vision, a sense of heaviness in the affected organ, excessive glossiness (of the eye), lachrymation, itching, sliminess and an aggravation of the Doshas are the features which mark a case of severe and **excessive** Tarpana. A sense of dryness in the affected organ, cloudiness of vision, profuse lachrymation, sensitiveness to light and an aggravation of the disease are the evils which follow an act of **defective** Tarpana (of the eye). 5.

Treatment of excessive and defective Tarpana :—Cases of defective and excessive Tarpana should be remedied with the application of medicinal snuffs, Anjanas, washes and inhalations of smoke and by adopting dry or emulsive measures, (as the cases may require). 6.

Cases for Tarpana :—Shrivelling and depilation of the eye-lashes, cloudiness and darkness of vision, archedness of sight, absolute want of lachrymation, parchedness of the eye, hardness of the eye-lid and a severely diseased condition of the eye are amenable to the application of the **Tarpana** measure as giving tone to the eye. The Tarpana measure should not to be applied in a cloudy day, nor in a day excessively hot or cold. It should not be applied to the eye of a person engrossed by anxiety or fear, nor before the subsidence of the supervening symptoms (Upadrava) of the eye-disease. 7-8.

The Puta-pa'ka :—The **Puta-páka** measure should be applied in the aforesaid cases. The Puta-páka is not applicable in cases where Nasya (errhines), Tarpana and the internal application of Sneha (Sneha-pána) are forbidden. After a complete subsidence of the Dosha, the Puta-páka should be applied to the (affected) eye in cases where the patient would be found capable of being treated with it. The Puta-páka measure may be divided into three classes, viz., Snehana (emulsive), Lekhana (scraping) and Ropana (healing) Puta-páka. The **Snehana** (emulsive) Puta-páka is recommended in cases marked by the extreme parchedness of the affected organ or locality, and **Lekhana** (scraping) ones are efficacious in cases of excessive applications of the Sneha to the eye ; while the eye-sight is invigorated by the **Ropana** (healing) Puta-páka, which restores the Váta, * the Pitta and the blood of the affected locality to their natural conditions, and (consequently) heals the ulcer. 9-10.

Preparation of Snehana, Lekhana, and Ropana Puta-pa'kas :—The **Snehana** (emulsive) Puta-páka should be prepared with the flesh (of animals frequenting marshy places) abounding in Sneha † and with the Vasá (lard), Majjan (marrow), and Medas (fat), and the drugs of the *Madhura* group and it should be retained in the eye so long as one would take to utter two hundred syllables. The scraping or **Lekhana** Puta-pàka should be prepared with the flesh and the liver of an animal of the Jángala species and the drugs possessing the *Lekhana* or scraping properties, as well as powders of black iron (steel), copper, conch-shells, *Vidruma* (corals), *Saindhva* salt, *Samudra-phena*, *Kásisa* (sulphate of iron) and *Srotonjana* (pasted together) with the cream of curd. The affected locality should be exposed to a Lekhana Puta-páka as long as

* A different reading, mentioned by Dallana, does not read "Váta."

† In place of "स्नेहमांस" meaning flesh abounding in Sneha, a different reading "सर्पिर्मांस" (i. e. clarified butter and flesh) is quoted by Dallana.

one would take to utter a hundred syllables at most. The healing or **Ropana** Puta-pâka should be prepared by cooking the flesh of an animal of the Jángala group with breast-milk, honey*, clarified butter and the bitter drugs, and should be retained in the affected eye for a period three times as much as the Lekhana-Puta-páka should be retained i.e., for a period as long as one would require to utter three hundred syllables. 11-13.

The fumigating measures mentioned in connection with the Tarpana of an affected eye, as well as the appli cations of Sneha and Sveda, should be resorted to in the cases of the application of the Puta-pâka measures, except in cases of the application of the Ropana Puta-páka. Puta-páka applications may be made on one day only or may be continued for two or three days.†. A strict regimen of diet and conduct should be observed for a period twice as long as the preparatory period (beginning with the time of administering the Sneha to the patient for preparing him for the application of the Puta-páka till the time of actually administering the Putapáka itself). 14-15.

Prohibition and Remedies for infringement :—After the application of Tarpana and Puta-páka (to the affected eye) the patient should not catch glimpses of the light, fire, sky, looking-glass or any other luminous object ; nor he should expose the eye

* In place of 'मध्वाज्य" (honey and clarified butter) Dallana quotes a variant "मेध्याज्य"—lit. sacred clarified butter i e., clarified butter prepared from cow's milk.

† Dallana explains that the application of the Puta-páka measure should be made for one day only in Kaphaja eye-diseases, or if the Puta-páka be a Lekhana one ; and it should be continued for two days in Pittaja eye-diseases, or if it be a Snehana one ; and for three days in Vátaja eye-diseases, or if it be a Ropana Puta-páka.

to the blast of the wind. The unfavourable symptoms incidental to and induced by an infringement of the rules to be observed after the application of these two (Tarpana and Puta-pâka) measures should be remedied with the applications of Anjana (collyrium), A'schyotana and Sveda (fomentation) to the deranged bodily Doshas, underlying each particular case. 16–17.

Satisfactory, excessive and defective application of Puta-páka :—Freshness and clearness of the colour (of the cornea), capability of the organ (eye) to bear heat, light and wind, refreshing sleep and an unembarrassed gladsome wakening and a lightness of the organ are the benefits which are derived from **Satisfactory** Puta-páka applications. Darkness of vision, pain and swelling of the eye and the appearance of eruptions (Pidaká) in the affected organ, are the evils which mark an **excessive** application of the Puta-páka measure ; while suppuration and lachrymations of the eye and a thrilling sensation (Harsha) in the affected organ, as well as a further aggravation of the Dosha (involved) are the characteristic features of a **deficient** Puta-páka application. 18.

Mode of preparing Puta-páka :—Now I shall describe the mode of preparing a **Puta-páka** remedy. Two *Vilva* (Pala) measures of cleansed and pasted meat, one *Pala* measure of the medicinal drugs pasted together and one *Kudava* (half a seer) measure of liquid ingredients should be mixed together (and made into a ball), well covered with the leaves of *Kadali*, *Kásmari*, *Eranda*, *Kumuda* or of *Padma* plant. Coated with clay, it should be duly scorched in the burning charcoal (fire) of catechu wood or in that of *Kataka*, *As'mantaka*, *Eranda*, *Pátalâ*, *Vásaka*, *Vadara*, *Kshira*-exuding trees, or in the fire of the dried cakes of cow-dung. When well cooked the ball should be taken out of the fire and broken and its contents withdrawn and squeezed. The fluid extract should then be collected and applied (to the affected organ) in the manner of applying a Tarpana. 19.

The mode of application :—The patient being laid on his back at the time, the fluid extract in both the cases (Tarpana and Puta-páka) should be dropped cold into the Kaniniká (Cornea) of the eye in cases of derangement of the blood and the Pitta ; it should be used lukewarm when the Váyu and the Kapha would be found to have been aggravated. A burning sensation in the affected eye as well as its consequential inflammation would result from the use of too hot (warm) or strong or keen-potencied (Tikshna) extract for the purpose. A thrilling sensation (Harsha), pain and numbness in the locality and lachrymation from the affected organ originate from the use of a cold and mild-potencied Puta-páka or Tarpana eye-drop. Redness and contraction of the eye attended with a jerking and throbbing sensation therein are the effects of an excessive (over-dose) application of the Puta-páka and Tarpana, whereas a deficient (under-dose) use of them produces an aggravation of the deranged bodily Doshas in the locality. Properly applied, they alley the burning and itching sensation, swelling, pain, lachrymation and mucous secretion, as well as the (unnatural) coating and redness in the affected eye. As every one is desirous of avoiding the aggravation of Doshas, so the Puta-páka and Tarpana measures should be applied in such a way as would give health and happiness (to the eye). The evils resulted by a course of injudicious application of Puta-páka or Tarpana, are to be remedied with the application of errhines (Nasya), Dhuma and Anjana remedial to the specific deranged bodily Dosha or Doshas involved in each case. 20.

The affected eye should be fomented before the use of a Puta-páka or a Tarpana measure with a piece of cloth soaked in hot water (and rinsed). Fumigation of the affected organ in the end should be prescribed in a case marked by an aggravation of the deranged Kapha of the locality. 21.

Ás'chyotana and Seka:—Properly prepared and applied, the **Ás'chyotana** and **Seka** measures would respectively subdue cases of slight and violent attacks of the eye. Like the Puta-páka measure these two also are devided into **three** classes *viz.*, (Lekhana, Snehana and Ropana). Seven or eight drops of the medicinal fluid should be used in **Lekhana**-Ás'chyotana (for the purpose of scraping the affected eye); ten drops in the **Snehana** (for emulsive purposes) and twelve drops in the **Ropana** Ás'chyotana (for the purpose of setting up a granulative process in a local sore or wound). The maximum period for which an (affected) eye should be subjected to the **Seka** measure is twice as long as is enjoined in respect of a Puta-páka measure,* or until the disease is gradually and wholly removed.† Both the Ás'chyotana and the Seka applications should be made in the morning or evening or at noon (in accord-

* The period for which an affected eye should be subjected to the Ás'chyotana measure, is not given in the text, but Dallana says that it should be the same as observed in cases of **Puta-páka**. Some, however, hold that in cases of both Seka and Ás'chyotana the period would be twice as that for Puta-páka.

† This rule for subjecting the affected eye to the measure till the disease is gradually and wholly removed is for Seka and Ás'chyotana only; but according to some it is a general rule which applies also to cases of Puta-páka and Tarpana, etc.

ance with the aggravation of the deranged Doshas),* or whenever there would be pain (in the affected eye). † The symptoms of proper and improper (excessive and deficient) applications of a Sneha (emulsive) Seka are identical with those of Tarpana. 22-23.

Śiro-vasti :—The serious diseases peculiar to the head readily yeild to and are conquered by the application of **Siro-vasti,** which also produces the very good effects known as the Murdha-tailika ones peculiar to the use of (emulsive) Śiro-vasti. The patient having been treated with purgatives and emetics (according to requirements) should be given a proper diet according to the nature of the disease, and made to sit erect in the evening, when an animal bladder (the bladder of a goat being usually used for the purpose) filled with the proper Sneha, should be placed on his crown and firmly tied up with a bandage. The Sneha-filled bladder should be so retained on the head ten times as long as is necessary for Tarpana measure, according to the nature of the disease. 24-25.

Anjana :—Proper Anjana for Lekhana (scraping), Ropana (healing), or Prasádana (invigorating) purposes should be applied after the cleansing (purging, etc.) of the system in cases where the deranged bodily Doshas would manifest themselves in the region of the eye only. 26.

A **Lekhana-Anjana** should be prepared with the

* The Lekhana-seka and Ás'chyotana should be applied in the morning in the aggravation of **Kapha,** while the Snehana one should be applied in the afternoon in the aggravation of **Váyu,**—the Ropana ones being applied at noon in the aggravation of **Blood** and **Pitta**.

† Dallana holds, that both the Seka and Ás'chyotana measures may be applied whenever there is pain in the affected eye, but others hold that this rule applies only in cases of Seka.

drugs of one or more tastes (Rasa) except the sweet one and should be used in five different ways according to the nature of the Dosha or Doshas involved in each case.* The Dosha accumulated in the regions of the eye and the eye-lids, in the ball, the passages, and in the capillaries of the eye, as well as in the gristle of the nose would be secreted through the mouth, the nostrils and the corners of the eyes by the application of a Lekhana Anjana. A **Ropana-Anjana** should be prepared with the drugs of bitter and astringent tastes (Rasa) mixed with (a little quantity of) clarified butter and is good for healing purposes. Owing to the presence of the Sneha, it is cooling in its effect and consequently gives natural colour and vigour to the eye. A **Prasádana-Anjana**, prepared with the drugs of sweet taste and with (a profuse quantity of) Sneha, imparts tone and vigour to the eyesight and should be used with advantage for all soothing purposes connected with the organ. The application of the different kinds of Anjana should be made in the morning, evening or in the night † in accordance

* In cases of the derangement of the local **Váyu**, the Anjana should be prepared with the drugs of acid and saline tastes (Rasa) ; in the derangement of the **Pitta** with those of astringent taste ; in **Kapha** with those of astringent, bitter and pungent tastes In cases of the derangement of the **blood**, the Anjana should be like that in the derangement of Pitta, and in cases of the derangement of two or three Doshas simultaneously, the Anjana should be prepared with drugs of two or three of the tastes required.

† The Anjana should be applied in the morning, in the evening and in the night respectively in the cases of the derangement of the Kapha Váyu and the Pitta. According to the others, the S'odhana, the Ropana and the Snehana Anjanas should be respectively used in the morning, in the evening and in the night. Others, however, are of opinion that these different times should be judiciously selected in the different seasons of the year according to requirement.

with the nature of the deranged bodily Dosha or Doshas involved in each case. 27–30.

Forms of Anjana :—The forms in which an Anjana may be, are those of pills, liquid (Rasa-kriyá) and powder * each succeeding, one being more efficacious than the one preceding it, in the order of enumeration. 31.

Their sizes and doses :—The size (dose) of a Lekhana, Prasádana and Ropana Varti (Pill) should be equal to that of one and a half and twice as much as a *Kaláya* pulse for ocular affections in general. As regards the application of Rasa-kriyá-Anjana in these disorders the quantity to be used in a dose should be equal to that of the Varti in the different cases respectively. As regards the dose of the powders (to be used in eye-diseases) it should be respectively twice, thrice and four times as much as would be contained at the end of a Śalâkâ (rod). 32.

The materials of the vessel and rod for the use of an Anjana :—The vessels containing the different kinds of Anjana should be according to the different kinds of Anjana themselves, and these vessels as well as the Śaláká (rod) for the use should be made of gold, silver, horn, copper, *Vaidurya* (a kind of precious stone), bell-metal and iron respectively (in accordance with the different tastes of the drugs the Anjanas are made of). † The end of the

* Dallana says that Pill-Anjanas, Liquid-Anjanas and Powder-Anjanas should be prescribed in cases of severe, intermediate and mild attacks respectively.

† According to Dallana the Anjana of sweet taste should be placed in a golden vessel, that of acid taste in a silver vessel, that of saline taste in a vessel made of horn (of a sheep), that of astringent taste, in a vessel either of copper or iron, that of pungent taste in a vessel made of Vaidurya,

rod should terminate in a bud-shaped ball with the girth of that of a *Kalâya* pulse, its entire length measuring eight fingers only. It would be well polished, slender at the middle and capable of being easily handled. A rod prepared of copper, precious stones such as *Vaidurya*, etc., and horns or bones, etc.,* will prove beneficial. 33.

How to apply an Anjana :—The lids of the affected eye (of the patient) should be slantingly drawn apart with the left hand, and the **Anjana** should be carefully applied by holding the rod with the right hand and by constantly moving the rod from the Kaniniká to the Apânga and *vice versa* (along the inner side of the eye-lid). This process should be repeated (twice or thrice) according to requirements. The Anjana should be applied with the finger when it would be necessary to use it on the outer side of the eye-lid. The Anjana in no case should be thickly painted in the corners of the eye (i.e., in the Kaniniká and the Apánga from fear of hurting them), nor the organ should be washed till all the aggravations of the deranged (bodily) Dosha in the locality are completely removed thereform, in as much as it might bring on a fresh aggravation and impair the strength of the eyesight. After the subsidence of the deranged local Dosha

and that of bitter taste should be placed in a vessel made of bell-metal. The S'aláká (rod) for the use of the different kinds of Anjana should be also accordingly prepared.

According to Nimi, however, as quoted by Dallana and S'rikantha Datta, in their commentaries, the Ropana, Lekhana and Prasádana Anjanas should be placed in a vessel and used with a rod prepared respectively of iron, copper and gold. The other materials may be, however, used with discretion by an experienced physician.

* The word 'आदि' in the text shows that a rod of gold may also be used with benefit—Dallana.

and of lachrymation, the eye should be first washed with water, and **Pratyanjana** should then be used in accordance with the nature of the specific deranged bodily Dosha or Doshas underlying in each case. 34.

Forbidden Cases :—The application of Anjanas is prohibited in cases of persons suffering from fever, Udávarta, and the diseases of the head and during fits of anger, grief, fear, weeping and intoxication, as well as in cases of the retention of stool and urine, in as much as it might produce (in these cases) lachrymation, Śula (aching pain), redness, pain, blindness (Timira), swelling in the locality, as well as giddiness. An application of the Anjana in a case of insomnia might be followed by the loss of the eyesight*. The application of an Anjana in a windy day may impair the eye-sight. Application to the eyes affected with dust or smoke, may bring on redness, Adhimantha (Ophthalmia) and local secretion. Applied after the use of an errhine (Nasya) it may usher in an aching pain and swelling in the eyes. It leads to the aggravation of the disease, if applied in any disease of the head. The application of an Anjana would be abortive, nay, it would rather aggravate the Dosha, if applied before sun-rise, after a bath, or in a very cold day, owing to the fixedness of the deranged bodily Dosha. Similarly, the application of an Anjana would fail to produce any effect in a case of indigestion, owing to the sluggish condition of the internal passages of the body (during the continuance of the disease).

* In some editions there is an additional text—"निद्राक्षयं च कुरुते निषिद्धे युक्तमञ्जनम्" which supplies a complete verb and makes the sense complete. The line means—the application of an Anjana in a forbidden case produces loss of sleep (insomnia) in addition (to redness, pain etc, mentioned in the preceding line).

The application of an Anjana in an aggravated stage of the deranged bodily Doshas, ushers in the distressing symptoms peculiar to each of them. Hence, the application of an Anjana should be carefully made in such a manner as not to induce any of the aforesaid evils, and these rules should be specially observed in connection with a **Lekhana-Anjana**. These distressing symptoms should be treated with washes (lotions), Áśchyotana, plasters, Dhuma (fumigation), Nasya and Kavala (gurgle) with due regard to the specific nature of the deranged bodily Dosha or Doshas involved in each case. 35-36.

Symptoms of satisfactory, excessive and deficient use of a Lekhana-Anjana :—Lightness, whiteness and pristine clearness of the eye, marked by the improved power of vision and absence of secretion and all other distressing symptoms, are the indications which point to the fact that the eye has been **satisfactorily** purged of the accumulated Doshas (by the proper application of a Lekhana Anjana). An **excessive** purging of the eye (by the excessive use of a Lekhana Anjana) begets such local evils as the deep discolouration of the external coat of the eye, its sense of looseness in the socket, lachrymation, archedness of the organ and a sense of constant dryness in its cavity. The medical treatment in such instances consists in the employment of soothing (Santarpana) and other Váyu-subduing remedies. An insufficient or **deficient** application of the Lekhana Anjana leads to the aggravation of the local deranged bodily Dosha which should be fully secreted out by employing medicinal errhines, Anjana and local fumigation. 37-39.

Symptoms of satisfactory, excessive and deficient use of Prasádana

(Snehana) and Ropana Anjanas :—The action of the **satisfactory** application of a **Prasádana** (Snehana) Anjana is to soothe the eye, to impart a healthy tone to the organ of sight, to restore its natural colour and gloss, and to make it strong and unclouded and free from the aggravation of any Dosha. Any **excess** in the application is followed by results identical with those of excessive application of Tarpana (soothing measures)* to the organ, and the remedy consists in employing mild but parching remedies antidotal to the deranged bodily Dosha (Kapha) involved in the case. The symptoms which mark a satisfactory and excessive application of a **Ropana** (healing) Anjana, as well as the medical treatment to be applied in cases of excess, are identical with those mentioned in connection with the satisfactory and excessive application of the Prasádana (soothing) Anjanas (respectively). **Deficient** applications of both the Snehana (soothing) and the Ropana (healing) Anjanas (in respect of ocular affections) are sure to prove abortive in their effects. Care should, therefore, be taken to apply it properly, if it is hoped to get the wished-for result. 40-43.

Thousands of remedial measures and remedies may be devised and employed in the manner of the Puta-páka and other measures on the basis of the fundamental principles herein inculcated. 44.

Now we shall describe the recipes and preparations of several principal Anjanas fit for the use of kings and crowned heads for the purpose of giving strength to the eye-sight and for the amelioration of ocular affections (Kácha, etc.) amenable only to the palliative measures. Eight parts of *Rasánjana* (Antimony) having the hue of

* See S'loka 5 of this Chapter.

a (full-blown) blue lotus flower, as well as one part each of (dead) copper, gold and silver should be taken together and placed inside an earthen crucible. It should then be burnt by being covered with the burning charcoal of catechu or *As'mantaka* wood, or in the fire of dried cakes of cow-dung and blown (with a blow-pipe till they would glow with a blood-red effulgence) after which the expressed juice (Rasa) of cow-dung, cow's urine, milk-curd, clarified butter, honey, oil, urine, lard, marrow, infusion of the drugs of the *Sarva-gandhá* group, grape-juice, sugar-cane-juice, the expressed juice of *Triphalá* and the completely cooled decoctions of the drugs of the *Sárivádi* and the *Utpaládi* groups, should be separately sprinkled over it in succession alternately each time with the heating thereof, (or to put it more explicitly, the crucible should be taken down after being heated and then one of these draughts should be sprinkled over its contents and then again heated and again sprinkled over with another draught, and so on). After that, the preparation should be kept suspended in the air for a week, so as to be fully washed by the rains. The compound should then be dried, pounded and mixed together with proportionate parts (quarter part) of powdered pearls, crystals, corals and *Kálanu-sárivá*. The compound thus prepared is a very good **Anjana** and should be kept in a pure vessel made of ivory, crystal, *Vaidurya*, *S'amkha* (conch-shell), stone, gold or silver or of *Asana* wood. It should then be purified (lit. worshipped) in the manner of the purification of the Sahasra-Páka-Taila described before. It may then be prescribed even for a king. Applied along the eye-lids as a collyrium, it enables a king to become favourite with his subjects and to continue invincible to the last day of his life free from ocular affections. 45.

Bhadrodaya-Anjana :—The drugs known as *Kushtha*, *Chandana*, *Elá*, *Patra*, *Yashti-madhu*, *Rasánjana*, flowers of *Mesha-s'ringi*, *Chakra* (Tagara), the seven kinds of jewels*, the pollens of the flowers of *Utpala*, *Brihati*, *Kantakári* and of lotus, *Nága-kes'ara*, *Us'ira*, *Pippali*, the shells of hen's eggs, *Dáru-haridrá*, *Haritaki*, *Gorochoná*, *Maricha*, marrow or kernel of *Vibhitaka*-seeds and the flesh of lizards (which are found to scale the walls of rooms), should be powdered together in equal parts and should be preserved in a vessel and purified (sanctified) in the preceding manner. This Anjana is called the **Bhadrodaya-Anjana** and should always be used by a king. 46.

Equal parts of *Chakra* (Tagara), *Maricha*, *Jatá-mámsi* and *S'aileya* with *Manah-s'ilá* equal to the combined weight of the preceding drugs, four parts of Patra with *Rasánjana* (antimony) twice the combined weight of all the preceding drugs and *Yashti-madhu* of equal† weight with the last-named drug (Rasánjana) should be powdered together and used as an Anjana in the foregoing manner. 47.

Manah-s'ilá, *Deva-dáru*, the two kinds of *Rajani*, *Triphalá*, *Trikatu*, *Lákshá*, *Las'una*, *Manjishthá*, *Saindhava*, *Elá*, *Mákshika*, *Sávaraka Rodhra*, dead iron and copper, *Kálànu-sárivá* and the outer shells of hen's eggs taken in equal parts should be powdered together, resolved into a paste with milk and made into pills of adequate size. Diseases of the eye such as the itching sensation in the eye, Timira, Śuklárma and Raktaráji readily yield to the curative efficacy of this Anjana. 48.

* The seven kinds of gems are (1) Padmarága, (2) Marakata, (3) Nila, (4) Vaidurya, (5) Muktá (pearl) (6) Praválа and (7) Hema (gold).

† According to some the weight of the *Yashti-madhu* to be used in this Anjana should be equal to that of all the other drugs combined.

An Anjana should be prepared by collecting lamp-black on a vessel made of Indian bell-metal, and mixing it with one part each of *Yashtimadhu*, *Saindhava*, *Tagara* and roots of *Eranda*, as well as two parts of *Brihati*. This compound should be pasted together with goat's milk and thinly plastered on a copper plate. This process should be continued for seven times in succession and dried in the shed. It should then be made into **Vartis** and (used as such) would relieve pain in the eye. 49.

One part each of *Haritaki*, *Yashti-madhu* with sixteen parts of *Maricha* should be pounded and pasted together with cold water. It should then be made into **Vartis** and would be efficacious in all sorts of ocular affections. An experienced physician may with care and discretion prepare **Pindánjanas** with the drugs antidotal to the specific Dosha or Doshas involved in the case, in the manner of preparing the Rasa-kriyá preparations. 50-51.

Thus ends the eighteenth chapter of the Uttara-Tantra in the Sus'ruta Samhitá whieh deals with the preparations and uses of the medicinal measures to be used in different ocular affections.

CHAPTER XIX.

Now we shall discourse on the medical treatment to be adopted in cases of hurt or injury to the eye **(Nayanábhigháta-Pratishedha).** 1.

A violent and intolerable pain in the eye accompanied by redness and swelling therein, resulting from a blow or from any sort of hurt or injury to the organ, should be remedied with the application of medicinal Nasya (errhines), plasters, sprinkling and Tarpana (soothing measures), and other measures mentioned before, as well as the measures prescribed in cases of Pittaja and Raktaja Abhishyanda—lit. remedial to the pain (Śula) caused by the deranged blood and Pitta in the locality. The affected eye (Drishti) should also be soothed with the help of cool, sweet and fatty drugs. This kind of treatment should also be followed in cases where the eye would be hurt or oppressed by (excessive) fomentation, smoke or glare-fire, or affected on account of fear, mental agony, pain or injury. These measures should also be resorted to in the **first stage** (*i. e.*, during the first week) of the hurt or injury in the eye. After this period the affected eye should be treated as a case of an Abhishyanda with due regard to the nature of the specific deranged bodily Dosha or Doshas involved in the case. A slight hurt in the eye may be instantaneously relieved by the application of warm breath-fomentation. 2-4.

Prognosis :—Any ulceration restricted to one Patala (coat) only of the eye may be easily cured ; an ulcer invading two Patalas of the organ may be healed only with the greatest difficulty, while the one affecting three Patalas should be regarded as incurable.

Palliative measures are all that are possible in cases of looseness, dislocation, sunkenness and the thrashed condition (Pichchita) of the eyes as well as in a case of Hata-drishti (loss of eye-sight). Cases of wrong or erroneous vision, marked by the dilation of the pupil, absence of any considerable redness and those cases where the eye (eye-ball) is in its proper place and is not affected in its power of vision prove amenable to medical treatment. 5-6.

A sunken eye may be uplifted either by holding the breath (Prána-váyu) or by inducing vomiting or sneezing, or by throttling or obstructing the wind-pipe. Where the eyes would be found to be hanging down from the sockets, the measures and remedies prescribed before* should be resorted to, and the patient should be made to take in long breaths of air (through the nostrils) and cold water should be poured on his head. 7.

Symptoms and treatment of Kukunaka :—The seventy-six kinds of eye-diseases herein mentioned before, occur to adults as well as to infants, but a peculiar disease, due to the action of deranged Váyu, Pitta, Kapha and blood, sometimes manifests itself in (the inner lining of) the eye-lids of an infant and this is known as **Kukunaka.** Its exciting cause is the vitiated condition of the breast-milk of the mother. In this disease, there is excessive itching in the eyes, and the child frequently rubs his eyes, nose and forehead with his fist ; there is constant lachrymation and the child cannot bear the least light of sun's rays. The organ should, in such cases, be speedily bled (by applying leeches) and be scraped (with rough leaves). The organ should further be rubbed with *Tri-katu* and honey pasted together,

* See Chikitsita-sthána, Chapter II, Para 29.

The mother (or the nurse) should also be treated in the manner prescribed before (in cases of an affection of the breast-milk). Compounds of *Saindhava* salt, honey and powdered *Khara-manjari* (Apámárga) seeds, as well as those of powdered *Pippali, Saindaava*-salt and honey with the vehicle of breast-milk should be given to the child for emetic purposes, but this should be discontinued as soon as vomiting would set in. 8–10.

To a child who takes both breast-milk and other solid food, the emetic should be administered with the admixture of *Vachá*, and to a much older child (*i.e.*, one who has given up taking breast-milk) the emetic should be given with the admixture of *Madana* fruit. 11.

Decoction of the tender leaves of *Jambu, Ámra* and *Ámalaki* should be used for washing and sprinkling purposes. Clarified butter duly cooked with *Tri-phalá* or with *Guduchi* should be dropped into the eye as an Ás'chyotana measure. 12.

Anjanas composed of *Manah-s'lá, Maricha, S'amkha* (conch-shell), *Rasánjana* and *Saindhava* pounded together and pasted with honey and treacle should be applied to the affected organ. Compounds of *Murvá*, honey and powdered copper should also be used as Anjana. The compound prepared by burning black iron (steel), clarified butter, milk and honey mixed together should be similarly used as an Anjana. As an alternative, the **Gutikánjana** made up of *Trikatu, Palándu* (onion), *Yashti-madhu, Saindhava, Lákshá* (lac) and *Gairika* (earth) pasted together, should be used. The Anjana made of *Nimba*-leaves, *Yashti-madhu, Dárvi,* *

* "*Dárvi*" generally means *Dáru-haridrá* ; but, here, on the authority of Videha, Dallana takes it to mean the two kinds of *Haridrá*, viz., Haridrá and *Dá'ru-haridrá*.

copper (powdered) and *Lodhra* taken in equal parts and pounded together, is also efficatious. 13.

An Anjana prepared with *Rasánjana* (Antimony), *S'amkha*, curd and *Saindhava* kept together for a period of half a fortnight, * should be applied to thc affected organ of the child in cases of **S'ukra**, and the directions given under the head of Kaphaja-Abhishyanda should also be followed by experienced physicians in such cases of the eye-disease of children. 14.

Conclusion :—The Science of medicine is as incomprehensible as the ocean. It cannot be fully described even in hundreds and thousands of verses. Dull people who are incapable of catching the real import of the Science of reasoning would fail to acquire a proper insight into the Science of medicine if dealt with elaborately in thousands of verses. The occult principles (of the Science of medicine), as explained in these pages, would, therefore, sprout and grow and bear good fruits only under the congenial heat of a (medical) genius. A learned and experienced (medical) man would therefore try to understand the occult principles herein inculcated with due caution and with reference to other Sciences. 15.

Thus ends the nineteenth chapter of the Uttara-Tantra in the Sus'ruta Samhitá which deals with the medical treatment to be adopted in cases of hurt or injury to the eye.

* The method of preparing this Anjana, as explained by Dallana on the authority of Videha, is as follows :—*S'amkha* (conch-shell) and *Saindhava* should be first pasted together with curd (Dadhi) and then a quantity of *Rasánjana* should be soaked with this preparation for seven days and a half and **Varti** should then be prepared therewith and applied to the eye as an Anjana.

CHAPTER XX.

Now we shall discourse on the chapter which treats of the causes and symptoms of the diseases peculiar to the ear—the organ of hearing **(Karna-gata-Roga-Vijnániya).** 1.

Classification :—Twenty-eight different forms of ear-diseases are noticed in practice, *viz.*, Karna-Śula (ear-ache), Pra-náda (ringing or noise in the ear), Vádhirya (deafness), Kshveda, Karna-Sráva (discharge of pus, etc., from the ear), Karna-Kandu (itching in the ear), Karna-gutha, Krimi-karna (vermin-infested ears), Prati-náha, the two kinds of Vidradhi (local abscess), Karna-páka (suppuration of ear), Puti-karna (fetor in the ear), four kinds of Arśas (Cysts or polypuses in the ear), seven kinds of Arvuda (tumour) and four kinds of Śopha (swelling). 2.

Symptoms of Karna-Śula and Pra-náda :—The violent aching pain in the region of the ear and inside the tympanum caused by the deranged local Váyu, aggravated and obstructed by the other deranged Doshas in the locality is called the **Karna-Śula** (ear-ache). Ringing and various other sounds in the ear are heard when the deranged Váyu of the locality gets into the wrong way and remains there stuffed in the sound-carrying channels of the organ. This disease is called the **Pra-náda**. 3-4.

Symptoms of Vádhirya and Kshveda :—**Vádhirya** (deafness) results from the continuance in the sound-carrying channels of the deranged local Váyu in combination with the deranged local Kapha in those localites without anyway being remedied or subdued. An attack of **Karna-kshveda** (expresing a peculiar sound in the ear) may be attributed to such causes, as to the use of any cold thing or exposure to cold after being treated with a head-purging remedy (errhines), or to the continuance of the deranged local Váyu in the sound-passage, aggravated by excessive labcur, by any wasting process in the system or by taking articles of fare of astringent taste or of parching (Ruksha) property.* 5-6.

Symptoms of Karna-Sráva and Karna-kandu :—Any discharge or secretion of pus from the ear caused by the deranged bodily Váyu stuffing the ear-cavity, owing to a blow on the head or a long immersion in water or a spontaneous suppuration (and bursting) of an abscess in the inner ear, is called **Karna-sráva**. The excessive itching sensation in the ear due to the aggravation of the local Kapha is called **Karna-kandu**. 7-8.

Symptoms of Karna-gutha and Karna-Prati-náha :—Any mucous accumulation in the ear dried and hardened by the heat of the local Pitta is called **Karna-gutha** ; when the dried accumulation of the ear in cases of Karna-gutha becomes liquefied, (and comes out through) the cavity of the nose † and produces head-disease ‡ it is called **Karna-Prati-náha**. 9-10.

* Tha difference in the "Karna-náda" and "Kshveda" is that in the former the sound in the ear is produced by the deranged Váyu alone and is of various kinds, whereas, in the latter it is of a special kind, *viz.*, that of a wind-pipe—the exciting cause being the deranged local Pitta, Kapha and blood.—Videha.

† Some explain "घ्राणमुखं" to mean the cavity of the nose and of the mouth.

‡ In place of "शिरसोऽभितापन:" (producer of head-disease) Mádhava in his Nidána reads "शिरसोऽर्द्धभेदकृत्" *i.e*,, producer of the head-disease known as Ardha-vedhaka (see chapter XXV).

Symptoms of Krimi-karna and Karna-Vidradhi :—Germination of vermins or of other local parasites in the cavities of the ear completely impairs the faculty of hearing and is called **Krimi-karna** from the existence of worms in the ear. Any abscess caused by any local ulcer or by a blow, as well as any idiopathic abscess in the cavity of the ear is known as **Karna-vidrathi.** It is marked by a choked and burning sensation, and piercing and sucking pain, and it secretes red, yellow or reddish bloody discharges. 11-12.

Symptoms of Karna-páka and Puti-karna, etc. :—A process of suppuration setting in (in any of these boils) in the ear through the aggravated condition of the deranged Pitta is marked by a blocked and putrid condition of the passage of the ear. The disease is called **Karna-páká** (suppuration of the ear). A discharge of condensed and fetid pus whether accompanied or not with pain is set up by the local mucous accumulation in the passage of the ear having been liquefied by the heat of the aggravated Pitta. This disease is called **Puti-karna** (pus in the ear). The symptoms of **swelling** (Śopha), **tumours** (Arvuda) and **polypoid growths** (Arśas) * in general as have been described before should be carefully understood by an experinced physicain to be the symptoms of these diseases in the region of the ear. 13-15.

Thus ends the twentieth chapter of the Uttara-Tantra in the Sus'ruta Samhitá which deals with the causes and symptoms of the diseases peculiar to the ear.

* See chapter VI, XVIII and XXIII, Chikitsita-Stháná.

CHAPTER XXI.

Now we shall discourse on the chapter which treats of the medical treatment of the diseases peculiar to the ear (**Karna-gata-Roga-Pratishedha**). 1.

General treatment :—Potions of clarified butter (after meal), use of Rasáyana-measures,* renunciation of all sorts of physical exercise, baths without immerging the head, absolute sexual abstinence and abstinence from talkativeness are the general remedies and rules to be prescribed in the affections of the ear in general. 2.

Treatment of the Vátaja Ear-diseases :—The course of medical treatment to be pursued in the four forms of the ear-diseases (all due to the action of Váyu) *viz.*, **Karna-s'ula**, **Pranáda**, **Vádhirya** and **Karna-kshveda** is the same and is as follows, Sneha should be first administered (both internally and externally) and the patient purged with emulsive purgatives after which the affected locality should be fomented with Váyu-subduing drugs administered in the manner of **Nádi-sveda** or **Pinda-sveda**. 3.

A case of **Karna-s'ula** (ear-ache), due to the concerted action of the deranged Váyu and Kapha of the locality yield to the application of fomentation to the affected part with (the fumes of) *Vilva*, *Eranda*-roots, *Arka*, *Varshábhu*, *Kapittha*, *Dhustura*, *S'igru*, *Ájagandhá*, *As'vagandhá*, *Jayanti*, barley and bamboo, boiled in *Áranála* (fermented rice-gruel) and administered in the manner of Nádi-sveda (fomentation through a pipe). An attack of Karna-s'ula (ear-ache) yieds to the application of

* In place of "Rasáyana" (use of tonic) some read "Rasás'anam" (use of meat-soup with meal).

Pinda-sveda made with pieces of boiled flesh of fish, cock or Láva (jointly or severally), or with (balls of condensed) milk. 4-5.

A bowl-shaped cup should be made of the leaves of the *As'vattha* soaked in oil and *Dadhi-mastu** and it should be heated by means of charcoal-fire. The oil, thus heated and made to drop into the affected organ, gives instantaneous relief in a case of **ear-ache.** The affected organ should be fumigated with the fumes of burning pieces of *Kshauma* (linen cloth) as well as with clarified butter, *Aguru* and *Guggulu* mixed together. Draughts of clarified butter as well as the application of **Śiro-vasti** after meal are also found beneficial. 6-7.

A rice diet should be foregone in the night, and draughts of clarified butter followed by potions of milk should be taken in its stead. The Śata-páka Valá-Taila† should also be prescribed as **Śiro-vasti**, errhine, as well as Mastikya-Śirovasti and sprinkling. It may also be given internally. Goat's milk first cooked with *Kanta-kári* (in the manner of Kshira-páka) and then with the fat (Vasá) of a cock is extremely efficacious (in cases of ear-ache) if used as an ear-drop. 8-9.

The four kinds of Sneha (oil, clarified-butter, lard and animal marrow) duly cooked together with the Kalka of *Tanduliyaka*, *Amkota* fruits, *Ahimsrá*, *Kendraká*-roots, *Sarala*, *Deva-Dáru*, *Las'una* (garlic), *S'unthi* and the scrapings of bamboo-skin and with the liquids of acid‡

* "Mastu" (curd-cream) is mentioned neither by Vrinda nor by Chakrapáni. According to Videha's recipe, clarified butter should be used in place of oil in cases of the aggravation of the Pitta.)

† For "Valá-Taila"—See chapter XV, Chikitsita Sthána.

‡ The liquid acids here are *Dadhi, Takra, Surá, Chukra* (a kind of Kánjika) and the expressed juice of *Mátulunga.*

taste (instead of water) should be used as an ear-drop in order to alleviate the aching pain therein. 10.

The expressed juice of *Las'una*, *S'igru*, *Árdraka*, *Murangi*, *Mulaka* and (branch of) *Kadali* jointly or severally poured lukewarm into the cavity of the organ acts as an excellent ear-drop (in case of acute ear-ache). As an alternative, the expressed juice of *S'ringa-vera* mixed with honey, *Saindhava*, and oil should be used lukewarm as an ear-drop to alleviate the pain therein. Clarified butter* duly cooked with the scrapings of bamboo-skin and the urine of a ewe and of a she-goat† should also be used as an ear-drop in cases of ear-ache. 11-13.

Dipiká-Taila :—Pieces of the roots of the major *Pancha-mula* measuring eighteen fingures in length should be covered (extending only to three-fourths of the whole) with a piece of linen and then soaked in oil. The stick so formed, should then be lighted and the oil pouring in drops therefrom should be used lukewarm (as an ear-drop). It instantaneously removes the pain, and is known as the **Dipiká-Taila.** Different kinds of Dipiká-Taila may be likewise prepared with pieces of *Deva-dáru*, *Kushtha* or *Sarala* wood, and used in the same manner in cases of ear-ache. 14-15.

Tender sprouts of *Arka* plants pasted with *Kánjika* (Amla) should be mixed with oil and salt. The paste thus prepared should be placed inside the hollow made in a branch of *Snuhi* tree and wrapped up with the

* Both Vrinda and Chakrapáni read "Taila" (oil) in place of "Sarpih" (clarified butter). But we have the authority of Videha (as quoted by S'rikantha Datta in his commentary on Vrinda) in favour of clarified butter.

† Clarified butter should first be cooked with the urine of a ewe and then with that of a she-goat.—Dallana.

leaves of the same plant. It should then be scorched in fire in the manner of Puta-pâka. The juice should then be squeezed out of it and used lukewarm as an **ear-drop** to alleviate the pain in the ear. 16.

Different kinds of Ear-drops:—The expressed juice of *Kapittha*, *Mátulunga* and *Árdraka* mixed together and made lukewarm, or the lukewarm *Chukra* (a kind of Kánjika) should be used as ear-drops in a case of ear-ache. As an alternative, the affected ear should be judiciously dusted with powdered *Samudra-phena* in such a case. As an alternative, the eight kinds of officinal urines made lukewarm and used as an ear-drop may prove efficacious in removing an ear-ache. Similarly, a case of an ear-ache yields to the curative virtue of an ear-drop, composed of the four officinal kinds of Sneha duly cooked with the different kinds of officinal urine and acids (wine, sour-gruel, etc.,) as well as with the Vâyu-subduing drugs. 17.

General and Specific treatment of Pittaja Ear-ache:—The above-mentioned mode of treatment (ear-drops and fomentations, etc.) with the Pitta-subduing drugs should be followed in **Pittaja-Karna-śula** (ear-ache). The use of the medicated Ghrita duly cooked with milk weighing ten times as much and with the drugs of the *Kákolyádi* group, as well as the Ghrita* duly cooked with the drugs of the *Tikta* (bitter) group would be found beneficial in such cases. Clarified butter duly cooked with the tender sprouts of *Kshira-vriksha* (milk-exuding trees), as well as with *Yashti-madhu* and *Chandana* wood, or that cooked with the decoction of *Vimbi* with (the Kalka of) sugar, *Yasthi-*

* Dallana says that Jejjatáchárya holds these two recipes as unauthoritative.

madhu and the purgative drugs would also be found beneficial. 18-20.

Treatment of the Kaphaja Karna-ŝula :—In cases of **Kaphaja-Karna-śula** mustard oil or *Ingudi* oil will be found beneficial if used as an **ear-drop**. Decoctions (Yusha) of the drugs of the bitter group, fomentation (Sveda) with Kapha-subduing drugs, as well as the oil cooked with the drugs of the *Surasádi*, or the major *Pancha-mula* group would be found beneficial. The expressed juice of *Mátulunga*, *Laśuna* and *Árdraka*, as well as *S'ukta*, or the oil cooked with any of them should be used as ear-drops in such cases. The use of strong head-purgatives (errhines), or of gurgles is, likewise, recommended in such cases. 21–24.

The medical treatment in a case of ear-ache due to the vitiated condition of the **blood** should be just the same as that in the case of a Pittaja Karna-śula. 25

Thus we have given a **general** outline of the course of treatment and remedial measures to be adopted in the four kinds of ear-affections, *viz.*, Karna-śula (ear-ache), Pra-náda, Vádhirya and Karna-kshveda. Now we shall deal with the **special** recipes and preparations of ear-drops to be employed in cases of deafness (**Vádhirya**). 26.

Treatment of deafness :—The oil duly cooked with water, milk and *Vilva* pasted with cow's urine (as Kalka) should be used as an ear-drop in cases of deafness. Oil should be first cooked with goat's milk or the decoction of *Vimbi* fruit with sugar and *Yashti-madhu* and *Vimbi* fruit (as Kalka). When cooled down (it should be churned with the hand and) the Sneha (oily portion) should be separated. This oily part, after being stirred in the decoction of

Vilva* should again be cooked with milk weighing ten times and with (the Kalka of) sugar, *Yashti-madhu* and (red) sandal wood. It should then be thickened and used as an ear-drop in cases of **deafness**. Measures and remedies, which will be mentioned in connection with Pratis'yáya† (catarrh) or have been already described in the chapter on Váta-Vyádhi ‡ Chikitsá may be as well employed with benefit in the present instances. 27-30.

Treatment of Puti-karna, Karna-sráva and Krimi-karna :—The **general** mode of treatment to be employed in cases of Karna-sráva, Puti-karna and Krimi-karna is the same as above. Now here (me describe) the **general** mode of treatment to be employed in them. Errhines, fumigating, filling up the cavity of the ear (as with an ear-drop), cleansing and washing should be employed according to the exigencies of each case. The affected ear should be washed with the decoction of the drugs of the *Rája-vrikshádi* or the *Surasádi* group and filled with the powders of those drugs. In a case of **Karna-Sráva**, the cavity of the affected organ should be filled in with the powders (D. R. decoction) of the *Pancha-Kasháya* § drugs mixed with honey and the expressed juice of *Kapittha*. 31-32.

* In place of "Vilvámbu-gádham" some read "Vimbi-gádham" ,*i e*,, mixed with an abundant quantity of powdered Vimbi fruit.—Dallana.

† Chap. XXIV, Uttara-Tantra.

‡ Chapter V and VI, Chikitsita-Sthána.

§ According to some, "Pancha-Kasháya" means the barks of *A'ragbadha*, *S'irisha*, *Jambu*, *Sarja* and of *Asvamára* (Palás'a), but Dallana, on the authority of the authors of the Tiká and the Panjiká, (the two commentaries) refutes this and holds that "Pancha-kasháya" means the barks of *Tinduka*, *Abhayá*, *Lodhra*, *Samanga'* and of *A'malaka* enumerated below in this chapter.

The use of the powders of *Sarja*-bark mixed with honey and expressed juice of the *Kárpási* fruit is recommended in cases of **Karna-Sráva**. A compound consisting of pulverised *Lákshá* and *Sarja-rasa* (D. R. Rasánjana) should be used in filling up the cavity of the affected organ in the said disease. The oil duly cooked with the tender sprouts of *S'aivála, Mahá-vriksha, Jambu* and of *Ámra*, as well as with *Karkata-S'ringi* honey and *Manduki* is highly efficacious in these cases. Powders of the barks of *Tinduka, Abhayá, Rodhra, Samangá* and of *Ámalaka* mixed with honey* and the expressed juice of *Kapittha* should be similarly used. 33–36.

The expressed juice of *Ámra, Kapittha, Madhuka* flower, *Dhava* and of *S'ála*, or an oil duly cooked with these is likswise recommended as ear-drops in these cases. The oil cooked with *Priyangu, Yashti-madhu, Ambáliká, Dhátaki, S'ita-parni, Manjishthá, Lodhra,* and *Lákshá* (as Kalka), and with the expressed juice of the sprouts of *Kapittha* as the liquid, if used as an ear-drop, arrests the secretion in a case of **Karna-sráva**. 37–38.

Treatment of Puti-karna :—*Rasánjana* rubbed and dissolved in the breast-milk and mixed with honey proves highly efficacious even in chronic and long-standing cases of **Puti-karna** attended with fetid discharge. The use as ear-drops of the compound composed of oil, the expressed juice of *Nirgundi* and honey mixed together arrests an attack of Puti-karna. 39–40.

Treatment of Krimi-karna :—Vermifuges should be employed for the treatment of a case

* S'rikantha Datta in his commentary on Vrinda quotes this couplet, but does not read 'honey' there. He reads "तथा" in place of "मधु" ।

Krimi-karna. Fumigation* of the affected parts with the fumes of (dried) *Vártáku*, or (the pouring of) mustard oil (into the cavity of the affected organ) is also beneficial in such cases. *Vidanga* and *Haritála* (yellow orpiment) mixed with cow's urine (and used as an ear-drop) as well as fumigating the affected organ with the fumes of (burnt) *Guggulu* tends to destroy the fetor in the ear due to local parasites. Administration of emetics, smoke-inhalation and gurgles are also beneficial in such cases. 41-42.

Treatment of Karna-Kshveda, Vidradhi, etc. :—Use of mustard oil as an ear-drop is efficacious in cases of **Karna-kshveda.**† An abscess (**Vidradhi**) in the ear should be treated as an ordinary abscess. The affected ear should be sufficiently fomented after being filled in with oil so as to soften the filthy deposit in the cavity of the ear, after which the filthy matter should be extracted with a probe or a director (Śaláká). 43-45.

Treatment of Karna-kandu and karna-pratináha :—Fumigation of the parts with the help of a tube (**Nádi-sveda**), exhibitions of emetics, smoke-inhalations, head-purging (errhines), as well as all kinds of Kapha-subduing measures should be resorted to in cases of **Karna-kandu.** Application of Sneha and of Sveda and then of head-purgatives (errhines) should be made in cases of **Karna-pratináha,**

* Dallana explains this to mean fumigation of the affected organ, as well as the use of the same in the manner of smoking.

† The use of oil is also recommended in cases of abscess in the ear. In cases of acute and painful Vâtaja Vidradhi sesamum oil should be used, whereas in cases of Kaphaja Vidradhi the use of mustard oil is recommended.—Dallana.

and the treatment thereafter should conform to the nature of the specific deranged Dosha of the body involved in the case. 46-47.

Treatment of Karna-páka, etc. :— Remedies and remedial measures described in connection with Pittaja Visarpa* should be used with equal profit in a case of **Karna-páka** (inflammatory suppuration of the ear). Any filth or vermin, etc., lodged in the cavity of the ear should be removed with the help of a probe, or (by cutting it) with a horn. Cures for the remaining cases of affections in the ear have been described before (in the Chikitsita-sthána, Chapters XVIII, VI and XXIII). 48-50.

Thus ends the twenty-first chapter of the Uttara-Tantra in the Sus'ruta Samhitá which deals with the treatment of the diseases peculiar to the ear.

* In place of 'Pittaja-Visarpa', both Vrinda and Chakradatta read 'Kshataja-Visarpa'.

CHAPTER XXII.

Now we shall discourse on the chapter which deals with the causes and symptoms of diseases of the nose **(Násá-gata-roga-Vijnániya).** 1.

Nomenclature and Classification :— Diseases which are specifically found to affect the organ of smell may be classified into **Thirty-one** different groups, viz.,—Apinasa, Puti-nasya, Násá-páka. Śonita-Pitta, Puya-śonita, Kshavathu, Bhramśathu, Dipta, Násá-náha, Pari-śráva, Násá-śosha, the four kinds of Arśas (polypoids), the four kinds of swelling, the seven types of tumours and the five types of Prati-śyáya which will be described hereafter with the specific treatment of each. Thus the diseases of the nose are said to be thirty-one in all. 2.

Symptoms of Apinasa and Puti-nasya :—Chokedness and burning sensation in the nostrils attended with dryness and deposit of filthy slimy mucus in their passages, thereby deadening the faculty of smell and taste for the time being, are the specific indications of **Apinasa**, (obstructions in the nostrils) which are identical with the symptoms (of the same type) of Pratiśyáya (catarrh). It is due to the concerted action of the deranged Váyu and Kapha. The disease in which the fetid breath is emitted through the mouth and the nostrils owing to the presence of the deranged Váyu mixed up with the other Doshas (Pitta, Kapha and blood) in the throat and about the root of the palate is called **Puti-nasya.** 3-4.

Symptoms of Násá-páka, Rakta-Pitta and Puya-rakta :—A purulent inflammation and the presence of pimples (Arush) in the nostrils owing to the vitiated condition of the local Pitta attended with sliminess and fœtid odor is called **Násá-páka.**. The four kinds of **Rakta-Pitta** (hæmorrhages) with the two different origins and two different courses will be dealt with again later on.* The disease in which bloody or blood-streaked pus is discharged through the nostrils either as the effect of a blow on the region of the fore-head or through the highly heated condition of the local blood, Pitta and Kapha is called **Puya-rakta** (bloody pus). 5-7.

Symptoms of Kshavathu :—The disease in which the Váyu charged with Kapha repeatedly gushes out of the nostrils accompained by loud reports or sounds, owing to the fact of the nasal Marma being anywise affected, is called **Kshavathu** (sneezing).† A trickling sensation in the gristle of the nose owing to the insertion of a thread, etc., into the nostrils, or to the action of any strong (Tikshna) articles of fare, or of any pungent smell, or of looking to the sun causes sneezing. 8-9.

Symptoms of Bhramŝathu and Dipta :—The disease in which the deranged undigested thickened and saline Kapha previously accumulated in the region of the head is dissolved or disintegrated and dislodged from its seat through the heat of Pitta and is expelled (sneezed off) through the nostrils is called **Bhramśathu.** The affection in which

* The four kinds are due to vitiated Váyu, Pitta and Kapha as well as their concerted action. The two origins are (*a*) the spleen and the liver, or (*b*) the Ámàs'aya (stomach) and the Pakvàs'aya (intestines). The two courses are (*a*) the upper and the lower orifice, or (*b*) the mouth and the nostrils. (2)

† The sneezing is here said to be of two kinds (1) Doshaja and (2) traumatic. Here the former is Doshaja, while the latter is of traumatic origin.

the Váyu, in the shape of warm vapour-like breaths, comes out of the nostrils accompanied by an excessive burning sensation in the locality is called **Dipta**. 10–11.

Symptoms of Násá-Pratináha, Násá-parisráva and Násá-Parisosha:—The condition under which the up-coarsing Udána Váyu of the region of the head is deranged in its passage by a surcharge of Kapha, seems to stuff the passages of the nostrils, and is called **Násá-Pratináha**. The disease in which there is constant, transparent, slightly discoloured water-like secretion (of Kapha) through the nostrils, more particularly at night, is called **Násá-Parisráva** (fluent coryza). Difficulty of respirating (inhaling and exhaling) caused by the drying up and consequent thickening of the Kapha (mucus) accumulating in the passages of the nostrils, through the action of the deranged Váyu and Pitta, is called **Násá-Parisosha** (parchedness of the nostrils). 12–14.

Local **Arsas** (polypoids) as well as local **Sopha** (four each) are due to the action of the three deranged Doshas of the locality jointly and separately. The different kinds of **Arvuda** (nasal tumour) as mentioned in the Śálákya-Tantra, with the one of Sánnipátika origin are seven in all. The five types of **Pratisyáya** (catarrh) mentioned here will be dealt with in chapter XXIV. Remarks made in the chapter on the causes and symptoms of swellings in general (Sopha-Vijnána), as well as those of Arsas (hæmorrhoid growths) in the Nidána-sthána should be understood to apply to those diseases affecting the locality of the nose as well. 15–18.

Thus ends the twenty-second chapter in the Uttara-Tantra of the Sus'ruta Samhitá which deals with the causes and symptoms of the diseases of the nose.

CHAPTER XXIII.

Now we shall discourse on the chapter which deals with the therapeutics of nasal diseases **(Násá-gata-Roga-Pratishedha).** 1.

Treatment of Apinasa and Puti-nasya :—In cases of the first-mentioned disease (*i.e.* **Apinasa**) and in those of **Puti-nasya**, applications of Sneha and of Sveda to the affected part, and application of emetics and purgatives should be made. The **diet** should be light and moderate in quantity. The water for drinking should be boiled before use, and inhalation of smoke (Dhuma-pána) should be indulged in at the proper time. *Hingu*, *Tri-katu*, *Indra-Yava*, *S'iváti**, *Lákshá*, *Katphala*, *Vacha*, *Kushtha*, *S'obhánjana*, *Vidanga*, and *Karanja* should be used daily with benefit in the manner of **Avapida-Nasya**. Mustard oil should be duly cooked with the aforesaid drugs together with cow's urine and be used as an errhine (**Nasya**). 2–3.

Treatment of Násá-páka, etc. :—In cases of **Násá-páka**, all the Pitta-subduing measures both for internal and external use should be duly employed. Barks of the *Kshiri* (milk-exuding) trees mixed with clarified butter should be duly employed as wash and plaster after a local bleeding. The medical treatment of **Sonita-pitta** (Hæmorrhaege) from the nose shall be hereafter† described. A case of **Puya-Rakta** (discharge of bloody pus from the nose) should be treated

* *S'iváti* may mean either white *Punarnavá* or *S'éphálíká*. Neither Chakrapáni nor Vrinda reads it in the text.

† See ch. XLIV of the Uttara-Tantra.

as a case of sinus (Nádi) * for all practical purposes, and Avapida-nasya as well as inhalations of smoke (Dhuma) of keen-potencied drugs and Nasya (snuff or errhines) of drugs of correcting or purifying virtues should be used after the satisfactory exhibition of emetics. 4-5.

Treatment of Kshavatu and Bhramśathu :—Powders of head-purgaing drugs in the form of snuff should be administered into the nostrils through a pipe in cases of **Kshavathu** and **Bhramśathu**. The head should be duly fomented with Váyu-subduing drugs and inhalation of Sneha-Dhuma† as well as similar other medicinal measures remedial to the deranged bodily Váyu should be resorted to. All the Pitta-subduing measures should be employed in a case of **Dipta**, and all cooling remedies and the drugs of sweet taste should also be prescribed. 6-7.

Treatment of Násá-náha, etc. :—The internal use of Sneha (Sneha-pána) forms the principal remedy in a case of **Násá-náha**, in which fumigations with lardacious drugs as well as head-purgings may be likewise employed. The use of Balà-Taila or any other Vàyu-subduing remedy mentioned in the chapter on the treatment of Váta-vyádhi (Ch. V. Chikitsita Sthána) may be similarly used with beneficial results. Powdered snuff should be introduced into the nostrils through a pipe or tube, and strong and keen Avapida-Nasya should be used in cases of **Násá-Sráva**. Strong fumes of (burnt) *Deva-dáru* and *Chitraka* should be applied to the affected part. Goat's flesh is also found beneficial in such cases. 8-9.

* See ch. XIV of the Chikitsita-Sthána.

† See ch. XVII of the Chikitsita-Sthána.

Treatment of Násá-Śosha :—The use of clarified butter churned out of milk, as well as that of the oil as an errhine prepared in the manner of Anu-taila are pre-eminently the best cures in a case of **Násá-Śosha**. Potions of clarified butter, meals with Jángala meat-soup, applications of Sneha and of Sveda, and fumigating the affected part with lardacious drugs may be similarly prescribed with best advantage. The remaining nasal diseases should be duly treated according to the specific treatment of each case as described before. 10–11.

Thus ends the twenty-third chapter of the Uttara-Tantra in the Sus'ruta Samhitá which deals with the treatment of the diseases of the nose.

CHAPTER XXIV.

Now we shall discourse on the chapter whlch deals with the (symptoms and) medical treatment of catarrh **(Pratiŝyáya-Pratishedha).** 1.

Causes:—Excessive indulgence in sexual intercourse, heating of the head, entrance of the minute particles of dust or smoke into the nostrils, excessive application of cold or heat, voluntary retention of stool and urine are the causes which may instantly usher in an attack of nasal catarrh (Pratiśyáya). The fundamental principles of Váyu, Pitta and Kapha, jointly and separately, as well as of blood becoming aggravated by various aggravating causes, bring on an attack of nasal catarrh in course of time. 2–3.

Premonitary Symptoms:—Heaviness of the head, sneezing and aching in the limbs, appearance of goose-flesh upon the body, as well as many other different kinds of supervening symptoms are seen to precede an attack of nasal catarrh (Pratiśyáya). 4.

Specific Symptoms:—Hoarseness of voice, a sense of stuffedness and obstruction in the nostrils accompanied by a thin mucous secretion, dryness of the throat, of the palate and of the lips, a pricking, and piercing pain in the region of the temples, as well as excessive sneezing and a bad taste in the mouth are the characteristlcs of **Vátaja type** of catarrh (Pratiśyáya). A hot and yellowish secretion from the nose, heated skin, thirst, emaciation and yellowness of the complexion, as well as the secretion being sudden, hot and smoky—these are the characteristics which mark the **Pittaja type** of catarrh. Constant running at the nose, the secretion being white and cold, paleness (of the skin) and swelling (D. R.

whiteness) of the eyes, heaviness of the head, flabbiness of the face* and tickling and itching sensation in the regions of the head, throat, lips and of the palate are the features which mark the **Kaphaja type** of the disease. 5-7.

The spontaneous disappearance, as well as re-appearance of Pratis'yáya—be it acute or chronic—is the charracteristic symptom of **Tri-doshaja Pratis'yáya**, wherein the specific symptoms of all (the three) kinds of Apinasa are present. 8.

Symptoms of Raktaja Pratiŝyáya:—Discharge of blood (from the nose), redness of the eyes, a bruised pain in the chest which seems as if struck with a blow, fetid smell in the breath and the mouth, and loss of the faculty of smelling are the characteristic symptoms of the **Raktaja** type of Pratis'yáya which has its origin in the deranged condition of the **blood**. In these cases † hosts of extremely small worms of whitish or blackish ‡ hue are found to infest the affected localities (*viz.*, the nostrils) which show symptoms identical with those of the head-disease due to the germination of parasites in that region. 9.

Prognosis:—The malignant nature of the disease (Dushta-Pratis'yáya) should be inferred from the constant alternate sliminess and dryness, as well as constant alternate contraction and expansion of the nostrils,

* In place of "भवेद्गुरु शिरोमुखः"—some read "भवेद्गुरुशिरा नरः"—*i. e.* "the man (patient) gets heaviness of the head." In this case the flabbiness of the face is not seperately mentioned.

† According to some this is the characteristic symptom of another kind of Pratis'yáya, and not one of the symptoms of the Raktaja type as appears at the first sight.

‡ Mádhava Kar reads 'श्वेताः स्निग्धाः' *i. e.*, glossy white in hue, in place of 'श्वेताः कृष्णाः' *i. e.* whitish and blackish in hue.

fetour in the breath and loss of the faculty of smell. Such a case of Pratis'yáya should be regarded as extremely hard to cure. Neglected and not properly remedied at the outset of an attack, any type of catarrh (Pratis'yáya) may bring on cases of malignant Pinasa, which in time gives rise to a number of diseases and produces in its train deafness, blindness, loss of smell, violent ocular affections, cough, dulness of appetite, and S'opha (swelling). 10–11.

General Treatment of Pratis'yáya :— Potions of clarified butter, various sorts of emetics, and fomentations (Sveda) may be prescribed in nasal catarrh (Pratis'yáya), except in fresh and acute cases. Errhines (Nasya) of Avapida type may also be employed in time, if required. Fomentation should be applied and diet should be taken in a tepid state with articles of acid taste, and draughts of milk should be administered with green ginger* and with any modification of the expressed juice of sugar-cane† for the purpose of thickening and maturing the secreted mucus, in cases where that maturing process has not already spontaneously set in. The mucus found matured, thick and pendent should be made to secrete by applying head-purgatives (S'iro-vireka). Purgatives, Vasti of the Ásthápana kind, smoke-inhalations and medicinal gurgles should also be prescribed according to the exigencies of each case under treatment and in consideration of the nature and intensity of the deranged Dosha involved therein. 12–14.

* Some explain "A'rdraka" to mean the expressed juice of *fresh* ginger, while others explain it to mean the powder of *dried* ginger.

† In place of "इक्षुविकारयोगैः"—with any modification of the expressed juice of sugar-cane, such as treacle, sugar, etc , some read "कटुकोपयोगैः" *i. e.*, with articles of pungent taste.

Regimen of diet and conduct :—In a case of Pratiśyáya the patient should sit, lie, or move about in closed and windless rooms and wear warm and thick turban on his head. He should take *Vijayá* (Haritaki) and partake of meals consisting of *Palánna** cooked without clarified butter. He should also be subjected to a course of strong head-purging as well as of smoke-inhalations. Use of new wine and cold drink, cold baths, sexual intercourse, anxious cares, lamentations, voluntary retention of stools and urine, as well as partaking of fares which are excessively dry (and beget dryness in the system), should be foregone by a person suffering from an attack of Pinasa. 15-16.

Fastings and employment of digestive (Páchana) and appetising (Dipaniya) remedies should be the medical treatment in cases of Pinasa (nasal catarrh) accompanied by such distressing symptoms as vomiting, aching, heaviness in the limbs, feverishness, non-relish for food, apathy, and Atisára (diarrhœa). In case of an adult person suffering from an attack of Pinasa due to the concerted action of Váyu and Kapha, the patient should be made to vomit by taking in a large quantity of any liquid substance. The complications (Upadrava) involved therein should be remedied by appropriate diet and remedial agents and after their subsidence, the patient should be treated according to the instructions given before. 17-18.

Treatment of Vátaja Type :—In cases of **Vátaja-Pratiśyáya** clarified butter duly cooked with the drugs of the *Vidári-gandhádi* group or with the five officinal salts should be prescribed for internal

* Palánna is generally prepared by cooking together rice, meat and clarified butter as well as other spices, but in this case clarified butter should not be used.

use, according to the rules of taking **Sneha** (see chapter XXXI., Chikitshita-Sthána). The process of snuffing, etc., should also be resorted to, if necessary, as in a case of Ardita (Facial paralysis). 19.

Treatment of Pittaja and Raktaja types :—In the **Pittaja** and **Raktaja** types (of Pratis'yáya) the patient should be given draughts* of clarified butter duly cooked with the drugs of the *Kákolyádi* group. Cold† washes and plasters should also be used. *Sarjarasa* (Resin), *Pattanga* (red-sandal), *Priyangu*, honey, sugar, *Drákshá*, *Madhuliká* (Guduchi), *Goji*, *S'ri-parni* and *Yashti-madhu* should be prescribed as gurgles, and purgings (errhines ?) should be induced with the help of the drugs of sweet potency (such as *Drákshá*, *Áragbadha*, honey, sugar, etc.). Oil duly cooked with (a paste composed of) *Dhava*-bark, *Tri-phalá*, *S'yámá*, *Tilvaka*, *Yashti-madhu*, *S'ri-parni*, *Rajani*, and with milk weighing ten times as much as oil, should be preserved for a time and used as an errhine (Nasya) in either of these cases. 20.

Treatment of Kaphaja Type :—In a case of the **Kaphaja-Pratis'yáya**, emulsive measures (Sneha-karma) should be performed with clarified butter, and the patient should be made to vomit by using **Yavágu** (gruel) prepared with *Másha*-pulse and *Tila*, (sesamum-seed), after which the general Kapha-subduing measure should be employed. Oil duly cooked with the two kinds of *Balá*, the two kinds of *Brihati*,

* Some read 'तिक्तैः' in place of 'पेयम्.' This word means that the clarified butter for use in this case should be duly cooked with the तिक्त (bitter) drugs, viz., the leaves of *Patola*, etc.

† Both the commentators of Vrinda and Chakradatta explain the term शीतलेन (cold) to mean 'prepared with the drugs of cold potency such as the drugs of the *Nyagrodhádi* and *Utpaládi* groups.'

Vidanga, *Tri-kantaka*, *S'vetá*-roots, *Sahá* (Mudgaparni), *Bhadrá* (Gámbhári) and *Varshábhu* should be employed as an errhine. *Saralá*, *Kinihi*, *Dáru*, *Nikumbha* (Danti) and *Ingudi* should be pasted together and duly formed as **Vartis**. These Vartis should be duly used for the purposes of smoking (Dhuma-pána) 21–22.

Treatment of Tri-doshaja Type:—Clarified butter duly prepared with the drugs of bitter and pungent tastes, inhalation of the smoke of strong-potencied drugs as well as the use of articles of pungent taste and other appropriate medicinal preparations would prove curative in a case of **Tri-doshaja** Pratis'yáya (nasal catarrh) brought about by the aggravation of all the **three Doshas**. An intelligent physician should prescribe as an errhine the medicated oil duly cooked and prepared with the admixture of *Rasánjana*, *Ati-vishá*, *Musta* and *Bhadra-dáru*. Gargles prepared with the decoction of *Musta*, *Tejovati*, *Páthá*, *Katphala*, *Katuka*, *Vachá*, *Sarshapa* (mustard), *Pippali-mula*, *Pippali*, *Saindhava*, *Agnika* (Ajamodá), *Tuttha*, *Karanja*-seeds, *Salt* and *Bhadra-dáru* should be prescribed. Oil duly cooked with the preceding drugs is recommended for purging (Śiro-vireka) the head of the patient. 23-24.

Flesh of birds and beasts of the Jángala group, aquatic flowers and the Váyu-subduing drugs (Bhadra-dárvádi) should be duly cooked in milk mixed with water weighing half as much as the milk. * The liquid in this case should be reduced to the original quantity of milk, when it should be taken down and allowed to cool. Clarified butter should then be prepared from this milk and should be again duly cooked with the drugs of the *Sarvagandhá* (Eládi) group, sugar, *Anantá*, *Yashti-*

* Some say that milk and water in equal parts should be taken.

madhu and (red) *Chandana* and with a quantity of milk ten times its own weight. All types of nasal catarrh, yield to the curative efficacy of this medicated Ghrita, if used as an errhine (**Nasya**). Oils medicated with the drugs remedial to the specific deranged Dosha involved in each case under treatment should also be prescribed. 25–26.

All the foregoing preparations should be surcharged with the urine and bile of a cow and used in cases due to the existence of local parasites, and vermifuges (*e. g.*, drugs of the Surasádi group) should be administered as a palliative measure.* 27.

Thus ends the twenty-fourth chapter of the Uttara-Tantra in the Sus'ruta Samhitá which deals with the (symptoms and) medical treatment of Pratis'yáya.

* In places of "यापनार्थं' Chakradatta reads '"नावनार्थं' *i e.*, as an errhine. He also reads "समूत्रपिष्टाः" *i.e.*, pasted with the urine (of a cow), and thus does not read the bile of a cow (पित्त) in the text. Vrinda, however, reads "धावनानि" in place of "यापनार्थं" which means that vermifuges should be used for washing purposes.

CHAPTER XXV.

Now we shall discourse on the chapter which deals with the symptoms of diseases peculiar to the region of the head (**Śiro-roga-Vijnániya**). 1.

Classification :—Diseases which are peculiar to the region of the head number eleven in all, *viz.*, the four kinds respectively due to the action of the deranged Váyu, Pitta, Kapha, and their combination, as well as those which are respectively incidental to any bodily waste (Kshayaja), or to the vitiated condition of the blood (Raktaja), or to the existence of parasites (Krimija), the remaining four being known as Suryávarta, Anantaváta, Ardhávabhedaka and Śamkhaka. The symptoms of these eleven kinds of head-diseases are given below. 2.

Symptoms of Dosha-origined types :—A fit of violent headache without any apparent cause and which becomes worse in the night and is relieved by pressure or by being bandaged or by an application of fomentation round the head, should be ascribed to the action of the deranged **Váyu**, and is known as the **Vátaja-Śiroroga**. A violent burning and aching pain in the head, in which the scalp seems to have been strewn over with bits of live charcoal, accompanied by a sense of scorching vapour being emitted from the nostrils, and which ameliorates in the night or on the application of cold, should be ascribed to the action of the deranged **Pitta**, and is known as the **Pittaja-Śiroroga**. A fit of headache in which the head (palate) and the throat* seem to be covered with a coat of sticky

* In place of "शिरोगलं" some read "शिरो भवेत्". This reading is adopted by Mádhava. There seems to be no difference in the meaning s the word शिरस् (head) may include both the palate and the throat.

mucus, and feel cold and heavy, and cannot be turned about, and the face and the eyes look swollen or flabby, should be attributed to the action of the deranged bodily **Kapha**, and is called the **Kaphaja-Śiroroga.** A case marked by the concerted action of all the three preceding Doshas exhibits all the symptoms peculiar to all of them, and is known as the **Tri-doshaja-Śiroroga.** 2–6.

Symptoms of Ràktaja, Kshayaja and Krimija types of Śiro-roga :—A case of headache due to the vitiated condition of the local **blood** manifests all the symptoms of the Pittaja type, and the head becomes incapable of (bearing) the least touch. This is known as the **Raktaja-Śiroroga.** A case of headache incidental to the waste of the local Vasá (fat) or Kapha* is marked by an intolerable pain (Abhi-tápa) in the head which is aggravated by the application of fomentation, fumigation, errhine, emetic and blood-letting. This is known as the **Kshayaja-Śiroroga.** The disease of the head in which a pricking and tingling pain is felt inside the head as if being stung, (by some poisonous insect), and which is accompanied by a watery discharge mixed with blood (D. R. pus) from the nose, should be attributed to the existence of local parasites. This disease is a dangerous one and is known as the **Krimija** (Parasitic) **Śiro-roga.** 7–9.

Symptoms of Suryávarta Śiro-roga :—The disease of the head in which a severe pain is felt in the eye and the eyebrow just at sunrise, and

* Dallana here comments that the term "**Vasá**" means all the fatty substances in the body, *e. g*, the brain substance, Medas, semen, Majjan, etc. There is a variant which is not recognised by Gayi. That reading is असृग्वसाश्लेष्मसमीरणानां (*i. e.*, by the waste) of blood, Vasá Kaphá and Váyú. This, however, seems to be the better reading.

which goes on growing worse with the progress of the day and begins to abate only when that great luminary begins to set in the western sky, is called **Suryávarta.** It (generally) abates on the use of cold articles but sometimes on that of warm things as well. It is ascribed to the concerted action of the **three** Doshas. 10.

Symptoms of Ananta-váta Śiro-roga :—The disease of the head in which a violent pain is felt at the Manyá and the Ghátá (the two nerves on the backside of the neck) which ultimately affects the region of the eye, the eyebrow and the temples and specially produces a throbbing of the cheek, as well as paralysis of the jaw-bone and the eye. The disease is known as **Ananta-váta** and is due to the concerted action of the **three** Doshas. 11.

Symptoms of Ardhávabhedāka and Śamkhaka :—The disease of the head in which a violent and excruciating pain of a piercing or aching nature is felt in one half of the cranium which makes the patient feel giddy, and which either follows no distinct periodicity or recurs at a regular interval of ten days or of a fortnight, is called the **Ardháva-bhedaka** and is due to the concerted action of the **three** Doshas. A violent pain caused in the head and more especially in the temples by the local Váyu in combination with the deranged Kapha, Pitta and blood is designated by the holy sages of Áyurveda as the **Śamkhaka**. It produces a very great pain, and is very hard to cure even by the joint advice of thousands of physicians and is as fierce as death itself. 12–13.

Thus ends the twenty-fifth chapter in the Uttara Tantra of the Sus'ruta Samhitá which deals with the symptoms of the diseases of the head.

CHAPER XXVI.

Now we shall discourse on the chapter which deals with the therapeutics of the diseases of the head (**Śiro-roga-Pratishedha).** 1.

Treatment of Vátaja-Śiroroga :—Remedial measures described in connection with the treatment of Váta-Vyádhi should be employed in their entirety in the Váyu-origined types of the diseases of the head, and all medicinal compounds of oil or clarified butter should be followed by a potion of milk. *Mudga*, *Kulattha*, or *Másha* pulse, unmixed with any other thing, as well as pungent and heat-making articles, saturated with clarified butter and followed by potions of tepid milk should be taken in the night. Sesamum oil or the paste of sesamum may also be taken. Milk duly boiled with the Váyu-subduing drugs should be employed in a lukewarm state in washing the diseased locality, and a plaster composed of the powders of the same drugs boiled with milk should be applied lukewarm to the scalp. In the alternative, the scalp may be plastered over with the boiled flesh of fish or with *Kris'ará* (preparation of rice and sesamum) saturated with *Saindhava* salt, or with (the paste of) *Chandana*, *Utpala*, *Kushtha* and *Pippali*, finely powdered together (all in a lukewarm state). 2-3.

Oil duly prepared with *Kulira* (crabs) should be used for Nasya (snuffing) purposes subsequent to the employment of the (above) fomentation. A quantity of milk diluted with the addition of half as much of water should be duly boiled with the paste of the drugs of the *Varunádi* group and taken down from the fire when the water has evaporated. Butter should be skimmed out of it when cool and clarified butter prepared therefrom should be again duly cooked with the paste of the drugs of the *Madhura* group. The use of this Ghrita as a Nasya (snuff) is highly efficacious in the type under discussion. Clarified butter duly cooked with the decoction of the preceding drugs (of the Varunádi group) and with milk should be taken with sugar. Snaihika Dhuma (Chikitsá, XL.) should be administered in time when required, and Traivrita Ghrita and Balá Taila should be prescribed as a draught and as an errhine, as well as for the purposes of anointing, sprinkling and Vasti-Karma. The food in the present type of the disease should be taken with milk cooked with Váyu-subduing drugs and with meat-soup saturated with Sneha *(clarified butter).* *4–5.*

Treatment of Pittaja and Raktaja S'iro-roga :—Cooling plasters saturated with clarified butter should be applied to the scalp and cooling head-washes should be prescribed in the Pittaja and Raktaja types of S'iro-roga. Milk, the expressed juice of sugarcane, fermented rice-gruel (Dhányámla), curd-cream (Mastu), honey and sugar mixed in water—these should be used for sprinkling purposes. Plaster for the head should be prepared with *Nala*, *Vetasa*, *Kahlára* (red lotus), *Chandana*, *Utpala*, *S'amkha* (conch-shell), *S'aivála*, *Yashti-madhu*, *Musta* and *lotus* taken together and mixed with clarified butter, and the plasters described in connection with the treatment of Pittaja and Raktaja Visarpa (Erysipelas) should also be used. The drugs of the *Madhura* group should be used in a tepid state as plasters and the **Sneha** (oil or clarified butter) duly cooked with the same drugs should be used as an errhine, and appropriate medicines should be used as purgatives as well as in Ásthápana and Sneha-Vasti measures,

Clarified butter skimmed from milk, and fresh *Vasá* (lard)* of Jángala animals should be used as errhines, and, cooked with the drugs of the *Utpaládi* group, should be used in the manner of Ásthápana-vasti. **Food** should be taken with meat-soup of Jángala animals, and clarified butter should be used in the manner of an Anuvásana Vasti. Clarified butter skimmed from milk and du'y cooked with the drugs of the *Madhura* group and mixed with sugar should be used for emulsive purposes (Snehana), and all measures and remedies which are remedial to the deranged blood and Pitta may be likewise employed with profit in these cases. 6–7.

Treatment of Kaphaja Śiro-roga:—In a case of Kaphaja-Śiroroga, the Kapha-subduing measures, such as strong emetics, head-purgatives (Śiro-vireka) and gargling should be resorted to. The transparent upper part of clarified butter † should be given to drink, and fomentation should then be frequently applied to the head. Head-purgatives should then be administered with the pith of Madhuka wood, or with *Mesha-s'ringi* and *Ingudi* bark. Vartis (sticks) made of *Mesha-s'ringi* and *Ingudi* barks should be used in smoking. Snuffs of powdered *Katphala* should be taken, and gargles with Kapha-subduing drugs should be used. Plasters prepared with *Saralá*, *Kushtha*, *S'árngashtá*, *Deva-dáru*, and *Rohisha* pasted together with the alkaline water and mixed with *Saindhava* salt should be applied lukewarm to the head. The **diet** should consist of cooked barley or *Shashtika* rice, which should

* In place of 'वसा' (lard) some read 'रसा' which means meat-soup.

† According to a variant matured clarified butter should be used in this case.

be judiciously taken with *Yava-kshára* and powdered *Tri-katu* and with the soup of *Mudga*, *Patola* and Kulattha pulse. 8.

Treatment of Tri-doshaja and Kshayaja S'iroroga :—The Measures which are severally remedial to the three deranged Doshas of the body should be employed in a case of Śiroroga marked by the concerted action of the three Doshas (**Tri-doshaja**) and draughts of old and matured clarified butter are said to be specially efficacious in such instances. Employment of nutritive (Vrimhana) measures and remedies is recommended in cases of the diseases of the head due to any waste or atrophy of the local fat, etc. (**Kshayaja Ŝiroroga**). Clarified butter duly cooked with the admixture of the drugs of the Vâyu-subduing and the *Madhura* groups* should be given as drinks and errhines. Any medicated Ghrita which acts as a remedy in cases of consumptive cough would be found most efficacious in the present (Kshayaja) type. 9-10.

Treatment of Krimija S'iroroga :—In a case of head-disease (head-ache ?) due to the germination of parasites (Krimi) in the head, the patient should be made to snuff in a quantity of animal blood. The worms or parasites lured with the smell of the blood, would greedily come down (into the passages of the nostrils) when they should be carefully extracted (by means of tongs, etc). Head-purgatives composed of the pulverised seeds of *Hraswa* (small) *S'igru* mixed with *Kânsya* (dead brass) and Nili (indigo) pounded together should then be used, if necessary, or any vermifuge drug (Vidanga, etc.) pasted with the urine of a cow should be

* According to Videha the clarified butter in this case should be cooked with the decoction of the Váyu-subduing drugs and with the Kalka of the Madhura drugs.

stuffed into the nostrils in the manner of an Avapida Nasya. Fumigations should be applied into the nostrils with the fumes of burnt sordid fishes and vermifuge foods and drinks of various kind should be given. 11.

Treatment of Suryávarta and Ardhávabhedaka :—Errhines etc. (plaster, gargle, etc.) should be prescribed in cases of the **Suryavarta** type of Śiroroga. The diet should principally consist of boiled rice and milk with clarified butter and the essence or extract of the meat of Jângala animals. These and similar other suitable remedial agents should be employed in cases of the **Ardhávabhedaka** type of Śiroroga. Śirisha* and *Mulaka* seeds or bamboo-roots camphor, or *Vacha* and *Mágadhi*, or *Yashti-madhu* and honey, or *Manah silá*, pasted with honey, or (pasted) *Chandana* should be stuffed into the nostrils in the manner of an Avapida Nasya in a case of the Suryávarta type of Śiroroga as well as in a case of Ardhávabhedaka headache. After the use of the above, the patient should be made to snuff in the medicated clarified butter cooked with the drugs of the *Madhura* † (Kákolyádi) group, in both the above cases. Plasters composed of *Sárivá*, *Utpala*, *Kushtha* and *Yashti-madhu* pasted with Kánjika(acid gruel) and surcharged with oil and clarified butter are to be found efficacious in both the cases, if applied to the affected region. This may be employed with equal success in the cases of the Kaphaja type ‡ of Śiroroga. 12-14.

* Sripati Datta, the commentator of Vrinda, prescribes the bark and S'ivadása Sen, the commentator of Chakrapáni, prescribes the seeds of S'irisha.

† Some take "मधुरसा" to mean "मूर्वा" ।

‡ In place of the Kaphaja type some read the Kshayaja type. But it is not accepted by Jejjata. Others again read "Anilátmake" *i.e.* in the Vátaja type.

Treatment of Ananta-váta :—Cases of Ananta-váta Śiroroga should be treated like those of Suryavarta. Moreover blood-letting should be effected (by opening a local vein) and the diet should be such as to subdue the Váyu and the Pitta and should cossist of *Madhu-Mastaka*, *Sangyáva* and *Ghrita-pura* (different kinds of confectionery made of wheat, sugar, milk, clarified butter, etc.). 15.

Treatment of Śamkhaka :—Clarified butter churned from milk should be given for a drink and used as an errhine in a case of **Śamkhaka** and the diet should consist of (boiled rice mixed with) clarified butter and the essence of the meat of jángala animals. Plasters composed of *S'atávari*, black *sesamum*, *Yashti-madhu*, *Nilotpala*, *Durvá* and *Punarnavá* pasted together, or of *Mahá-sugandhá* (Utpla-asárivá) or *Pálindi* pasted with *Kánjika* should be applied to the affected locality. Cooling washes and plasters as well as different Avapida Nasyas prescribed in cases of Suryávarta should also be prescribed for this disease (Śamkhaka). 16.

Strong head-purgatives (errhines) composed of oil and honey should be first administered in cases of Śiroroga with the exception of the Krimija and the Kshayaja types. Then the patient should be made to snuff in drops of mustard oil. In cases where the preceding remedies would fail to produce any relief, the patient should be treated with Sneha and Sveda, and bleeding should then be effected by opening a local vein. 17-18.

The Conclusion :—The causes, symptoms and the therapeutics of the seventy-six kinds of ocular affection, of the twenty-eight kinds of the disease of the ear, of the thirty-one kinds of nasal disease, of the eleven kinds of the disease of the head as well as of the sixty-seven (sixty-five) kinds of the affection of the mouth have been described in detail in other treatises (*e.g.* those of Videha, etc. dealing with this special subject—the diseases of the over-clavicular region). The number, symptoms and therapeutics of these diseases of the over-clavicular region are herein briefly described in accordance therewith. 19.

Thus ends the twenty-sixth chapter of the Uttara-Tantra in the Sus'ruta Samhitá which deals with the treatment of the diseases of the head.

Here ends the Śálákya Tantra (Surgery Minor).

CHAPTER XXVII.

Now we shall discourse on the chapter which deals with the specific features (of the nine diseases of infant life, which are attributed to the influences) of the nine malignant Grabas (**Nava-Grahákriti-Vijná-nam**). 1.

Different Names :—Attentively hear me describe, Sus'ruta, the origin, cause and medical treatment of the diseases of infancy which are due to the influences of malignant stars (**Graha**) or demons as well as the characteristic symptoms by which each can be accurately diagonosed. The diseases number nine in all and are called Skanda-Graha, Skandápasmára, S'akuni, Revati, Putaná, Andha-Putaná, S'ita-Putaná, Mukha-mandiká and Naigamesha or Pitri-Graha. 2-3.

General course of attack :—These malignant stars (Graha) or demons affect the person of a child in the cases where the directions laid down before (in the S'árira-sthána) in respect of the conduct of the mother or the nurse during the time the child is brought-up on the breast are not followed, and consequently where proper benedictory rites are not performed and the child is allowed to remain in an uncleanly state, or where the child becoming anyhow uneasy gets frightened, is rebuked, or begins to cry. They (demons) make their appearance for the purpose of getting proper respect and worship. They being omnipotent and omnipresent are not capable of being seen by man when they enter the person of a child. I should, therefore, discourse on the symptoms of their presence, as derived from the authority of the sages of yore. 4.

Symptoms of attack by Skanda-graha and Skandápasmára-graha :—Swelling of the eyes and distorted features of the face and an aversion to the breast-milk are the indications of an attack by the **Skanda-graha**. The body of the chiid emits a bloody smell and one of the eyelids becomes fixed or motionless. The child looks frightened, closes his fists (as in a fit of convulsion) and moans a little. The eyes become highly rolling and the stool becomes hard and constipated. Alternate fits of fainting and consciousness, convulsive jerks of legs and hands like those in dancing, foaming (at the mouth), yawning and the passing of stool and urine with the passage of wind are the characteristic features of an attack by the **Skandápasmára-graha**. 5-6.

Śakuni and Revati :—Looseness of limbs which emit a peculiar bird-like* smell are the indications of an attack of the child by the **Śakuni Graha**. The child in such a case starts up in terror and its body is covered with a large number of secreting ulcers (Vrana), or of eruptions of vesicles attended with a burning sensation subsequently suppurating and bursting of themselves. The face assumes a blood-red hue, the stool (as well as the urine) becomes green and the body of the child looks as if of deep yellow or dark brown colour, fever ensues with an inflamation of the mouth, a bruised pain is felt all over the body and the child frequently rubs its nose and ears—these are the features which mark a sure attack of **Revati-Graha**. 7-8.

Putaná and Andha-putaná :—Looseness of the limbs, disturbed sleep whether by day

* By the word विहङ्ग (lit. a bird) in विहङ्गगन्धिः is here meant meat-eating aquatic birds.

or at night, loose stools, emission of a crow-like smell from the body, vomiting, appearance of goose-flesh on the skin and thirst are the specific symptoms of an attack of the child by the **Putaná-Graha.** Dislike for the breast-milk as well as an attack of dysentry, (Atisára), cough, hic-cough, vomiting, fever, discolouring of the complexion, and swelling in the skin as well as an inclination to lie always on the face are the symptoms which are exhibited in a case of an attack by the **Andha-Putaná-Graha.** 9–10.

Śita-putaná and Mukha-mandiká :— Constant and frightened startling up, excessive shivering, comatose sleep, constant diarrheic stools and bloody smell of the limbs are the symptoms which characterise a case of an attack by **Śita-Putaná.** The child in this case cries almost unceasingly, and a rumbling sound is heard in the intestines. Paleness (emaciation) of the body (trunk) and a glossy line (swelling) of the face and the extremities attended with frightfulness, voracious appetite, appearance of net-like veins on the abdomen and the emission of urine-like smell from the body are the symptoms of an attack of the child by **Mukha-mandiká Graha.** 11–12.

Naigamesha-Graha :—Frothy vomits, bending of the middle of the trunk, anxious appearance, loud crying, upward gaze of the eyes, constant emaciation (fever-D. R.), a fatty smell in the body and unconsciousness are the symptoms which mark a case of an attack by the **Naigamesha.** 13.

Prognosis :—A stupified state of the child attended with anaversion to breast-milk and constant fits of fainting as well as the full development of all the specific symptoms show the imminent fatal termination of the disease. Otherwise it may prove amenable to medical treatment, if it be not a case of long standing. 14.

Rules to be observed :—The child should be kept in a clean and purified chamber and its body should be rubbed or anointed with old and matured clarified butter. Mustard seeds should be strewn all over the floor (by a person) in a clean state and a lamp of mustard oil should be kept perpetually burning therein. Libations of clarified butter with the drugs of the *Sarva-gandhá* and *Sarvoushadhi* * groups and garlands of flowers as well as sandal paste should be cast into the fire and kept continually burning by reciting the following incantations, "Obeisance to thee, O fire-god, obeisance to thee, O goddess Krittiká, obeisance to thee, O Skanda, obeisance to thee, O lord of the Grahas (which has cast this malignant influence). With head down with deep humility, I supplicate thy favour. Dost thou accept the offerings I have made to thee. May my child get rid of the disease it has been suffering from. Makest it hale and hearty again." 15.

Thus ends the twenty-seventh chapter of the Uttara-Tantra in the Sus'ruta-Samhitá which deals with the specific features of an attack by the nine (malignant) Grahas.

* The drugs of the Eládi group are known as Sarva-gandha. Sarvaaushadhi drugs here mean *Yava, Dha'nya, Tila*, etc.

CHAPTER XXVIII.

Now we shall discourse on the chapter which deals with the Therapeutics (and remedial measures) of an attack by Skanda-Graha (**Skanda-Graha-Pratishedha**). 1.

Decoctions of the leaves of the trees (Vilvádi) possessed of Váyu-subduing virtue should be used for sprinkling purposes and oil duly cooked and prepared with the decoction of their roots and with the drugs of the *Sarvagandha*, group and with *Kaitaryya** and *Surá-manda* as Kalka should be used in anointing the body of the child laid up with an attack of Skanda-graha. Draughts of clarified butter duly cooked with *Deva-dáru*, *Rásná*, the drugs of the *Madhura* group and with milk, should be internally administered. 2–3.

Fumigation :—Moreover the body of the child should be fumigated with the fumes of the mustard seeds, the cast-off skin of a snake, *Vachá*, *Kákádani*, clarified butter and the hairs of a camel, a goat, a sheep or of a cow mixed together and burnt. 4.

The twigs of *Soma-balli* (Guduchi), *Indra-balli* (As'mantaka) and *S'ami* as well as the thorns of *Vilva* and the roots of *Mrigádani*, should be strung together (in the shape of a garland) and tied (round its neck). 5.

The physician (or any other person acting on his behalf) should bathe in the night and worship the god Skanda for three successive nights in the inner quadrangle of the house of the child or at the crossing of roads with various offerings, *viz.*, garlands of red flowers, red flags, red perfumes such as *Kumkuma*, edibles of various

* Kaitaryya, according to Dallana, means Nimba or Guduchi.

kinds and newly harvested barley grains, *Sáli* rice. A cock should be sacrificed on the occasion (to appease his wrath) and bells should be rung (for his propitiation). The water to be used for bath (in course of worship), should be consecrated by reciting the Gáyatri Mantra and the sacrificial fire should be duly lit with (three, seven or ten) libations (of clarified butter). 6.

Mantras :—The body of the child should be guarded by a careful physician against the influence of the malignant Grahas by reciting every day a Mantra which runs as follows :—"May Skanda, the eternal and changeless deity who is the receptacle of all sorts of energies produced by austerities, fame, valour, or organic combination (vital energy), be propitious to thee. May the almighty Guha protect thee from all evils—Guha who is the commander-in-chief both of the army of the gods and of the Grahas and is the destroyer of the enemies of the army of the gods (in which rank he has been installed, lit. wedded, with the suffrage of all the gods). May he who is the begotten son of the supreme deity—the god of the gods and who acknowledges severally the exalted motherhood of Gangá, Umá and the Krittikás, give thee health and comfort. May the beautiful god who pierced with a single shaft right through the heart of the mountain Krouncha and who is effulgent with the red rays of his own divine person smeared with the paste of red sandal-wood and decked with the garland of red flowers, protect thee from all perils." 7.

Thus ends the twenty-eighth chapter of the Uttara-Tantra in the Sus'ruta Samhitá which deals with the Therapeutics of Skanda-Graha.

CHAPTER XXIX.

Now we shall discourse on the chapter which deals with the Therapeutics of an attack by Skandápasmára **(Skandápasmára-Pratishedha).** I.

A decoction of *Vilva*, *S'irisha*, *Golomi* (*Durálabhá*), and the drugs of the *Surasádi* group should be employed in **sprinkling** the body of the possessed child in a case of the present disease. Medicated oil duly cooked with the drugs of the *Sarvagandhá* group should be used in **anointing** its body. Clarified butter duly cooked with milk and the decoction of the barks of the *Kshiri* trees together with the drugs of the *Kákolyádi* group as Kalka* should be prescribed for internal use. 2A.

The body of the affected child should be rubbed (**Utsádana**) with the paste of *Vachá* and *Hingu* taken together. The dungs of an owl and a vulture, human hairs, the nails of an elephant, clarified butter, and the hairs of a bull should be mixed together and used for **fumigating** the child's body. *Anantá*, *Vimbi*, *Markati*, and *Kukkuti* should be strung together and fastened (as a charm) to the body of the child. 2B.

The physician (or the votary officiating for him) should worship the presiding deity of the disease in a ditch (dug out for the purpose) with the offerings of both cooked and uncooked meat, fresh blood (of a goat), milk, and edibles prepared with the *Másha* pulse for the ghosts, and the possessed child should be bathed at the crossing of roads by physician observing the

* Although Dallana prescribes the drugs of the Kákolyádi group to be used as Kalka, we are inclined to take the sentence to mean that the decoction of those drugs should be used.

necessary fast, etc. with the recital of the following Mantra :—"O thou, the trusted and beloved friend of the god Skanda, O Skandápasmára, O thou ugly-faced one whom the world knows by the epithet of Visákha, may good befall this child in distress." 2.

Thus ends the twenty-ninth chapter of the Uttara-Tantra in the Sus'ruta Samhitá which deals with the Therapeutics of an attack by Skandápasmára.

CHAPTER XXX.

Now we shall discourse on the chapter which deals with the medical treatment of an attack by Śakuni (**Śakuni-Pratishedha**). 1.

A wise physician should **sprinkle** the body of the child possessed by Śakuni with the decoction (duly prepared) of *Vetasa*, *Ámra* and *Kapittha*. Oils duly cooked with the drugs of the sweet and astringent groups should be used in **anointing** its body. **Pradehas** (plasters) composed of *Madhuka*, *Us'ira*, *Hrivera*, *Sárivá*, *Utpala*, *Padmaka*, *Rodhra*, *Priyangu*, *Manjishthá* and *Gairika*, should be applied. 2A.

Various kinds of medicinal powders and diet and remedial measures in general described in connection with the medical treatment of Ulcers * as well as the fumigations (Dhupana) mentioned in the chapter on the treatment of Skanda-graha (vide ch. XXVIII.) should be prescribed for the disease under discussion. Drugs such as *S'atávari*, *Mrigádani*, *Erváru*, *Nágadanti*, *Nidigdhiká*, *Lakshmaná*, *Sahadevá* and *Vrihati* should be fastened (as a charm) to the body of the child (in the preceding manner). 2B.

The presiding deity of the disease (Śakuni Graha) should be worshipped by a physician of self-control inside a *Karanja* bower and be propitiated with offerings of huskless sesamum, garlands of flowers, *Haritála* (yellow orpiment) and *Manahs'ilá* (realgar) and the child should be bathed duly inside the bower (according to the rules laid down in the treatment of Skanda Graha). The medicated Ghrita prescribed for

* See Chapter I, Chikitshita Sthána.

the treatment of Skanda Graha may also be advantageously given in the present instance. 2C.

Various sorts of worship should be made with the offerings of various species of auspicious flowers. The **Mantra** to be recited on the occasion runs as folllows :—"May the ever down-looking sharp-beaked goddess, Śakuni, who (with her keen and far-seeing eyes) is decked with all sorts of ornaments and who traverses the ethereal sky in her flight, be propitious to thee. May the brown-eyed, fierce-looking, huge-bodied, large-bellied, and spike-eared Śakuni, who strikes terror into the heart of man with her terrible voice, be pleased with thee." 2.

Thus ends the thirtieth chapter of the Uttara Tantra in the Sus'ruta Samhitá which deals with the treatment of (an attack) by S'akuni.

CHAPTER XXXI.

Now we shall discourse on the chapter which treats of the Therapeutics of an an attack by Revati (**Revati-Pratishedha**). 1.

The duly prepared decoction of *As'vagandhá*, *Sárivá*, *Ajas'ringi*, *Punarnavá*, the two kinds of *Sahá* and *Vidári* should be employed in **sprinkling** (Sechana) the body of the affected child (in a case of an attack by Revati). Medicated oil duly cooked with *Kushtha* and *Sarjarasa* (resin) * should be used in **anointing** the child's body. Medicated Ghrita duly cooked with the decoction of *Dhava*, *As'va-karna*, *Kakubha*, *Dhátaki* and *Tinduka* and with the drugs of the *Kákolyádi* group (as Kalka) should be employed internally as a draught. 2A.

Kulattha, (burnt and) powdered *S'amkha* (conch-shell) and the drugs of the *Sarvagandha* group should be used as **Pradehas** (plasters), and the body of the child should be fumigated (*Dhupana*) morning and evening with the smokes of barley, *Yava-phala* (bamboo), and the dungs of vultures and owls mixed with clarified butter. Neck-ornament should be made with (the wood or pith of) *Varuna*, *Arishta* (Nimba), *Ruchaka*, *Sinduka* (Nirgundi), and *Putranjivaka* and should be always worn on the neck (as a charm) by the child. 2–3.

The presiding deity of the disease known as Revati should be worshipped in a cow-shed by a self-controlling physician with the offerings of white flowers, milk, parched

* There is an additional text in the Bhávaprakás'a which says that Guggulu (Palamkashá), Nalada (Khus-khus) and Giri-kadamba should also be used in the preparation of the medicated oil.

paddy and boiled *S'áli* rice and the nurse as well as the child should be bathed in a junction of rivers. The **Mantra** (to be recited in course of worship) runs as follows :—"May the goddess, Revati, of dark complexion who is clad in parti-coloured garments and garlands of flowers of various colours and painted with anointments of various kinds and with oscillating ear-rings, be pleassd with thee. May the goddess, Revati, who is tall, drooping and terrible-looking, and who is the mother of many sons be always propitious to thee." 2.

Thus ends the thirty-first chapter of the Uttara-Tantra in the Sus'ruta Samhitá which deals with the Therapeutics of an attack by Revati.

CHAPTER XXXII.

Now we shall discourse on the chapter which treats of the medical treatment of an attack by Putaná (**Putaná-Pratishedha**). 1.

A decoction of the barks of *Kapota-banká*, *Araluka*, *Varuna*, *Páribhadraka* and *A'sphotá* should be used in **washing**, and medicated oil duly cooked and prepared with (the Kalka and decoction of) *Vacha*, *Vayasthá*, (Bráhmi), *Golomi*, *Haritála*, *Manah-s'ilá*, *Kushtha* and *Sarja-rasa* (resin) should be used in **anointing** the body of a child possessed by Putaná. 2–3.

Clarified butter duly cooked with the *Tugá-kshiri*, *Kushtha*, *Tális'a*, *Khadira* and *Chandana*, and the drugs of the *Madhura* group would be found beneficial. 4.

Deva-dáru, *Vachá*, *Kushtha*, *Hingu*, *Giri-kadamba*, *Elá* and *Harenu* should be used in fumigating the body of the child. Fumigation of *Gandhanákuli*, *Kumbhiká*, marrow of *Vadara-fruits*, shells of crabs, and mustard-seeds pounded together and mixed with clarified butter may also be used. *Kákádani*, *Chitra-phalá*, *Vimbi* and *Gunjá* should be worn on the body (as a charm) by the child. 5–6.

Putaná, the presiding deity of the disease, should be worshipped in the interior of a lonely chamber with oblations and with the offerings of boiled rice prepared with the admixture of fish as well as those of *Kris'ará*, and *Palala* (meat or puddings of sesamum) placed in a saucer and covered with another, and the child should be bathed with the water left behind after worship. 7A.

The worshipping **Mantra** is as follows :—"May the slovenly shag-haired goddess, Putaná, who is dressed in dirty clothes, and who loves to haunt lonely

20

dwellings, preserve the child. May the fierce-looking, frightful goddess who is as black as a dark rain-cloud, who loves to haunt lonely and dilapidated human dwellings and whose body gives off filthy odours protect the child from all evils." 7.

Thus ends the thirty-second chapter of the Uttara-Tantra in the Sus'ruta Samhitá which deals with the medical treatment (of an attack) by Putaná.

CHAPTER XXXIII.

Now we shall discourse on the chapter which deals with the medical treatment of (an attack by) Andha-putaná **(Andha-putaná-Pratishedha).** I.

The decoction of the leaves of the trees of the *Tiktaka* gana (trees of bitter taste) should be used in **sprinkling** (the body of the possessed child). *Surá* (wine), *Souviraka* (a kind of acid gruel), *Kushtha*, *Haritála*, *Manah-s'ilá* and *Sarjarasa* (resin) should be used in due proportion in medicating the oil (for the child) and medicated Ghrita should be duly cooked with the Kalka and decoction of *Pippali*, *Pippali-mula*, the drugs of the *Madhura* group, *S'álaparni* and the two kinds of *Vrihati* with the addition of honey (as an after-throw). 2A.

Plasters of the drugs of the *Sarva-gandhá* (Eládi) group should be applied to the body of the child and its eyes should be soothed with cold applications. The feces of the the cock, its feather and skin*, the cast-off skin of a snake and the ragged garment of a (Buddhist) monk† should be used for **fumigating** the child's body. The child should be made to wear (the roots of) *Kukkuti*, *Markati*, *S'imbi* and *Anantá* as a charm. 2B.

Offerings of meat, cooked or uncooked, and of blood should be made (to Andhaputaná) at the crossing of roads or inside a house for the preservation of the

* Some explain "केशान्" (hair) and चर्म (skin) as those of man and not of a cock.

† Bhávaprakás'a reads "जीर्णश्चाभीक्ष्णशो वासः" *i. e.*, very old cloth. This reading does not suggest that the cloth to be used should have been worn by a Buddhist monk.

child, which (with its nurse) should also be bathed with the decoction of the holy drugs of the *Sarva-gandha* group. The **Mantra** runs as follows :—"May the dreadful, brown-coloured, bald-headed, goddess Andha-putaná, wearing a red-coloured garment be pleased to save this child." 2.

Thus ends the thirty-third chapter in the Uttara-Tantra of the Sus'ruta Samhitá which deals with the medical treatment of (an attack) by Andha-putaná.

CHAPTER XXXIV.

Now we shall discourse on the medical treatment of (an attack by) Śita-putaná **(Śita-putaná-Pratishedha).** 1.

The decoction of *Kapittha*, *Suvahá* (Rásná), *Vimbi*, *Vilva*, *Prachivala* (?), *Nandi* (Vata) and *Bhallátaki* should be used in **sprinkling** (the child's body). The urine of a cow and of a she-goat, as well as *Musta*, *Deva-dáru*, *Kushtha* and the drugs of the *Sarva-gandha* (Eládi) group should be used in duly preparing a medicated oil (for the purpose) and medicated Ghrita should be duly cooked with (three parts of) the decoction of *Rohini*, *Sarjarasa* (resin), *Khadira*, *Palásá* and barks of *Arjuna* and (one part of) milk. 2 A.

Dungs of an owl and a vulture, the cast-off skin of a snake as well as *Ajagandhá* and *Nimba* leaves and *Yashthi-madhu* should be used for **fumigating** purposes, and *Lambá* (Tiktálávu), *Gunjá* and *Kákádani* should be be worn (as a charm) by the child. 2B.

The goddess Śitaputaná should be worshipped with the offerings of the preparation of rice and *Mudga* pulse (cooked together) as well as with *Váruni* wine and blood, and the child should be bathed near a river or a tank. The **Mantra** is as follows :—"May the goddess Śita-putaná, who is fond of the preparation of rice and *Mudga* pulse, who delights in drinking wine and blood and who resides by the side of a river or a tank, preserve thee." 2.

Thus ends the thirty-fourth chapter in the Uttara-Tantra of the Sus'ruta Samhitá which deals with the medical treatment of (an attack by) S'itaputaná.

CHAPTER XXXV.

Now we shall discourse on the chapter which deals with the medical treatment of (an attack by) Mukha-mandiká (**Mukha-mandiká-Pratishedha**). 1

The decoction of *Kapittha*, *Vilva*, *Tarkári* (Jayanti), *Vams'a-lochana* (D.R. Vásá), *Gandharva-hastaká* (Eranda) and *Kuverákshi* (Pátalá) should be used in **sprinkling** (the body of the possessed child). Oil and fat (in equal parts) should be duly cooked with the expressed juice of the *Bhringarája*, *Ajagandhá* and *Harigandhá* (As'wa-gandhá) and be used in **anointing** the child's body. Medicated Ghrita should be duly cooked with *Madhuliká* (Murvá), *Tugá-kshiri* and the drugs of the *Madhura* and the minor *Pancha-mula* groups and with milk. 2. A.

Fumigation with *Vachá*, *Sarjarasa* and *Kushtha* mixed with clarified butter would be found beneficial and the child should be made to wear the tongue of a *Chása* bird, a *Chiralli* bird or a snake (as a charm). 2. B.

Offerings of *Varnaka* (Kampillaka), *Churnaka*, garlands of flowers, *Rasánjana*, *Párada* (mercury), *Manah-S'ilá*, *Páyasa* (rice boiled in milk) and puddings should be made (to the deity) inside a cow-shed and the child should also be bathed therein with water consecrated with Mantra. The **Mantra** runs as follows :—"May the beautiful and blessed goddess, Mukhamandiká, who is decked with ornaments, who can assume different forms at will and who resides in cow-sheds, preserve thee".

Thus ends the thirty-fifth Chapter of the Uttara-Tantra in the Sus'ruta Samhitá which deals with the medical treatment of (an attack by) Mukhamandiká.

CHAPTER XXXVI.

Now we shall discourse on the chapter which deals with the medical treatment of (an attack by) Naigamesha (**Naigamesha-Pratishedha**). 1.

The decoction of *Vilva*, *Agnimantha* and *Putiká* should be used in **sprinkling** (the body of the possessed child) and sprinkling with *Surá*, *Sauvira* and *Dhánydmla* (Kánjika) is also advisable in such cases. A medicated oil should be duly cooked with *Priyangu*, *Saralá*, *Anantá*, *S'ata-pushpá* and *Kutannata* and with cow's urine, the liquid of the milk-curd (Dadhi-mastu) and *Kánjika*. Medicated Ghritas should be duly prepared with the drugs of the *Madhura* group as Kalka, with the decoction of the *Dasámula* and with milk or with the head of a date-palm tree 2. A.

The child should be made to wear *Vachá*, *Vayasthá*, *Golomi* and *Jatilá* as a charm and the **utsádana** measures recommended in the treatment of Skandápasmára should be used in this case also. *Siddhárthaka* (white mustard), *Vachá*, *Hingu*, *Kushtha*, parched rice, *Bhallátaka* and *Ajamodá* should be used in **fumigating** the body of the child. In cases of attacks by Navagraha the dungs of a monkey, an owl and a vulture should also be used by persons wishing the good of the child for a fumigating purpose and that at the dead of the night when all persons are asleep. 2. B.

Offerings of huskless sesamum, garlands of flowers and various dishes should be made to the deity Naigamesha (the preserver of the child) at the foot of a *Vata* tree on the sixth day of the fortnight and the child should be bathed there at the foot of the tree.

The **Mantra** runs as follows :—"May the far-famed god, Naigamesha, the preserver of children, who has a goat's face with moving brow and rolling eyes and who can assume different forms at will, preserve the child." 2.

Thus ends the thirty-sixth chapter of the Uttara-Tantra in the Sus'ruta Samhitá which deals with the medical treatment of (an attack by) Naigamesha.

CHAPTER XXXVII.

Now we shall discourse on the chapter which deals with the origin of the (nine) Grahas **(Grahotpatti-Adhyáya).** 1.

The nine presiding deities—*viz.*, Skanda and others—of the nine diseases of infant life are all possessed of ethereal frames, divine effulgence and specific sex-distinction of their own. They were created by the gods Agni, Mahádeva and the goddesses Krittiká and Umá for guarding the person of the new-born Guha though protecting himself with his own divine prowess amidst the stems of *S'ara* grass. Of these Grahas the females who are possessed of various shapes as described before are considered as originally made of the Rájasa essence of the goddesses Gangá, Umá and Krittiká. 2A.

The Naigamesha Graha who is possessed of a sheep's face was created by the goddess Párvati as the friend and protector of the young god Guha and who was as dear to him as his own self. Skandápasmára, the presiding deity of the disease named after him, was created by Agni, the fire-god (Vulcan). He is as bright as fire itself and is a constant companion of the god Skanda and is also known by the name of Vis'akha. The god Skanda, the tutelar divinity of the disease of that denomination, was begotten by His Holiness, the Almighty Destroyer of Tripura and is otherwise known by the name of Kumára (lit. a child, *viz.*, of Mahádeva). 2B.

It is impossible that the god springing from Rudra and Agni, with his exalted parentage would find pleasure in such a dangerous disease even out of childish frolicsomeness and it has also been asserted by eminent authorities on the physical science that some unintelligent persons have been misled into holding, through a mistake due to the identity of the names, that the author of the disease under discussion (Skanda) is no other than the invincible Skanda. 2.

On the effulgent god Skanda's being elevated to the leadership of the armies of Heaven, the presiding deities of those diseases waited upon him and with folded palms asked him about the means of their subsistence. The god Skanda in his turn, referred them to His Holiness the god Śiva for the answer, whereupon they went to the latter in a body and made the same query. Mahádeva, the Destroyer of Bhaga's eyes, replied "Gods, men and other animals, O, ye Grahas, exist on the principle of reciprocal benefit*. The gods minister to the wants of men and beasts, etc., by marshalling different seasons of the year and by setting the air in motion and sending down the rain, and men, in their turn, propitiate the gods by duly and reverentially performing the sacrificial rites, by saying their prayers with blended palms, by bowing down in reverence, and by repetition of prayers, religious vows and other religious observances. All services and their emoluments in consequence have been filled up and settled and there remains nothing for you to fill. Your proper means of subsistence will, therefore, be in the life of an infant (though the emoluments you shall receive shall be stained with the tears of many an anxious, watchful and night-worn parent). 3A.

* Exchange or reciprocity of services underlies the foundation of all distinct and cognitive existences, whether beasts, men or gods. The worlds are linked to one another by bonds of service. Give-and-take is the law of the universe. Duty implies obligation.

Children of the families in which the gods, the Pitris (departed fathers), the Brahmans, the pious, the preceptors and the seniors and the guests are not properly worshipped and attended upon and wherein the rules of cleanliness and virtues are not observed and the members of which do not make daily offerings to the gods and give alms to beggars and live on food prepared by others and eat from broken bowls and plates of Indian bell-metal would be the proper persons whom you might strike with impunity, and by your malign influence lay them up with diseases peculiar to infant life. (It shall be your duty to see that iniquities of the parents are visited on their children. Attack them without least compunction of heart and ample means of subsistence will be thereby secured to you). There the parents of those children will worship you in their calamities and you shall get plenty to live upon." 3B.

Thus the Grahas came into being and began to attack the children (of iniquitious parents), and it is therefore that a child attacked by a malignant Graha becomes very hard to be cured. Death or permanent disfigurement of any limb or organ is sure to ensue from an attack of Skanda Graha, since he is the most dreadful of all the Grahas. A case of full-developed attack by any other Graha should be likewise held as incurable. 3.

Thus ends the thirty-seventh chapter of the Uttara Tantra in the Sus'ruta Samhitá which deals with the origin of the Grahas.

CHAPTER XXXVIII.

Now we shall discourse on the chapter which deals with (the symptoms and) the therapeutics of the diseases of the female* organ of generation **(Yoni-vyápat-Pratishedha).** 1.

Causes :—The bodily (as well as the local) Váyu of a girl of tender years, weakly constitution or build and dry organic temperament, is deranged and aggravated in consequence of her excessive indulgence with a man of abnormally developed reproductive organ, and on getting into her organ of generation (yoni) gives rise to different local vaginal diseases which become manifest through the presence of the symptoms of the aggravation of the three specific Doshas. 2.

In the chapter on the enumeration of diseases, the diseases which affect the female organ of generation (yoni) have been classified into twenty different kinds†. The injudicious conduct of life which is usually found in females, menstrual disorders, the diseased or defective nature of the seed (of the parents of the girl), or any accidental cause may be fairly set down as causes of these female diseases. Now hear them discussed separately. 3.

Enumeration and Classification :—Udávartá (dysmenorrhœa), Bandhyá (sterility), Viplutá (introversion of the uterus), Pariplutá (retroversion or retroflexion of the uterus) and Vátalá are the five kinds

* The term **"yoni"** is here used in a very comprehensive sense and means the whole female organ of generation, *i. e.*, Uterus, Vagina, etc.

† These three lines correspond *verbatim* with three lines in the Charaka Samhitá (vide Charaka Samhitá, Chapter XXX, Chikitsita-sthána).

of **Vátaja** vaginal diseases. Rudhirakshará (menorrhœa), Vâmini, Sramsini, Puttraghni and Pittalá are the **Pittaja** ones. Atyánandá (nymphomania), Karnini, the two kinds of Charaná and Ślaishmiki find their origin in **Kapha**, and Shandi, Phalini, Mahati, Suchivaktrá and Sarvajá are said to be due to the aggravation of the **three Doshas**. 4.

Symptoms of the Vátaja types :—An **Udávartá** yoni discharges painful and frothy menses and a **Bandhyá** yoni is marked by the absence or suppression of the catamenial flow. A local pain is always complained of in a **Viplutá** yoni and in a **Pariplutá** yoni an excessive local pain is experienced at the time of sexual congress. A **Vátalá** yoni is marked by an aching and piercing pain in the organ which seems rough and numbed. The peculiar pain due to the derangement of the Váyu is also felt in the first four types of the series. 5.

Symptoms of the Pittaja types :—Discharge of the menses with a burning sensation in the passage is the characteristic symptom of **Lohitakshará** or **Rudhira-kashrá** yoni. The yoni from which the semen charged with the menstrual blood, is ejected with Váyu (sound) is called **Vámini** ; the coming out (prolapsus) of the organ (uterus) when disturbed and a difficult or painful parturition are the symptoms of a **Prasramsini** yoni. The yoni in the case of repeated abortions due to the excessive discharge of catamenial blood during the period of gestation is called **Puttraghni**. An extremely burning sensation and suppuration in the organ attended with fever are the symptoms which mark a **Pittalá** yoni. The four previous vaginal diseases are also marked by the specific symptoms of the aggravated Pitta. 6.

Symptoms of the Kaphaja types :—An **Atyánandá** yoni knows no satisfaction in matters of sexual pleasures. Hæmorrhoid growths or polypii due to the aggravation of Kapha and vitiated blood appear on the living membrane of the organ in a **Karnini** yoni. In an **Acharaná** yoni a greater quantity of ovum is secreted before the completion of sexual act, and in the other *i. e.*, in an **Aticharaná** yoni the semen is not retained in consequence of over-indulgence. A **Śleshmalá** yoni is very cold and slimy and has a local itching sensation. The first four kinds of this series of vaginal disease (lit. diseased vagina) are also characterised by the actions of the deranged and aggravated Kapha in the locality. 7.

Symptoms of the Tri-doshaja types :—The yoni of a woman marked by the non-appearance of the menses, non-development of her breasts and the roughness of the vagina (vaginal canal) which is felt at the time of coition is called a **Shandhi**. A woman of tender years, who has just passed her girlhood, when ravished by a man with an abnormally developed genital organ, offers the illustration of a **Phalini** yoni. An extremely dilated vagina is called **Maháyoni**, while an extremely constricted one is called a **Suchivaktrá** (lit. a vagina with a needle-eyed vulva). The yoni marked with the symptoms of the aggravation of all the three Doshas is said to be a **Sarvajá** yoni. The four preceding kinds of vaginal malformations or diseases are also due to the concerted action of the three deranged Doshas in the locality and these last (five) kinds of Tridoshaja vaginal diseases are incurable. 8.

Medical Treatment :—The medical treatment of the curable types of vaginal diseases should begin with the administration of a **Sneha** according to the Dosha involved in each case and applications of properly charged vaginal enemas (Uttara-vasti) should be particularly resorted to. In cases where the yoni (vagina) would feel cold, rough, numbed and be marked by diminished sensibility of its mucous membrane during sexual action it should be fomented, in the manner of Kumbhi-sveda, with the flesh of aquatic and A'nupa animals ; and drugs of the *Madhura* group mixed with Ves'avára (all described before) should be applied (in the form of poultice) to the part, and plugs of oil-soaked cotton should be constantly retained in the yoni (vagina). Proper vaginal lotions and washes as well as the measures of Purana *i e.* medical injection (prepared with the Váyu-subduing drugs) should also be employed ; cooling measures should be adopted in the cases marked by dryness and sucking pain (Osha and Chosa) in the affected locality. The vagina should be filled up with the powders of the five officinal kinds of drug (*Pancha-kasháya*) in a case, marked by fetour and slimy mucous secretion, and the decoction of the drugs of Rájavrikshádi group should be used in washing. Pindas (balls) of disinfectant (S'odhona, lit. purifying) drugs pasted with cow's urine and saturated with salt, should be inserted into the vagina marked by the discharge of pus. 9—12.

A yoni (vagina) marked by an itch and impaired sensibility should be fumigated with the vapour of *Vrihati* and the two kinds of *Haridrá* taken together, which should be as well inserted and retained in the vagina (in the shape of a plug). A plug or stick composed of a paste of disinfectant (or S'odhana) drugs should be inserted into and retained in a **Karnini** yoni ; and a prolapsing (Prasramsini) yoni should be fomented with hot milk and rubbed with clarified butter. It should then be restored to its proper place and, being pasted with Ves'avára, should be duly bandaged 13—14.

Diet.—**Surá, Ásava, Arishta,** (wines of medicinal drugs) should be prescribed according to the Dosha involved in each case and the patient should be made to take the expressed juice of garlic (*Lashuna*) every morning and her diet should consist mainly of milk, meat-soup, etc. 15.

We have already described the nature of the medical treatment and the remedial agents to be respectively pursued in and prescribed for diseases of the semen, menstrual complaints, affections of the mammae, impotency, cases of false presentation of child and diseases during the period of pregnancy and motherhood, and all those may be employed with equal benefit in these diseases peculiar to the female sex. Other diseases (such as fever etc.) which may arise from immature delivery should be treated in the manner described in the respective treatment of those diseases in the Uttara Tantra. 16.

Thus ends the thirty-eighth chapter of the Uttara Tantra in the Sus'ruta Samhitá which deals with the therapeutics of the female organ o generation.

Here ends the Kaumárabhritya Tantra.

CHAPTER XXXIX.

Now we shall discourse on the (symptoms and) medical treatment of Fever (**Jwara-Pratishedha**). 1.

The Divine Dhanvantari, who in his first incarnation arose out of the primordial Ocean with a pitcher of ambrosia on his head, (when it was churned by the gods and the demons) and who conferred immortality on Indra and his brother celestials, was thus interrogated by his disciples, Suśruta and others "You have instructed us, O, you, the foremost of physicians, the subject on all the concomitant distressing symptoms (Upadrava) of **Ulcer** (Vrana). Now let us have a general outline and detailed description of the concomitant distressing symptoms, physiological and pathological conditions *e. g.* fever, dysentery, cough, etc. showing in an ulcer-patient. An ulcer attended with many a concomitant symptom (Upadrava) may be cured only with the greatest difficulty and such concomitant symptoms appearing in an emaciated and weak ulcer-patient, take time to be subdued because of the loss of his Doshas and Dhátus. Hence illumine us fully, O sir, on those diseases affecting the whole body (and not localised in any particular limb or organ) observed by the holy sages of yore, and instruct us the nature and application of the therapeutic agents to be employed in their cure". 2.

Description of Jwara:—To the query of the disciples, the divine physician, Dhanvantari replied as follows:—"First I shall discourse on the nature and origin of fever for it is the king of all bodily distempers in as much as it affects the whole orgainsm at a time. It was begotten by the fire of wrath of Rudra, and afflicted the whole animal world or organic kingdom. The different names by which it is designated amongst the different kinds of animals are well known. Its presence is perhaps an indispensable condition under which a creature can come into being or can depart from this life, and hence it is called the lord of ailments and none but a god or man can bear the heat of fever. Men may become gods by virtue of their good deeds (Karma) in life and would again revert to humanity (mortality) at the close of their blissful effects, and it is this divine or godly element in man that enables him to bear this abnormal heat of fever whereas the lower animals are simply lost under its influence. 3.

Definition and Classification of Fever:—The disease which is marked by the arrest of the flow of perspiration, by increased heat (of the skin), by pain all over the body and by a sense of numbness in the limbs, is called **Jwara** (fever). Cases of fever of which the causes are numerous, are divided into eight types according as they are brought on through the derangement of the three bodily Doshas separately, or through that of any two of them in combination or through their cencerted action, or by any extraneous causes.* 4-5.

When the Doshas of the body are deranged by their respective aggravating causes and in the hours of their specific dominance† they bring on an attack of fever by

* There can be three cases of fever due to the derangement of the three Doshas separately, three cases from the derangement of two of them at a time and one case only from the concerted action of the three Doshas These are the seven cases while that due to an extraneous cause is the eighth.

† Kapha is aggravated in the morning, Pitta, at noon and Váyu, in the evening. Fever follows a distinct periodicity determined by the

spreading through the whole organism. The deranged bodily Doshas augmented or enraged by their specific aggravating causes, enter into the Ámás'aya, and soon find lodgment in the Rasa (lymph-chyle) by virtue of their inherent heat (Ushman). The Doshas thus deranged and mixed with Rasa obstruct the Rasa-carrying and sweat-carrying ducts, impair the digestive fire and expelthe inherent heat (Ushman) out of its seat in the Pakvás'aya, and spreading all over the body during the period of their specific dominance, bring on fever and causes its rise and exhibit their specific colour on the skin, etc. (of the patient). 6—7.

Pathology :—The improper and excessive application of Sneha, etc., any kind of blow, the presence of any other affection in the organism, suppuration (of an existing boil or ulcer in the body), over-fatigue, any process of physical waste, indigestion, introduction of any extraneous poison or poisonous matter into the system, infringement of any habitual rule of diet and conduct, the sudden change or contrariety of seasons, the smelling of any kind of poisonous herb or flower, grief, the malignant influences of inaus picious stars or planets (at the time of birth), dynamics

time of aggravation of the deranged bodily Doshas ushering in the attack An attack of fever due to the deranged Kapha comes on in the morning or after dusk ; one due to the deranged Pitta comes on at noon or mid-night, one due to the deranged Váyu comes on in the afternoon or during the small hours of the night. In a case of Dvi-doshaja fever (due to the combined action of the two deranged bodily Doshas) the heat is aggravated during the specific hours of domination of the stronger Dosha and continues through those peculiar to each of them. All night attacks should be regarded as connected with the action of the deranged Pitta. In a Tri-doshaja case, the heat comes on with the specific hour of the strongest one and is abated on the approach of the time peculiar to the weakest. Váyu is aggravated in the Varshá (rainy) season, Pitta, in the S'arat (autumn) and Kapha, in the Vasanta (spring).

of deadly incantations or charms, curses (from Bráhmanas and superiors), any fancied dread or anxiety, effects of miscarriage or untimely parturition, injudicious conduct of life on the part of a woman after delivery, and the first accumulation of the milk in the breast (after delivery) are the causes which lead to an attack of fever, the derangement and aggravation of the fundamental vital principles (Doshas) of the body being the existing origins of the disease. The stomachic heat is propelled by the extremely deranged and aggravated Doshas of the body, and, coursing through the wrong channels in the orgainsm, tends to escape through the surface (the skin of the body) and, by incarcerating the vitiated Rasa Dhátu generally causes a rise in the bodily temperature and puts a stop to perspiration. 8—9.

Premonitory Symptoms :—A sense of fatigue or physical languor, aversion to all sorts of work, paleness of complexion, bad taste in the mouth, tearfulness of the eyes, alternate liking and dislike for heat, cold and air, constant yawning, aching of the limbs, a sense of heaviness of the body, horripilation, disrelish for food, darkness of vision, depression and a feeling of creeping cold in the body are the general **premonitory symptoms** which usher in an attack of fever Constant yawning, burning of the eyes and aversion to food are the special premonitory symptoms of the derangement of Váyu, Pitta and Kapha respectively. The derangement of all the three Doshas is marked by the presence of all the symptoms, while, in the derangement of any two of these, the special symptoms of those two Doshas appear. 10.

Symptoms of Vátaja fever :—Shivering,

irregular fits of fever, dryness of the throat, lips and of the mouth, loss of sleep, stoppage of sneezing, parchedness of the skin, pain in the head, chest and limbs, distaste in the mouth, suppression (D. R.—hardness) of stool and aching pain (in the abdomen) are the characteristics of a case of fever due to the action of the deranged **Váyu** of the body.. 11.

Symptoms of Pittaja fever :—High fever (hyperpyrexia), diarrhœa, scanty but disturbed sleep, vomiting, inflamation in the throat, lips, mouth and nostrils, perspiration, delirious talks, swoon or fainting fits, burning sensation in the body, loss of consciousness, pungent taste in the mouth, yellowness of the stool, urine and of the eyes and vertigo are the symptoms which mark the **Pittaja** type of fever. 12.

Symptoms of the Kaphaja fever :—Heaviness of the limbs, shivering, nausea, appearance of goose-flesh, excessive sleep, obstruction of the internal passages of the body, slight pain (in the limbs), water-brash, sweet taste in the mouth, slight heat in the body, vomiting, lassitude, mal-assimilation (Avipákatá), whiteness (glossinss) of the eyes are the indications which point to the **Kaphaja** origin of the disease. 13.

Symptoms of the Tri-doshaja fever :—Insomnia, vertigo, laboured or difficult breathing, drowsiness (somnolence), a sense of innertness in the limbs, aversion to food, thirst, swoon, delirium, numbness, burning sensation and shivering of the body, pain about the region of the heart, delayed assimilation of the deranged bodily Doshas, (temporary) insanity, blackish yellow coat on the teeth, blackness and roughness of the tongue, pain in the head, in the joints and in the bone, dilation of the pupil and cloudiness of the eyes, pain and ringing in the ears, delirious talks, inflamation of the living membranes of the channels (of the nose and of the mouth), indistinct sound in the mouth, coma (loss of consciousness) as well as perspiration, scanty emission of urine and fæcal matter at long intervals, are the symptoms which are exhibited in a case of fever due to the concerted action of all the three deranged Doshas of the body (**Tri-doshaja** or **Sannipátaja**) 14.

Abhinyása fever :—Now hear from me about the peculiar forms of this type of fever the symptoms whereof are as follows :—Where a slight or imperceptible rise of the bodily heat, or a slightly subnormal temperature attended with a subcomatose state, erroneous vision, loss of voice, injured or cracked condition of the tongue, dryness of the throat, suppression of stool, perspiration and urine, tearful eyes, hardness of the thorax *, aversion to food, dulness of complexion, difficult breathing and delirious talks and other concomitant symptoms are the specific indications in a patient always confined to his bed, it is known by the name of **Abhinyása**, while others call it a case of **Hataujasa** fever. 15.

An attack of Sannipátaja fever can be cured only with the greatest difficulty, while others hold it to be almost incurable. A case of Sannipátaja fever attended with somnolence is called **Abhinyása**, it is called **Hataujasa** when the vitality of the patient is greatly diminished and it is called **Sannyása** when there is an innertness of the limbs. 16

* "साश्रुनिर्भुग्ननयन:" is a different reading in place of 'सास्रो निर्भुग्नहृदय:"। The term निर्भुग्न is more appropriately applicable to नयन than to हृदय both grammatically and in sense.

When (in a case of Sannipátaja fever), the Ojo-dhátu (one of the fundamental principles) of the organism being disturbed or agitated by the deranged and aggravated Pitta and Váyu, gives rise to shivering and numbness of limbs and makes the patient drop into fits of unconsciousness whether asleep or awake, and when there are somnolence, delirious talks, horripilation, looseness of the limbs and slight pain (in the body)—this kind of fever is called **Ojo-nirodhaja** fever (due to an obstruction or an overwhelmed condition of the Ojo-dhátu) by the experts. 17.

The disease, (in such cases) finds aggravation on the seventh, the tenth or on the twelfth day * when the case takes either a favourable turn or ends in death. 18.

Symptoms of Dwandvaja fever :— A case of fever which involves, and is due to the combined action of any two deranged Doshas of the body, is called **Dwandvaja** fever and such cases are classified into three different types (*e. g.* Vâta-pitta-fever, Vâta-s'leshma-fever and Pitta-s'leshma-fever). Yawning, distension of the abdomen, loss of consciousness, shivering pain in the joints, emaciation of the body, thirst, delirium and heat or increased temperature of the skin, are the characteristic symptoms of **Váta-pitta fever** (due to the action of the deranged Pitta and Váyu). Aching pain (S'ula), cough, the vomiting of Kapha, shivering, coryza, cold, sense of heaviness of the limbs, aversion to food, and a feeling of general numbness, are the

* The fever in which Váyu predominates gets aggravated on the 7th, that in which Pitta predominates becomes aggravated on the 10th and that in which Kapha predominates comes to be aggravated on the 12th day. According to some authority, however, Abhinyása, Hataujasa, and Sannyása types of fever are pacified on the 7th, 10th and 12th. day respectively.—*Dallana*,

symptoms of a case of **Váta-śleshma-fever** (due to the action of the deranged Váyu and Kapha). Sensation of cold and heat, aversion to food, numbness, perspiration, epileptic fits, unconsciousness, vertigo, cough, lassitude and nausea are the symptoms which characterise a case of **Pitta-śleshma-fever** (due to the action of the deranged Pitta and Kapha)* . 19—21.

Even a small residue of the deranged bodily Doshas in a patient just cured of an attack of fever but still sufferring from weakness and indulging in injudicious regimen of diet and rule of conduct, is apt to be augmented and aggravated by the deranged Váyu of the body, and thus begets five different types of fever lodged in any of the five specific locations of Kapha †. These five types are known as the Satata, Anyedyushka, Tritiyaka, Chaturthaka and the Pralepaka ‡. The (residue of the) deranged Dosha of the body, shifting from one location of Kapha to the next in the course of the entire day

* Dallana in his commentary has quoted in eight lines with different wordings the symptoms of these kinds of **Dwandvaja** fever and these lines have been adopted by Mádhava in his Nidána The lines when translated would be thus :—Thirst, unconsciousness, vertigo, burning sensation, somnolence, pain in the head, dryness of the mouth and of the throat, vomiting, horripilation, disrelish for food, giddiness, pain in the joints, and yawning are the symptoms of **Váta-pitta-fever**. Sensation of moisture (स्तिमित) all over the body, pain in the joints, excessive sleep, heaviness of the limbs, pain in the head, catarrh, cough, scanty perspiration, slight sensation of heat, and pulsation not too quick nor too slow, are the symptoms of **Váta-śleshma-fever**. A bitter taste, a coating on the mouth, somnolence, unconsciousness, cough, disrelish for food, thirst, alternate and varying sensation of heat and cold are the symptoms of **Śleshma-pitta-fever**.

† The five locations of Kapha are the Ámás'aya, chest, throat, head and the joints.

‡ There is another kind of Vishama Jwara named Santata (cf. S'loka 31 of this Chapter) and Dallana remarks that it is begotten when the residue of the deranged Dosha is lodged in all the five seats of Kapha.

and night, ultimately finds lodgment in the Ámáśaya (stomach) and thus brings on the virulent attack of (those) fevers. Of these the type known as the **Pralepaka** appears in cases of Śosha (consumption) and though its attak is a mild one, it puts almost insurmountable difficulties in the way of its cure, brings about a loss or waste of Dhátus (the seven fundamental principles of the organism) and thus ultimately ends in death. There are cases of Vishama-jwara known as the **Viparyyaya** type (reverse of the above type) which are the result of the deranged bodily Doshas being simultaneously located in two or four specific seats of the deranged bodily Kapha and are hard to cure. 22—23.

Several authorities hold Vishama Jvara to be *sui-generis* in its origin. But whether spontaneously idiopathic or not, an extraneous fact (either a passing psychic condition such as fear, grief, etc. or the presence of any foreign poisonous matter in the system) is always involved in and intimately connected with a case of Vishama fever. The pre-dominance of the deranged and aggravated Váyu is marked in cases of **Tritiyaka** (tertian) and **Chaturthaka** (quartan coming on every fourth day) fevers. A case of fever due to the abuse of any wine or ardent spirits as well as the one occuring in a low land at the foot of a mountain, should be supposed to involve a predominant action of the deranged and aggravated Pitta. A case of **Pralepaka** fever is due to the concerted action of the deranged and aggravated Váyu and Kapha, of which the action of the latter should be regarded as more dominant. Cases of Vishama fever ushered in by epileptic fits should be regarded as the result of the concerted action of any two deranged Doshas of the body. 24—25.

The deranged Kapha and Váyu of the body, if located under the surface of the skin, produce cold (shivering) during the first stage of fever, while the deranged Pitta brings on the characterstic burning sensation at its latter stage after the subsidence of the deranged Kapha and Váyu. In certain cases the burning sensatlon is engendered by the deranged Pitta at the outset, cold (shivering) being brought on by the deranged Kapha and Váyu at the latter stage after the subsidence of the deranged Pitta. Both these two types of fever are brought on through the combined action of two deranged Doshas of the body and of these two, the type which is ushered in by a burning sensation in the body is extremely hard to cure. A case of continued fever resulting from an abnormal psychic condition (such as anger, grief, desire, etc.) or due to any blow or hurt is likewise hard to cure. 26—28.

Fever of the Vishama type attacks a man in various ways and follows a distinct periodicity, it being aggravated during the six specific times of dominance of the deranged bodily principles (Doshas) as mentioned before * in the course of day and night. This Vishama fever never finds complete remission, (but lurks in the deeper organic principles of the body) and produces a sense of physical langour and heaviness of the limbs as well as the characteristic emaciation. It is called Vishama-jwara because its abatement is always confounded with its cure and remission, and this confounding is due to the fact that the disease (fever) lies dormant in a very small degree in the deeper principles of the vital organism to be patent only at the slightest exciting cause, just as a feeble fire fed with an insufficient supply of fuel, becomes patent at the slightest exciting cause. 29.

* See chapter XXI.—Sutra-sthána.

Seat of Vishama Jwara :—Even a small residue of the deranged bodily Dosha, lurking in the system after the apparent cure of fever, is aggravated by a course of injudicious conduct and indifference to strict regimen of diet, and thus invites a fresh attack * which is known as the **Vishama Jwara**. A case of **Santata** (remittent or continuous) fever has its seat in the vitiated Rasa (serum) and blood † of the organism ; while a case of **Anyedyuh** finds location in the contaminated flesh of the body. The type known as the **Tri-tiyaka** (tertian-fever coming on every third day) affects the principle of Meda (fat), while the one called **Cháturthaka** (quartan-fever coming on every fourth day) affects and is infiltrated into bones and marrow. The last named type is very dangerous. It brings on a simultaneous attack of several other diseases and often terminates fatally. Several authorities include cases of fever due to the malignant influence of evil spirits within the category of Vishama Jwara. 30.

Duration of Vishama Jwara :—The type of fever which continues for seven, ten or twelve days without any break or remission, is called **Santata**. A case of **Satataka** fever is characterised by two distinct aggravations in the course of day and night. Fever of the **Anyedyushka** type comes on only once a day and one of the **Tri-tiyaka** type comes on every third *i. e.* on every alternate day, while a case of **Cháturthaka** fever sets in every fourth day. 31.

* A case of fever may lapse into a Vishama type even from the very commencement of the attack.

† Vijaya Rakshita, the commentator on Mádhava Nidána, says, on the authority of Charak, that by the term **Santata** are meant here both Santata and Satataka and that they have their origin in the vitiated Rasa and blood respectively.

Influence of Váyu on Vishama Jwara :—Just as the ocean is overflown when its water is swollen up by the gusts of wind (Váyu), so the bodily Doshas are aggravated by the bodily Váyu, and give rise to different kinds of fever. Just as the water of the occean floods the shore at flow-tide and rolls back to its former place during ebb-tide, so fever being augmented by the deranged Doshas of the body, rushes out of its lurking place in the organism and manifests itself (or comes to the surface of the skin) during the hours of the specific aggravation of the Doshas, only to be driven back into the deeper tissues and vital principles of the body during the period of their specific abatement, or to be expelled from the organisim at the completion of their perfect assimilation in or elimination from the system. 32.

Ágantuka Jwara :—A case of fever due to any extraneous blow or injury should be treated in the light of its periodicity and aggravation or in other words the nature of the deranged bodily Doshas under-lying, or involved in such a case should be ascertained from the periodicity of its aggravation. A case of fever due to the effects of **poison** is marked by such symptoms, as blackness of the face, burning sensation, diarrhœa, catching pain in the region of the heart, aversion to food, thirst, piercing pain in the limbs, epileptic fits and extreme weakness. A case of fever caused by smelling the pollens of any kind of (strong smelling) herbs (as **Hay fever**) is marked by fainting fits, pain in the head and sneezing. A case of fever incidental to an un-gratified amorous longing of the heart, or due to any such ardent passion is characterised by aberration or a distracted state of the mind, drowsiness, languidness, aversion to food, pain at the cardiac region and a speedy emaciation of the body. Delirium marks a case of fever due to grief or terror and shivering characterises one due to a fit of anger. Thirst and fainting fits are the concomitants of a case of fever due to any curse, or ushured in through the dynamics of deadly incantations. Anxiety, laughter, shivering and weeping mark a case due to the malignant influence of evil genii. 33—34.

The bodily Váyu deranged and aggravated by fatigue, physical waste or by a blow spreads through the entire organism and begets **(traumatic)** fever. There is another kind of fever which is due to any extraneous cause or which results from the acute stage of any other disease attendant on the body. It exhibits all the symptoms characteristic of each of the deranged bodily Doshas involved therein * 35—36.

Gambhira fever and its prognosis :— A case of **Gambhira** fever is characterised by a feeling of internal burning sensation in the body (which is not complained of in the surface), thirst, suppression of the stool, laboured or painful breathing and cough. Paleness of the complexion, dulness of the sense-organs, emaciation of the body, depression of the mind † and presence of supervening symptoms (e. g. hard breathing, cough, etc.) in cases of both Gambhira (inward or latent) and

* "Abhichár,' means incantations or Atharvan rites by which disease, death and any other injuries are brought about.

"Abhis'ápa" means the curse pronounced by Bráhmins, preceptors, seniors and alters possesed of puissance.

† Dallana says in his commentary that some read a few additional lines after this. He, however, does not comment on those lines and further adds that Jejjata does not read them. So we, too, refrain from translating those lines.

Tikshna (high) fever are the indications which point to the hopeless nature of the case. 37—38.

A slightly, middling or excessively aggravated condition of the deranged Doshas of the body forebodes the continuace of fever for three, seven and twelve days respectively, each succeeding one being more difficult to cure than the one immediately preceding it in order of enumeration. Thus we have done with the description of (the nature, causes and symptoms of) the different types of fever. We shall now deal with the remedial measures or therapeutic agents to be employed in these cases. 39.

Treatment:—Draughts of filtered (matured but non-medicated) clarified butter should be given as soon as the premonitory symptoms would make their appearance and the patient would get relief thereby. This is applicable only in a case of the **Vátaja** type of fever while purgatives should be administered in a case of the **Pittaja** and mild emetics, in a case of the **Kaphaja** type under similar conditions. In cases of **Dwi-doshaja** and **Tri-doshaja** fevers, the foregoing measures should be adopted according to the Doshas involved in each case. In the cases in which emulsive measures (Sneha-Karma) and exhibition of purgatives and emetics are forbidden, such measures should be employed as would tend to lighten the system such as fasting, (Langhana) etc. 40.

Fasting:—The premonitory and the actual stages of fever are of various forms like those of fire and its fume. **Fasting** is pre-eminently the best remedy as soon as the characteristic symptoms of the disease make their appearance distinctly and **vomiting** is most efficacious in a case marked by the presence of the deranged bodily Dosha in the Ámásaya (stomach) and attended with nausea, thirst, water-brash.

Fasting should be continued as long as the least quantity of the deranged Dosha or Doshas would remain intact in the organism, and light food should then be given with discretion after the Doshas have been fully assimilated in (to) the sysmtem. 41.

Prohibition of Fasting :—Fasting is prohibited in a case of fever due to a wasting process in the body or incidental to the action of the deranged bodily Váyu or appearing in consequence of any serious state of the mind (e. g. lust, anger, grief, etc,) as well as in cases in which fasting has been forbidden as in the chapter on Divi-vrana (Chapter I, 25—Chikitsá-sthána). 42.

Effect of Fasting :—Fasting in the case of a patient in whom the bodily Doshas have been deranged and of whom the digestive fire has become dull, lead to an assimilation of the deranged Doshas and kindles the digestive fire, produces remission of fever, lightness of the body and relish for food. 43.

Satisfactory and excessive fasting :—Easy and natural passing of Váyu and stool and urine, intolerable keenness of thirst and appetite, lightness of the body, sprightly, action of the mind and the sense-organs and a weakness of the body are the results which spring from **Satifactory** fasting ; while such symptoms as loss of strength, thirst, dryness (of the mouth), insomnia, vertigo, doziness, fatigue and such other supervening symptoms (as difficult breathing, cough, fever, hic-cup) mark an **excessive** fasting. 44—45.

Tepid water :—**Tepid** (boiled) water is appetising and it tends to disintegrate the accumulation of Kapha and restores the deranged bodily Pitta and

Váyu to their normal condition. The use of tepid water which allays thirst is highly efficacious in cases of fever due to the actions of the deranged bodily Kapha and Váyu, as it tends to cleanse the internal passages of the body and helps in the easy movement of the deranged bodily Doshas in the organism. The effect of **cold water** is just the reverse and its inherent cold tends to aggravate fever. 46

Peyá :—A potion consisting of water boiled with the admixture of the following bitter drugs viz. *Gángeya* (Musta), *Nágara*, *Us'ira*, *Párpata*, *Udichya* (Bálaka) and red sandal-wood should be given, when cooled, for drinking in a case of Pittaja fever, as well as in one due to the effect of any liquor or poison *. A **Peyá** prepared with digestive drugs should be given to the patient when hungry in as much as it is digestive, appetising, light and febrifugal. Tasteful decoctions of digestive drugs, which alleviate thirst, remove bad taste in the mouth, bring about a fresh relish for food and prove remedial for fever, should be given after the seventh day in a case of fever which, in consequence of a plethora of deranged Dosha in the system, would not abate even after the observance of fasting and the subsequent use of **Yavágu** and where the digestive power of the patient has been impaired. 47—49.

A decoction of *Pancha-mula* assimilates the bodily Dosha in a case of Vátaja fever, while a decoction of *Musta*, *Katuka* and *Indra-yava* mixed with honey (when cold) proves curative in a case of Pittaja fever, and a decoction of the component drugs of the *Pippalyádi* group helps the assimilation of the deranged bodily Dosha in a case of Kaphaja fever. Decoctions reme-

* According to different authorities purely boiled water, when cooled, may also be given in such cases.

dial to each of the deranged bodily Doshas should be administered in combination in a case of fever due to the concerted action of any two deranged Doshas of the body. A decoction should not be given to a patient immediately after eating, drinking or fasting, nor to a patient afflicted with thirst, extreme weakness, emaciation and indigestion. 50.

Symptoms of Pakva-Jwara :—Abatement of the bodily heat, lightness of the body and an easy passing of stool and urine are the indications from which the **assimilation** of the deranged bodily Doshas should be presumed, and it is then that febrifuges should be administered according to the nature of the deranged bodily Doshas underlying the case under treatment *. Some, however, believe that the assimilation of the deranged Doshas should be presumed from the changes in the symptoms characteristic of the Doshas. 51.

Symptoms of Áma-Jwara :—A crushing sensation in the region of the heart, drowsiness, salivation, aversion to food, non-assimilation of the deranged bodily Doshas, suppression of stool (and wind), copious discharge of urine, laziness, sense of heaviness in the abdomen, stoppage of perspiration, undigested stool, dissatisfaction, somnolence, heaviness and numbness of the limbs, dulness of appetite, bad taste in the mouth, a sense of physical languor and increased virulence and continuity of the attack of fever (abnormal rise in the bodily temperature) are the symptoms by which a learned physician should ascertain the

* Some read these two lines in a different way. They would mean that the non-assimilation (A'ma) of the deranged Doshas would be presumed by the presence of high fever, heaviness of the body and stoppage of the excreta (Mala), and the reverse is the sign of their assimilation (Páka).

undigested state of the deranged bodily Doshas ushering in an attack of fever. 52.

Time for administering Febrifuge:—According to several authorities, medicines (febrifuges) should be given in a case of fever after the seventh, or according to others after the tenth day of the attack. Febrifuges may be administered earlier in the cases of Pittaja fever, or in the event of the deranged bodily Doshas being digested earlier. An administration of (febrifugal) medicine in an undigested stage of the fever is sure to produce a recrudescence of the disease. Corrective, purifying and soothing (Śamaniya) remedies (in a case of fever with undigested Dosha) helps the lapse of the disease (fever) into a Vishama type. 53—54.

The spontaneous motions of the bowels (Mala) of a patient suffering from fever should not be stopped unless they are excessive, when the case should be medically treated as one of Atisára (Diarrhea). 55.

Preliminary Treatment:—A suitable purgative should be administered even in a case of acute fever if the digested Malas (fæcal matter etc.) are accumulated in the internal passages of the Koshtha (abdomen), in as much as their presence in the organism in that undigested state may usher in an attack of Vishama Jwara attended by distressing symptoms, or may produce loss of strength. Hence they should be eliminated from the system with the helf of emetics, etc. Emetics, Ásthápana-enemas, purgatives, Śiro-virechana and errhines should be successfully employed for the purpose. **Emetics** should be at the outset exhibited in a case of Kaphaja fever where the patient would be found to be a person of considerable physical strength, and **purgatives** should be given in a case of fever marked by the predominant action of the deranged Pitta in the event of there being laxity of the bowels (intestines). **Nirudha-vasti** should be applied in a case of Vátaja fever attended with aching pain in the limbs and with Udávarta (obstinate constipation of the bowels), whereas **Anuvásana-vasti** should be prescribed for a patient with a strong appetite, if there be pain in the regions of the back and the waist. **Śiro-virechana** (head-purgative) should be adiministered in cases marked by the accumulation of the deranged Kapha in the head, as the pain in and heaviness of the head would be relieved, and the sense-organs roused up thereby to their normal functions. 56-A.

A **plaster** composed of *Deva-dáru*, *Vacha*, *Kushtha*, *S'atáhvá*, *Hingu* and *Saindhava* pasted together with *Kánjika* should be applied lukewarm to the abdomen in a case of fever attended with painful tympanites if the patient be weak, whereas a medicated **plug** (Varti) prepared with the above drugs should be applied into the anus in a case marked by the upward coursing of the bodily Váyu attended with suppression of stool and urine, and **Yavágu** prepared with *Pippali*, roots of *Pippali*, *Yamáni* and *Chavya* should be given to the patient as a potion, it being remedial for the deranged bodily Váyu. 56.

Administration of Ghrita:—The residue of the deranged bodily Dosha having lurked in the system (of a patient) even after the exhibition of proper emetics and purgatives, the fever should be remedied by draughts of medicated clarified butter, if the system of the patient be sufficiently dry (Ruksha). 57.

A weak patient with only a small quantity of the deranged bodily Dosha should be treated with the help of soothing (Śamaniya) remedies. **Fasting** should be the principal cure for all types of fever due to (Santarpana) over-eating etc., provided the patient be found to possess sufficient strength. 58.

Diet :—Diluted barley gruel (Yavágu) should be given to a patient constantly feeling thirsty and with impaired digestion. Powdered parched corn (paddy) mixed with honey and water should be given in copious quantity to a patient suffering from the after-effect of liquor, and afflicted with vomiting, thirst, burning or perspiration and it should be followed, when duly digested, by meals of rice-soup and meat-soup. A diet consisting of boiled rice mixed with meat-soup should be given to a patient suffering from an attack of fever marked by the preponderance of the bodily Váyu, as well as in a mild type * of fever due to fasting or over-fatiguing physical labour. The diet in a case of Kaphaja fever should consist of boiled rice and of *Mudga* pulse. In a case of Pittaja fever it should consist of boiled rice and a soup of *Mudga* pulse and be taken, when cold, with the admixture of sugar. In a case marked by the concerted action of the deranged Váyu and Pitta, the diet should consist of *Mudga* soup mixed with (the expressed juice of) *Ámalaka* or *Dádima*. In a case of Váta-s'leshmá fever the diet should be prescribed to be taken with the soup of tender radish, while in one of Kapha-pitta type it should consist of the soup of the leaves of *Nimba* and *Patola*. 59—60.

Lája-tarpana—powdered parched corn (paddy) mixed with a copious quantity of water and with honey (and sugar)—should be given, instead of any other diet (e.g

* This passage is quoted by S'reekantha Datta in his commentary on Chakra-datta wherein he does not read यीषे (mild type), and his reading appears to be the better one, it being supported by Charaka as well.

boiled rice) to a patient suffering from fever marked by burning sensation, vomiting, thirst and weakness. *Yavágu* is not beneficial in summer as a diet in a case of Kapha-pittaja fever or in a case of Rakta-pitta (Hemoptysis ?) or in the case of a habitual drunkard. Such a case should be treated with the soup of any pulse or of the meat of Jángala animal with or without any acid juice. 61—62.

Prepared barley mixed with any old wine would prove beneficial in cases of (fever accompained by) a dullness of appetite. *Takra* (butter-milk or whey) mixed with the powdered *Tri-katu* should be given in case of disrelish for food due to the action of the deranged Kapha. 63-A.

Milk as a diet :—Milk may be given with advantage in a case of chronic or lingering fever marked by the scanty presence of the deranged bodily Dosha in the system, by emaciation of the frame and by mental depression as well as in a case of Váta-pittaja fever accompained by dryness of the organism and non-emission or otherwise of the deranged bodily Doshas as well as in a case of fever marked by thirst or burning sensation. But milk taken in a case of fever in its acute stage is highly injurious. 63.

A spare and light diet for a weak person should be observed in all cases of fever, when its intensity abates, as, otherwise by a heavy diet, it is aggravated. A proper and wholesome diet should be given in a case of fever even if the patient would show a positive aversion to it since the want of food at the proper time or when the system craves for it, is sure to be followed by the waste of the body, and may bring about death in the end. A food which is heavy of digestion (Guru), or secreting (Kapha-producing) in its effect should by no means be taken nor should food be taken at an improper time, since such a food which is not beneficial, is neither conducive to longevity nor to happiness (in a case of fever). 64—66.

A light diet (such as milk or essence of meat) may be given in copious quantity and with advantage to a patient emaciated through a long and protracted attack of Satataka or Vishama fever. The soup of such pulses as *Mudga*, *Masura*, *Chanaka (gram)*, *Kulattha* and *Makushtaka*, etc. may be given with benefit as diet to the hungry patient suffering from fever. 67. A

Meat-diet :—The meat of *Láva*, *Kapinjala*, *Ena*, *Prishata*, *S'arabha*, *Kála-puchchha*, *Kuranga*; *Mriga-mátriká* (different kinds of deer) or *S'as'a* (hare) may be prescribed as diet for a fever-patient accustomed to the use of animal food *. Several authorities, however, † do not recommend the use of the meat of *Sárasa*, *Krouncha*, *Mayura* (peacock), *Kukkuta* (cock) and of *Tittira* in cases of fever, owing to its heaviness (as regards digestion), as well as to its heat-making potency. (We, too, subscribe to this opinion with a certain limitation) The use of the flesh of these animals may, however, be recommended in a case of fever in moderate quantitiy and at proper time provided the fever is marked by a preponderance of the deranged bodily Váyu. 67.

Prohibitions in fever :—A fever-patient should forego baths, washing (Parisheka), plunge-bath (Avagáha. D. R. Pradeha—plaster), anointments, emulsive potions, day-sleep, physical exercise, sexual intercourse and any cold articles or any emetic or purgative

* According to Charaka, the meat-soup, in cases of fever, may be given with or without the addition of an acid juice (e.g. Dádima, A'mlaki, etc)

† Charaka also holds the same opinion as Sus'ruta.

medicine (for a time even after his recovery) till he is restored to his wonted strength and vigour. * 68.

Any of the preceding prejudicial acts done in a weak state of health, closely following a recovery from fever may bring on a relapse which invariably consumes the body just as fire does a dried and sapless tree. These rules, therefore, should be strictly followed after recovery from fever till the fundamental Principles of the body have returned to their normal condition and the health and strength is fully regained. 69.

A very small amount of physical exertion, in cases of fever, is likely to usher in an attack of fainting fit and hence the patient in such cases should be supported when he sits taking his food or passing urine or stool. An emetic or purgative (Śodhana) remedy should be resorted to even after the subsidence of fever in the case where the continuance of a residue of the deranged Doshas in the organism would be apprehended from such symptoms as aversion to food, weariness of the limbs, discoloration of the body, its evacuations, etc. A fever-patient emaciated through prolonged suffering should not be largely fed at a time (D. R. should not have a bath) and in haste *i.e.* until the patient recruits his strength in as much as it might lead to a fresh attack of the disease. 70—72.

All cases of fever should be remedied with therapeutic agents antidotal to the exciting factors. The principal pathogenic cause or causes should be first removed and remedied in a case of fever due to bodily

* **Additional text** :—A patient suffering from acute fever should forego also the use of astringent, heavy and dry food as well as fatty and secreting food. In short he should also discourage mental emotions of anger, grief, etc. as well as the use of newly collected corns. This is evidently Dallana's reading.

exhaustion, waste or hurt. An attack of (peurperal) fever incidental to miscarriage or to the spontaneous accumulation of milk in the breast of the mother after delivery, should be medically treated by an experienced physician with Dosha-subduing (Sams'amana) remedies according to the deranged bodily Dosha involved therein. Now we shall deal with the recipes of Dosha-subduing (Sams'amana) decoctions which may be advantageously employed in all types of fever. 73—74.

Sams'amana decoctions for Váta-J'wara:—A decoction duly prepared of *Pippali, Sárivá, Drákshá, S'atapushpá* and *Harenu* should be given with the admixture of treacle in a case of *Vátaja* fever or a cold infusion ‡ of *Guduchi* should be taken by the patient. Similarly a decoction of *Valá, Darbha* and *S'wa-danshtrá* boiled down to a quarter part of the original quantity of water and mixed with sugar and clarified butter ; or a decoction of *S'atapushpá, Vachá, Kushtha, Devadáru, Harenuká, Kustumburu Nalada* and *Musta* mixed with sugar and honey should be given to a patient in a case of Vátaja fever. A decoction of *Drákshá, Guduchi, Kás'marya, Tráyamáná* and *Sárivá* mixed with treacle should be prescribed in a case of Vátaja fever. A potion of the expressed juice of *Guduchi* mixed with an equal quantity of that of *S'atávari* and with treacle proves almost instantaneously efficacious in a case of fever of the same type. Rubbing of the

‡ According to Dallana the cold infusion of *Guduchi* should be given in a case of Vátaja fever involving the action of vitiated Pitta also ; whereas the decoction duly prepared of *Guduchi* should be prescribed if, in a case of Vátaja-fever, the vitiated Kapha is also involved. Cold infusion is prepared by keeping over-night a quantity of the drugs immersed in hot water. The infusion thus prepared is used in the morning.

body with clarified butter as well as fomentation (Sveda) and plaster should also be prescribed under certain conditions in the present disease. 75—81.

Samśamana decoctions for Pittaja Jwara:—A decoction of *S'riparni*, red sandal wood, *Us'ira*, *Parushaka* and *Madhuka* (Moul) flowers duly boiled and mixed with a proportionate quantity of sugar (when cold), or a decoction of the drugs of the *Sárivádi* group duly mixed with sugar, or a decoction of the drugs of the *Utpaládi* group and *Yashti-madhu*, * or a cold infusion of the drugs of the same group mixed with sugar would cure a case of **Pittaja** fever. A similar preparation of *Guduchi*, *Padmaka*, *Rodhra*, *Sárivá* and *Utpala* taken, when cold, with sugar would prove beneficial in cases of Pittaja fever. 82-84.

A decoction of *Drákshá* and *Áragvadha*, or of *Kás'marya*, or of the drugs of sweet, bitter or astringent groups mixed with sugar and used, when cold, would alleviate thirst and the severe burning sensation of the body (in a case of Pittaja fever). The contents of the stomach should be vomited out by large draughts of cold water saturated with honey whereby thirst (in a case of Pittaja fever) would be alleviated. Milk duly cooked with the decoction (of barks or twigs) of the *Kshiri-Vriksha* (milk-exuding trees), or with Chandana or with any other cooling drugs should be used cold (both internally and externally) as a relief for an internal sensation of burning in a case of Pittaja fever. 85—87.

Draughts of water with *Padmaka*, *Yashti-madhu*,

* *Yashti-madhu* is comprised in the drugs of the *Utpalàdi* group. Hence in preparation of this deeoction, two parts of *Yashti-madhu* should be taken.

Drákshá, *Paundarika* (white lily), *Utpala*, parched barley, *Us'ira*, *Samangá* and *Kás'mari* fruit steeped therein and stirred and kept overnight and then mixed and taken with honey (in the morning) would give relief from fever and burning sensation and a plaster of the same drugs should be applied over the scalp in a case of fever accompained by dryness of the tongue, the palate, the throat and of the Kloma. Pastes of the polens or filaments *(Kes'ara)* of *Mátulunga* mixed with honey and *Saindhava* salt, or of *Dádima* mixed with sugar, *Drákshá* and *Kharjura* (date) as well as gargles prepared from these drugs should be retained in the mouth with a view to removing its bad taste. 88—89.

Sams'amana decoctions for Kaphaja Jwara :—A decoction of *Saptachchhada*, *Guduchi*, *Nimba* and *Sphurjaka* mixed with honey, or of *Trikatu*, *Nága-Kes'ara*, *Haridrá*, *Katurohini* and *Indrayava*, or of *Chitraka*, *Haridrá*, *Nimba*, *Us'ira*, *Ativishá*, *Vacha*, *Kushtha*, *Indra-yava*, *Murvá* and *Patola* mixed with honey and pulverised *Maricha* (black pepper) should be given in a case of **Kaphaja** fever. A decoction of *Sárivá*, *Ativishá*, *Kushtha*, *Puru* (Guggulu), *Durálabhá* and *Musta*, or of *Musta*, *Vrikshaka-seeds* (Indra-yava), *Tri-phalá*, *Katurohini* and *Parushaka* will be found to be equally efficacious in the case of Kaphaja fever. 90—94.

Treatment of Kapha-Vátaja Jwara:—A decoction of the component members of the *Rája-vrikshádi* group mixed with honey and taken in due course, would readily prove curative in a case of fever due to the concerted action of **Váta** and **Kapha**. The exhibition of the decoction of *Nágara*, *Dhanyáka*, *Bhárgi*, *Abhayá*, *Devadáru Vachá*, *Parpataka*, *Musta*, *Bhutika*, and *Katphala* mixed with honey and *Hingu* (asafœtida) would be attended by almost instantaneous benefit in the present type of fever accompanied with bronchitis, cough, asthma, constriction of the throat, hic-cough, swelling in the throat and aching pain at the chest and at the sides. 95—96.

Pitta-S'leshmaja Jwara:—A decoction duly prepared with *Elá*, *Patola*, *Tri-phalá*, *Yashtyáhva*, and *Vrisha* (Vásaka) and mixed with honey, or one of *Katuka*, *Vijayá*, (*Haritaki*), *Drákshá*, *Musta* and *Parpataka*, or of *Bhárgi*, *Vacha*, *Parpataka*, *Dhanyáka*, *Hingu*, *Abhayá*, *Ghana*, *Nágara* and *Kás'marya* mixed with honey would prove efficacious in a case of fever due to the combined action of the deranged **Pitta** and **S'leshmá**. Similarly two Tolá-measure of powdered *Katuka* and sugar dissolved in warm water proves curative equally in a case of the present type. 97—100.

A decoction of *Bhu-nimba*, *Guduchi*, *Drákshá*, *Ámalaki* and *S'athi* mixed with treacle, or of *Rásná*, *Vrisha* (Vásaka), *Tri-phalá* and fruits of *Rája-vriksha* proves curative in a case of fever due to the combined action of the deranged **Váyu** and **Pitta** 101—102.

Drugs and therapeutic agents remedial to each of the specific deranged Doshas involved in a case of the **Tri-doshaja** type should be employed in combination for cure according to the predominance of each Dosha. A potion of milk duly boiled with *Vris'chika* (white Punarnavá), *Varshábhu* (red Punarnavá), *Vilva* and water, but from which the water has entirely evaporated would prove curative in Tri-doshaja fever. The pith and marrow of a *S'irisha* tree duly mixed with milk (weighing eight times that of the drug) and with water weighing three times that of the milk, should be boiled down to the quantity of the milk which, if administered as a drink would prove curative in Tri-doshaja fever. A potion of the decoction* duly prepared with the roots of *Nala* and of *Vetasa* (cane) and *Murvá* and *Devadáru* would prove remedial to this form of fever. † Clarified butter mixed with the decoction of *Tri-phalá* should be given to a patient suffering from an attack of Tri-doshaja fever. ‡ 103—106.

Two-Tolá-measure of powdered *Anantá* (Durálabhá), *Válaka*, *Musta*, *S'unthi* and *Katuka* should be given with (one Pala of) tepid water with benefit to a patient before sun-rise in Tridoshaja fever. Moreover, it acts as a good appetiser. Any one or two of the (groups of the) drugs of the purgative or appetising properties can be employed with benefit in a case of (chronic) fever. A lambative composed of *Abhayá* pasted together with honey and mixed with oil and clarified butter should be licked by the patient in a case of Tri-doshaja fever. *Trivrit* with honey would pacify a case of high fever. 107—109.

Medical treatment of Vishama-Jwara:—Purgatives and emetics should be exhibited in a case of **Vishama Jwara** and the medicated clarified butter described under the treatment of Plihodara (chapter XIV Chikitsá-sthána), or pulverised *Tri-phalá* § with the addition of treacle may be advantageously used in the type under discussion. A decoction of

* The decoction should be prepared with water only or with milk and water according to the rules of Kshira-páka, if the exigencies of the case so require —Dallana.

† **Additional text**:—A potion of the decoction of *Haridrá*, *Bhadra-musta*, *Tri-phalá*, *Katuka*, *Nimba*, *Patola*, *Devada'ru* and *Kanta-ka'ri* would cure a case of Tri-doshaja fever with indigestion, water-brash, dropsy, cough and disrelish for food.

‡ Dallana includes this line also in the additional text.

§ According to Dallnaa the decoction of *Tri-phala'* should be used.

Guduchi, *Nimba** and *Dhátri* duly mixed with honey, may be likewise prescribed (in a case of Cháturthaka fever). The patient should be likewise made to take *Las'una* (garlic) with clarified butter. The three decoctions duly prepared with three, four or all of the following drugs, viz :—*Madhuka*, *Patola*, *Katuka*, *Mustaka* (D. R.—*Batsaka*) and *Haritaki* † should be likewise administered. 110—111.

A potion consisting of milk, clarified butter, sugar, honey and *Pippali* should be administered according to the strength of the patient. Similarly *Pippali* should be taken with the decoction of *Das'a-mula*. **Pippali-Bardhamána** (see chapter V, Chikitsita-sthána) should be likewise used by a patient who should then be made to take only milk or meat-soup. The use of good wine with the meat of fowl is also recommended. 112

Use of medicated Ghrita in cases of Vishama Jwara :—Clarified butter duly cooked with the decoction of *Kola*, ‡ *Agnimantha* and *Triphalá*, with milk-curd (Dadhi), with *Tilvaka* as Kalka would be found to be highly efficacious in a case of Vishama Jwara A potion of clarified butter duly cooked with the Kalka (and decoction—Dallana) of *Pippali*, *Ativishá*, *Drákshá*, *Sáriva*, *Vilva*, *Chandana* (red), *Katuka*, *Indra-yava*, *Us'ira*, *Simhi*, *Támalaki*, *Musta*, *Tráyamáná*, *Sthirá* (S'ála-parni), *A'mlaki*, *S'unthi* and *Chitraka* would be found highly beneficial to irregular (Vishama) appetite and would cure cases of chronic

* Chakradatta reads "*Musta*" in place of "*Nimba*".

† Dallana says that some commentators are inclined to use the decoction of the 16 different combinations of the five drugs taken three, four or five at a time.

(25) Kola is here used for Pancha-kola, viz :—*Pippali*, *Pippali-roots*, *Chavya*, *Chitraka* and *Na'gara*.

fever, headache, Gulma, Udara (ascites), Halimaka, consumption, cough, burning sensation in the body and pain at the sides. 113—114

Guduchyádi Ghrita :—The use of a medicated clarified butter duly cooked with the decoction of *Guduchi*, *Tri-phalá*, *Vásá* (*D. R. Rásná*), *Tráyamáná* and *Durálabhá* together with the Kalka of *Drákshá*, *Mágadhiká*, (Pippali), *Ambhoda* (Musta), *Nágara*, *Utpala* and *Chandana* would be attended by good results in cases of consumption, asthma, cough and Jirna-Jwara (chronic fever). 115.

Kalaśyádi Ghrita :—Cases of chronic fever, headache, pain at the sides, cough, and of consumption (lit.—any wasting disease of the body attended with fever) would readily yield to the curative efficacy of a medicated clarified butter duly cooked and prepared with the decoction of *Kalas'i* (Priśni-parni), *Vrihati*, *Drákshá*, *Tryánti*, *Nimba*, *Gokshura*, *Valá*, *Parpataka*, *Musta*, *S'ála-parni* and *Yavásaka* and with the Kalka of *S'athi*, *Támalaki*, *Bhárgi*, *Medá*, *Kataka* (D. R.—Ámalaka) and *Pushkara-roots* and with milk twice as much as the clarified butter. 116.

Patoládi Ghrita :—Clarified butter duly cooked with the Kalka of *Patola*, *Parpata*, *Arishta* (Nimba), *Guduchi*, *Tri-phalá*, *Brisha*, *Katuka*, *Ambuda* (Musta), *Bhu-nimba*, *Yavása*, *Yashti-madhu*, *Chandana*, *Dárvi*, *Indra-yava*, *Us'ira*, *Tráyamáná*, *Kaná* and *Utpala* and with the expressed juice of *Dhátri*, *Bhringa-rája*, *Abhiru* (Śatávari) and *Káka-máchi* readily proves curative in cases of Apachi (scrofula), Kushtha, fever, Śukra and Arjuna (two optical diseases), ulcer and in diseases of the mouth, ears, nose and the eyes. 117.

Kalyánaka Ghrita :—Clarified butter duly cooked with the Kalka of *Vidanga*, *Tri-phalá*, *Musta*,

Manjishthá, Dádima, Utpala, Priyangu, Elá, Elaváluka, Chandana, Devadáru, Varhistha (Válaka), *Kushtha, Haridrá,* the two kinds of *Parnni* and of *Sarivâ, Harenuka, Trivrit, Danti, Vacha, Tális'a, Kes'ara* and *Málati* flowers with milk twice as much as clarified butter, is called the **Kalyánaka Ghrita**. The range of its therapeutic application includes such diseases as Vishama Jwara, asthma, Gulma, insanity and diseases due to the effect of any poison. It is auspicious and it removes affections due to the evil influences of malignant spirits and demons, etc., dulness of appetite, epileptic fits, senile decay, sterility and diseases of the seminal cord. It invigorates the eye-sight and imparts memory and longevity to the person who uses it. 118.

Mahá-Kalyánaka Ghrita :—A Prastha measure of clarified butter made from the milk of a cow of Kapila species and duly cooked with the Kalka of the preceding drugs and the drugs known as *Sarvagandhá* (Elâdi-gana) and with (dead) gold and gems should again be duly cooked with the Kalka of *Sumanah, Champaka, As'oka* and *S'irisha* flowers and with *Nalada* and *Padma* (red lotus) and the polens of *Dádima* flowers with the milk of a cow of the same species. It should be prepared under the auspicious of favourable astral combinations and lunar planes of both the physician and of the patient and then be duly consecrated by Brámhanas. It is called **Mahá-Kalyánaka Ghrita** aud may be prescribed for a king. It proves curative in all forms of fever. Its very touch and sight confers bliss and destroys disease. Its use enables a man to live to three hundred years free from disease and decay and to remain invincible against the attacks of all created beings. 119.

Pancha-Gavya-Ghrita :—Fqual parts of milk, curd, clarified butter and urine of a cow and the expressed fluid of cow-dung duly cooked with the Kalka of *Tri-phalà*, *Chitraka*, *Musta*, the two kinds of *Haridrá*, *Ativishâ*, *Vachá*, *Vidanga*, *Tri-katu*, *Chavya* and *Suradáru* prove curative in Vishama Jwara. It is called **Pancha-Gavya-Ghrita**. The same five substances obtained from a cow (e.g., milk, curd, clarified butter, urine and the expressed liquid of cow-dung) may be duly cooked without the addition of any Kalka as also with the above Kalkas and the expressed juice of *Vâsaka* or of *Valá*, or of *Guduchi*. * All of these medicated Ghritas are efficacious in cases of Jirna Jwara (chronic fever), chlorosis and edema. The same five substances (e. g. milk, curd, clarified butter, urine and the expressed fluid of dung) of a she-sheep, a she-goat or a she-buffalo and the four substances (e. g. milk curd, clarified butter and urine) of a she-camel may be prepared (and used) in the same manner. 120—122.

Tri-phaládi Ghrita :—Clarified butter duly cooked with the Kalkas † of *Tri-phalá*, *Us'ira*, *Sampáka*, *Katuka*, *Ativishá*, *S'atávari*, *Sapta-parna*, *Guduchi*, the two kinds of *Rajani*, *Chitraka*, *Trivrita'*, *Murvá*, *Patola*, *Árishta*, *Válaka*, *Kiráta-tikta*, *Vachá*, *Vis'álá*, *Padmaka*, *Utpala*, the two Kinds of *Sárivá*, *Yashti-madhu*, *Chaviká*, *Rakta-chandana*, *Durálabhâ*, *Parpataka*, *Tráyamáná*, *Atarushaka* (Vásaka), *Rásná*, *Kumkuma* (saffron), *Manjishthá*, *Mágadhi* and *Nágara* with the

* Dallana says that the expressed juice of *Vásaka*, *Balá* or *Guduchi*, should be separately used along with the ordinary Kalkas (Tri-phalá, etc.) of the Pancha-gavya Ghrita. But we are inclined to take the lines to mean that *Vásaka*, *Vala'* and *Guduchi* should be separately used as Kalkas in place of the ordinary Kalkas.

† Some here add *Ghana* (Musta) with the other Kalkas,

expressed juice of *Dhátri* weighing twice as much as clarified butter proves curative in Parisarpa (erysipelas), fever, Asthma, Gulma, Kushtha, Chlorosis, enlargement of the spleen and dulness of appetite. 123.

One Pala weight each of *Patola*, *Katuka*, *Dárvi*, *Nimba*, *Vásá*, *Tri-phalá*, *Durálabhá*, *Parpataka* and *Tráyamáná* and a Prastha measure of *Ámalaka* should be boiled in one Drona measure of water down to its quarter measure. A Prastha measure of Ghrita should then be cooked with the above decoctions.* The Ghrita thus prepared proves curative in cases of Rakta-pitta, diseases due to Kapha, perspiration, muco-purulent discharges, atrophy of the limbs, fever, chlorosis, erysipelas and Ganda-málá (scrofula). 124.

Pancha-s'ara :—Boiled milk, sugar, *Pippali*, honey and clarified butter should be taken by stirring them together with hands. The compound is called **Pancha-sára** and may be employed with advantage in cases of Vishama-Jwara, Kshata-Kshina, consumption, asthma and affections of the heart. 125.

Medicated Tailas :—A medicated oil duly prepared by cooking it with *Lákshá*, *Vis'va*, *Nis'á*, *Murvá*, *Manjishthá*, *Sarjiká* and *Ámaya* (Kushtha) as Kalka and with *Takra* weighing six times as much as oil acts as a febrifuge. A medicated oil duly cooked and prepared with *Kshiri-Vriksha*, *Asana*, *Arishta*, *Jambu*, *Sapta-chchhada*, *Arjuna*, *S'irisha*, *Khadirá*, *Ásphotá*, *Amrita-valli*, *Atarushaka*, *Katuka*, *Parpata*, *Us'ira*, *Vacha*, *Tejovati* and *Ghana* as Kalka may be employed

*__Additional text__ :—Some recommend the use of *Kutaja*, *Bhu-nimba*, *Ghana* (Musta), *Yashti-madhu*, *Chandana* and *Pippali* as Kalka in the preparation of this Ghrita and that it proves efficacious in the diseases of the eye, nose, ear, mouth and of the white part of the eye and of the eye-lid and in ulcer.

in anointing the body of the patient in a case of Jirna-Jwara with benefit. 126—127.

The patient should be frightened with a non-venomous snake, trained elephants and bogus thieves (or rebuked with a thievish act falsely supposed to have been committed by him before) at the appointed date and hour of the paroxysm and be kept in empty stomach for the day. In the alternative, he should be fed with heavy and extremely secreting articles (milk, milk-curd, etc.) and be made to continually vomit out the contents of his stomach afterwards, or he should be made to drink any strong liquor, or febrifugal medicated clarified butter or simply matured clarified butter in copious quantity or be treated with drastic purgatives, or with fomentations followed by Nirudha-Vasti application on the date of the expected attack. 128.

Fumigation and Anjana:—The body of the patient should be **fumigated** with the fumes of the skin and hairs of a goat and a sheep mixed with *Vachá, Kushtha, Palankashá (Guggulu), Nimba* leaves, and honey and burnt together. The excreta of a cat should be similarly used in fumigating the body of the patient in a case of fever marked by shivering. *Pippali, Saindhava* and *Naipáli* (Manah-śilá) should be pasted together and mixed with oil and be applied along the eye-lids as an **Anjana**. 129—130.

The medicated Ghritas mentioned in conection with the treatment of Udara (ascites), as well as the Ajita Ghrita mentioned in the Kalpa-sthána (Chapter II.) may be likewise employed with benefit in fever. 131.

A case of fever due to the malignant influence of the spirits, etc. should be remedied with the help of magical incantations (Áveśana), binding and beating (D. R.—adoration) mentioned in the treatment of Bhuta-vidyá (demonology—Chapters LX—LXII). A case of fever due to any mental condition should be cured with psychic (hypnotic) measures ; while the one due to over-fatigue or exhaustion should be treated with diets of Rasaudana * after anointing the body of the patient with clarified butter. Fever due to any curse or to deadly incantations (exorcism) may be cured by performing Homa (offering oblations to the gods) and such other ceremonies ; while the cases due to the malignant influence of any hostile planet, or of any unearthly sound may be cured by practising charity, hospitality and peace-giving rites (Svastyayana). All heat-engendering (Ushna) measures are prohibited in a case of traumatic fever and sweet and astringent drugs charged with oil or clarified butter should be prescribed. Other therapeutic agents should also be employed according to the nature of the specific derangement of Dosha involved in the case. In a case of fever caused by the smell of any herb or cereals or in one due to the effect of any sort of poison, the treatment should consist in such measures as would alleviate the poison and the aggravated Pitta in the system. † Decoction of *Sarva-gandhá* (the drugs of the Eládi-gana) is also beneficial in these cases. A decoction of *Nimba* and *Deva-dáru* or of *Játi* flowers may be prescribed as well. Clarified butter, wine and preparations of barley grains are wholesome in a case of Vishama-Jwara which may be got rid of as well

* Rasaudana is a kind of food prepared by boiling rice in meat soup (instead of in water). The term may, however, mean rice simply mixed with meat-soup.

† In place of "विषपित्तप्रसादनैः" some read "विषपीतप्रसादनैः" and that would mean that the measures and remedies prescribed in cases of poisoning (see Kalpa-sthána) should be applied. This variant seems to be the better one.

by worshipping Bráhmans, cows, the god Is'ána, and Ambiká. 132—133.

The body of the patient overwhelmed with coldness (shivering) in cases of fever due to the action of the aggravated Kapha or Váyu, should be plastered with a paste of the drugs of the heat-making group * and heating measures should then be resorted to. In the alternative, a compound of *Árandla*, *S'ukta*, cow's urine and *Mastu* (curd-cream) made lukewarm should be sprinkled over the body. Plasters of the leaves of *Surasa*, *Arjaka* and *S'igru* pasted together with water would prove beneficial. The body may be rubbed with Kshára-taila (oil cooked with alkali) mixed with *S'ukta*. A decoction of the drugs of the *Áragva-dhádi* group proves highly efficacious particularly in the present case, and decoction of Váyu-subduing drugs should be used tepid as a bath. The shivering having been thus relieved with the foregoing measures and by the sprinkling of tepid water over the body, the languid body of the patient should be smeared with pasted *Káláguru* and wrapped up in a silk, woolen or linnen cover and then the patient should be made to lie in a bed. 134.-A.

Damsels young, beautiful and skilled in the sport of love, with faces glowing like the full moon of autumn and darting forth beams of love from their languid blue-lotus-like eyes, with eye-brows moving in the ardour of desire and with dreary foreheads throbbing with the gentle pulsations of love, with girdles sliding down from their slender waists, with their splendid buttocks naturally making them lazy in their steps, with their lips vying with the ripe *Vimba* fruit in their luscious

* Dallana explains the Ushna-varga (heat-making group) to mean the Bhadra-dárvádi, Surasádi and the Eládi groups.

redness, with their elevated thickest breasts, and smeared with saffron and *Aguru* pastes and clad in thin transparent garment, fumigated and scented with the vapours of burnt *Aguru*, should be asked to take the patient into a firm embrace like a forest-creeper entwining itself around a sylvan tree, and the girls should be told to keep off as soon as the patient would feel himself heated. The patient thus cured of the disease (cold-fever) by the fond embrace of these beautiful damsels should be treated to such a wholesome repast as would be welcome to him. 134.

Measures which alleviate the burning sensation should be employed in a case of fever marked by sever burning sensation of the body. Vomiting should be induced in such cases with honey and treacle mixed with the (cold) infusion of *Nimba* leaves. The body of the patient should be anointed with Śata-dhauta * Ghrita and then plastered with a paste formed by mixing powders of barley, *Kola* and *Ámalaka* with the fermented boilings of *S'uka* paddy, or with the cold paste of tender leaves of *Phenilá* (soap-berry) mixed with *Kola* and *A'malaka* and pasted with *Amla* (Kánjika), or with the cold paste of the leaves of *Palás'a* pasted with *Amla* (Kánjika), or with the froth (produced by stirring in *Kánjiká* the paste) of the leaves of *Vadara* or *Arishta*, † whereby thirst, swoon and burning sensation would be relieved and removed. 135.

A Prastha measure of oil duly prepared by cook-

* Clarified butter washed hundred times in water is known as **Śata-dhauta Ghrita**.

† *Arishta* according to Dallana and S'rikantha (the commentator of Vrinda) may mean either *Nimba* or *Phenila'* (soap-berry). But S'ivadása, the commentator of Chakradatta, explains *Arishta* to mean (leaves of) *Nimba*. The practice, however, is, to use the leaves of *Nimba*.

ing it with half a Kudava measure of *Yava* (barley), half a Pala weight of *Manjishthá* and a hundred Prastha measure of *Amla* (Kánjika). The oil is called **Prahládana** (refreshing) Taila and it relieves the burning sensation of the body due to an attack of fever. 136.

In the alternative, the body of the patient should be plastered with the pasted drugs of the *Nyágrodhádi*, *Kákolyádi* or *Utpaládi* groups, or anointed with a Sneha duly cooked with the decoction of the drugs of the preceding groups and with *Amla*, or the patient should be given a bath (Avagáha) in the Śita-kasáya * of these drugs. On the alleviation of the burning sensation, the patient should be raised out of the tub and then washed with the spray of cold water and smeared with soothing sandal pastes, etc. Young, gay, beautiful and lotus-faced damsels with their youthful cooling breasts profusely smeared with sandal pastes, wearing garlands of beautiful lotus flowers as well as necklace of pearls, etc., and clad in fine silken clothes should be asked to hold the depressed patient in their firm embrace and to kiss him. These damsels should be removed as soon as the patient would exhibit symptoms of exhilaration. He should be given wholesome (Pitta-subduing) food which would give him much relief. Purgative and pacifying (soothing) medicines described in connection with the Pittaja fever are likewise beneficial in the present case. 137.

General treatment of the Complications :—The deranged Pitta should be crushed and remedied first of all in a case of fever, involving therewith the co-operation of any of the deranged Doshas of the body, in as much as it is extremely hard

* "**Śita-kasáya**" may here mean either the **cold** infusion of the drugs or only the cold decoction.

to subdue the deranged Pitta especially in a case of fever. Such distressing symptoms as vomiting, epileptic fits, thirst, etc. should be remedied with such therapeutic agents as are not hostile or aggravating to the principal disease (fever) but are antidotal to the exciting factors. 138.

Specific treatment of the complications :—Now hear me tell you other specific remedies for the complications. A plaster composed of *Yashti-madhu*, *Rajani*, *Musta*, *Dádima*, *Amla-vetasa*, *Rasánjana*, *Tintidika* (tamarind), *Nalada* (Mánsi), *Patra*, *Utpala*, *Tvak* (cinnamon), *Vyághra-nakha*, the expressed juice of *Mátulunga*, honey and *Madhu-s'ukta*, * if applied to the head, would alleviate heat in the head, delirium, vomiting, hic-cough, and shivering—concomitants in cases of fever. Vomiting would yield to the use of a compound consisting of *Madhuka* flower, *Hrivera*, *Utpala* and *Madhuliká* mixed with honey and clarified butter and used to be licked up with the tongue as a lambative. It is equally efficacious in water-brash, hic-cough, Rakta-pitta (hemoptisis) and asthma. Fits of cough and asthma in cases of fever readily yield to the use of the electuary prepared with *Tri-phalá*, *Pippali* and *Mákshika* † and mixed with honey and clarified butter. 139—141.

A plaster of *Vidári*, *Dádima*, *Lodhra*, *Dadhittha* and

* *Madhu-s'ukta* is prepared by preserving the expressed juice of *Jambira*-lemon, *Pippali* and honey in an earthen pot formerly used in keeping honey. It should be laid for a month under the heap of paddy before use. (Dallana) For an alternative mode of preparation see शाङ्गधर, Chapter X—मध्य खण्ड.

† Dallana takes "*Mákshika*" in the sense of honey and comments largely on the seperate use of honey (मधु) in the compound. But we are inclined to take "Mákshika" as the mineral of the same name.

Vijapuraka pasted together may be applied with advantage to the scalf of a fever-patient afflicted with thirst and burning sensation. Pastes of *Dádima* and sugar, and of *Drákshá* and *Ámalaka*, if kept in the mouth, or a gargle (Gandusha) of milk, expressed juice of sugar-cane, *Mádhvika*, * clarified butter, oil and warm water, according to the exigency of the case, would remove the bad taste in the mouth in fever. An empty feeling in the head in fever would be relieved by using as an errhine (Nasya) the medicated clarified butter prepared with the drugs of the Jivaniya group. 142—144.

A pulverised compound consisting of *Tri-phala'*, *S'ya'ma'*, *Trivrit* and *Pippali* mixed with honey and sugar, can be given for purgative purposes with benefit after the digestion of the derangsd Dosha in a case of chronic Pittaja fever, in an up-coursing Raktapitta and in shivering. The system of the patient should be cleansed with similar purgatives and lardaceous lubrications in cases of Kaphaja and Vátaja fever. Lambative of honey, sugar and *Abhaya'* should be given in a case marked by vertigo (Bhrama) even after the subsidence of the aggravated Dosha. 145.

Application of Vastis :—Nirudha-vastis charged with the decoctions of sweet (Kákolyádi) or Váyu-subduing (Bhadra-dárvádi) drugs, should be applied in fever due to the derangement of the bodily Váyu, according to the nature and intensity of the specific deranged Dosha in the case and to the strength of the patient ; in the alternative, Anuvásana Vasti should also be similarly applied. The decoction of the drugs

* Dallana seems to read "*Ma'kshika,*" and explains it as honey. "*Madhvika*" which generally means the wine made of honey, may however, also mean honey.

of the *Utpalâdi* group mixed with *Chandana* and *Us'ira* and sweetened with the addition of sugar should be similarly applied cold (as a Nirudha Vasti) in cases of Pittaja fever. A Vasti (in the manner of Nirudha) charged with a compound consisting of *Âmra*-barks, etc., *S'amkha* (conch), *Chandana*, *Utpala*, *Gairika*, *Rasânjana*, *Manjishthâ*, *Mrina'la* and *Padma-kâshtha* pasted together and dissolved in milk saturated with sugar and honey should be passed through a piece of linen and then applied cold in a case of (Pittaja) fever marked by intolerable pain. The characteristic burning sensation due to fever may be relieved by applying Vasti charged with a decoction of the preceding drugs in the manner of an Ânuvásana-vasti. A Nirudha Vasti charged with the decoction of the drugs of the *Âragvadhâdi* group mixed with (the powders of) the drugs of the *Pippalâdi* group and with honey should be applied in cases of Kaphaja fever and the decoction of the Kapha-subduing (Âragvadhádi) drugs should also be injected into the rectum in the manner of an Anuvásana Vasti. In cases of fever due to the aggravation of two or three Doshas, the Vastis (Nirudha and Anuvásana) to be applied should be charged with the decoction of the drugs respectively antidotal to the deranged Doshas involved in each case. 146—150.

All the medicated lardacious substances with the exception of oil, which have been prescribed as being efficacious (in the use of Vastis) in diseases of the deranged Váyu, are equally applicable (in Anuvásana Vastis) in a case of fever due to the same cause. But all of them (including also oil) are equally applicable to anointing, etc. Lubrication of the body with oil at the close of the acute stage i.e., on the thirteenth or fourteenth day of the attack would be attended with beneficial results in a case of Váta-śleshma fever, where fomentations have utterly failed to relieve the distressing symptoms of the deranged Váyu. Clarified butter duly cooked with sweet and bitter drugs should be used (for the purpose of annointing) in Pittaja fever; while in Kaphaja fever, the Ghrita should be cooked with bitter and pungent drugs. In the cases of fever due to the concerted action of two or three Doshas, the Ghrita should be cooked with the drugs of two or more of the above groups according to the nature of the Doshas involved in each case. 151—152.

The presence of even a small residue of the deranged Pitta in the organism maintains the heat of the skin up to the fever-point, so the remedy consists in taking the expressed juice of sugar-cane, or sweet cordials or *Sarvats* (sugar dissolved in water), and the diet in such a case should consist of cooked Śáli and Shashti rice and milk. Fomentations and anointments should be employed in cases of Kaphaja and Vátaja fevers. Draughts of clarified butter should be given in all forms of fever at the close of twelve days, for by that time the aggravated Doshas return to their respective Áśayas (places in the system). The Dosha involved (in a case of fever) becomes aggravated by affecting, at the time of the remission of the fever, the other fundamental vital principles (Dhátus) of the body and thereby makes the patient weak and dejected at this time. 153—155.

Symptoms of remission:—The features or indications which mark a complete remission of fever, are lightness of the head, flow of perspiration, pale and yellowish colour of the face, sneezing and desire for food. 156.

Fever originating from the wrath-fire of the god Śambhu, is a dangerous disease. It affects appetite and the strength as well as the complexion of the body and is virtually the sum-total of all the other diseases. It is, therefore, called the lord of all bodily diseases. It is common to all created beings (men and animals), affects the whole of the organism (including also the mind), is extremely hard to cure and is present in all cases at the time of the death of all creatures. Hence it is rightly called the destroyer of created beings. 157.

Thus ends the thirty-ninth chapter of the Uttara Tantra in the Sus'rutra Samhitá which deals with the (symptoms and) medical treatment of fever.

CHAPTER XL.

Now we shall discourse on the (causes, symptoms and) medical treatment of diarrhœa, etc. **(Atisára-pratisheda).** 1.

Causes of Atisára:—The excessive use of extremely heavy (hard to digest), oleaginous, dry, hot, cold, fluid, thick, and incompatible articles of food, eating irregularly and at improper time (or unaccustomed articles of fare), indigestion, eating before the digestion of the previous meal, excessive use or misuse of any lardacious substances, etc., (Sneha, Sveda, etc.), use of any poison, fright, grief, drinking impure water, the excessive drinking of liquor, change of season or physical contrarieties, indulgence in aquatic sports, voluntary repression of any natural urging (of the body) or germination of parasites in the intestines are the causes which bring on an attack of diarrhœa (**Atisára**) the symptoms whereof will be dealt with presently. 2.

Pathology:—The liquid part (Ap-dhátu) of the body, if aggravated and carried downward by the bodily Váyu, impairs the fire in the stomach (fire of digestion) and mixing with the fecal matter, is painfully and constantly emitted through the anus. This dangerous disease is named **Atisára** from the constant oozing out (Ati and Sarana) of the liquid fecal matter from the anus. It is usually classified into six different types, *viz.*, those due to the predominance of the deranged bodily Doshas severally involved therein, that due to the concerted action of the three Doshas, one due to grief and that due to the indigested mucous accumulations (Áma) in the intestines. Some authorities hold that Atisára is of many kinds but the holy Dhanvantari, on the contrary, holds that it is not so but that the physical conditions of a diarrhœic patient undergo changes and become manifold. 3.

Premonitory Symptoms :—Piercing pain in the regions of the heart, umbilicus, rectum, abdomen and in the Kukshi (sides of the abdomen), a sense of numbness in the limbs, stoppage or suppression of flatus and of stool, distension of the abdomen, and indigestion are the premonitory symptoms of the disease. 4.

Symptoms of Vátaja, Pittaja, Kaphaja and Tri-doshaja Types :— The **Váyu**-origined type of the disease is marked by Śula (colic), suppression of urine, rumbling sound in the intestines, looseness (constant movement in the intestines) of the abdominal (Apána) wind, a gone feeling in the waist, in the thighs and in the legs, and frequent emissions with flatus of a scanty, frothy, dry (Ruksha) brown-coloured (yellowish black) stool. The specific features of the **Pitta**-origined type are that the stool is fetid, hot, yellow, blue or slightly red-coloured, or resembles the washings of meat, and is emitted with sharp or acute force and is accompanied by thirst, epileptic fits (fainting), burning sensation, perspiration, suppuration and inflamation (Páka) of the affected organs, and fever. In the **Kapha**-origined type of the disease the stool becomes loose and constant, gets mixed with the lump of mucus and looks white. The stool comes out without any sound. A sense of constant urging is complained of and each motion only creates the apprehension of a fresh one in the mind. The patient becomes drowsy or sleepy, and feels a sense of heaviness in the limbs, nausea, disrelish for food, horripalation and lassitude. The symptoms which mark a case of **Tri-doshaja** type (due to the concerted action of the three simultaneously deranged bodily Doshas) are drowsiness, swoon, lassitude, dryness of the mouth, thirst and a varied colour of the stools. A case of Tri-doshaja type, if attended with all the symptoms, is very hard to cure and if occurring in an infant, or an old person, is scarcely amenable to medical treatment. 5-8.

Symptoms of Śokaja and Ámaja Atisára :—The suppressed tears of a bereaved person of sparing diet, on quenching the digestive fire, reach down into the Koshtha (intestines) and there freely mix with, and vitiate the local blood which becomes dark-red like *Kákananti* (Gunjá). It then passes through the rectum, charged with a peculiar fetour imparted to it by the fecal matter in case of its combination with the latter or without any fetid smell, when passing out unmixed. Such an attack ushered in by the **grief** of bereavement of a person is accordingly considered very hard to cure. The local bodily Doshas in the Koshtha (abdomen) are aggravated and deranged when they come in contact with the **Áma** (unassimilated chyle), and are brought down into the Koshtha (bowels), where they are more agitated and emitted in combination with the undigested fecal matter in various ways, and are attended with pain and characterised by a variety of colour. This is the **sixth** type of Atisára. 9—10

Symptoms of Áma and Pakva Atisára :—A case of Atisára (diarrhœa) would be said to be in the **Áma** (acute) state, if the stool of the patient suffering from any of the foregoing Doshas would be found to sink in water and to emit a very fetid smell and to pass in broken jets (D. R.—to be slimy). A contrariety of the preceding symptoms and a sense of lightness of the body and in the affected cavity would indicate that the disease has passed the acute stage and it is then called **Pakva** (chronic) Atisára. 11.

Prognosis :—If the colour of the stool (in a case of Atisára) resembles that of clarified butter, fat, the washings of Veśavára, oil, goat's milk, honey, *Manjishthá*, brain-matter, or *Rasánjana*, or if the stool is cold or hot to the touch, or if it is charged with a fleshy or fetid smell, or marked with lines or specks of variegated colours, or if it looks like pus or clay, or if just the opposite or reverse symptoms or other distressing symptoms would be exhibited, the case is likely to end fatally in case the patient be weak. A patient suffering from an attack of Atisára would be given up (as incurable) if he be weak, if the orifice of his anus become suppurated and cannot be closed, if there be distension of the abdomen (D. R.—if the patient be not self-restrained), if there be distressing symptoms and if the patient be found destitute of thermal heat. 12-13.

An attack of Atisára ushered in by whatsoever cause, is sure to be marked by the specific symptoms of the deranged bodily Dosha or Doshas complicated with it. All cases of Atisára whether due to the indigestion of any oleaginous food or drink (Ghrita, oil, etc.), whether with (or without) the symptoms of Praváhiká and the accompanying colic, as well as those due to Visuchiká or any other kind of indigestion as also those due to the effect of any poison (affecting the digestive system), hœmorrhoids (Arśas), or worms in the intestines,—all of them are marked by the symptoms of the specific Dosha involved therein. The treatment of Atisára varies according to its acute or matured stage, the characteristic symptoms of those therefore are to be carefully observed and noted in each case under treatment. 14-15.

The patient should be kept without food as soon as the premonitory symptoms of Atisára would appear, and then the dietic gruels (Yavágu) prepared with the admixture of digestive drugs should be given in their proper order. In a case marked by colic and flatulent distension of the abdomen, fasting should be first advised. And then vomiting should be induced with draughts of water mixed with powdered *Pippali* and Saindhava salt. A light diet in the shape of a *Khada-yusha*, *Yavágu*, etc., prepared with the admixture of the drugs of the *Pippalyádi* group, should then be prescribed after the cessation of vomiting. A decoction of the drugs of the *Haridrádi*, or *Vachádi* group, should be be taken in the morning where the preceding remedies would fail to relieve mucous accumulations in the intestines (**Ámátisára**). No astringent or costive medicine in the acute or immature (Áma) stage of the disease should be administered in as much as by obstructing the passage of the Doshas it might bring on an attack of enlarged spleen, chlorosis, distension of the abdomen with suppression of stool and urine, Meha (urinary complaints), Kushtha (cutaneous affections), ascites, fever, œdematous swellings of the limbs, Gulma (abdominal gland, etc.,) diarrhœa, piles, colic, Alasaka and catching pain at the heart. 16-17.

Purging should be induced with *Haritaki* in a case marked by constant and scanty motions (of mucus and) attended with griping and pain (Śula) or by an incarceration of the deranged bodily Doshas (in the intestines). Emetics should be first exhibited and followed by fastings and digestive or assimilative (Páchana) remedies in a case marked by watery and copious motions. Powdered *Haritaki* and *Pippali* with tepid water should be administered for purgative purposes in a case marked by scanty emissions of stool at times attended with pain and colic (S'ula). Fasting is the first remedy to be prescribed in cases of **Áma** (acute) Atisára, or in the alternative, digestive remedies should be prescribed. The recipes of digestive medicinal compounds which are curative in the disease under discussion (Ámátisára) are described below. 18—19.

Twenty different Recipes for Ámátisára :—(1) *Deva-dáru*, *Vacha*, *Musta*, *Nágara*, *Ativishá* and *Abhayá* ; or of (2) *Kalinga* (*Indra-yava*), *Ativishá*, *Hingu*, *Sauvarchala*-salt, *Vachá* and *Abhayá*, or of (3) *Abhayá* (D. R.-Nágara), *Dhanyáka*, *Musta*, *Válaka* and *Vilva* ; or of (4) *Musta*, *Parpataka*, *S'unthi*, *Vacha*, *Ativishá* and *Abhayá* ; or of (5) *Abhayá*, *Ativishá*, *Hingu*, *Vachá*, and *Sauvarchala*-salt ; or of (6) *Chitraka*, *Pippali-mula*, *Vacha*, *Katuka-rohini*, or of (7) *Páthá*, *Vatsaka*-seeds (Indra-yava), *Haritaki* and *Mahaushadha* (S'unthi), or of (8) *Murvá*, *Nirdahani*, (Chitraka), *Páthá*, *Tryushana* (*Tri-katu*) and *Gaja-pippali* ; or of (9) *Siddhárthaka*, *Bhadra-dáru*, *S'atáhvá* and *Katu-rohini* ; or of (10) *Elá*, *Sávaraka* (Lodhra), *Kushtha*, the two sorts of *Haridrá*, *Kutaja*-seeds (Indra-yava) ; or of (11) *Mesha-s'ringi*, *Tvak*, *Elá*, *Krimighna* (Vidanga) and *Vrikshaka* (Indra-yava) ; or of (12) *Brikshádani*, *Virataru*, the two kinds of *Vrihati* and the two kinds of *Sahá* (Mudga-parni and Másha-parni) ; or of (13) barks of *Eranda*, *Tinduka*, *Dádima*, *Kutaja* and of *S'ami*; or of (14) *Páthá*, *Tejovati*, *Musta*, *Pippali* and *Indra-yava* ; or of (15) *Patola*, *Dipyaka* (Yamáni), *Vilva*, the two kinds of *Haridrá* and *Deva-dáru* ; or of (16) *Vidanga*, *Abhayá*, *Páthá*, *S'ringavera*, *Ghana* (Musta) and *Vacha* ; or of (17) *Vacha*,

Vatsaka-seeds (Indra-yava), *Saindhava* and *Katu-rohini*; or of (18) *Hingu*, *Vatsaka*-seeds (Indra-yava), *Vacha* and dried green *Vilva*; or of (19) *Nágara*, *Ativishá*, *Mustá*, the two kinds of *Pippali* and *Vatsaka*-seeds (Indra-yava); or of (20) *Mahaushadha*, *Prati-vishá* and *Mustá*,—these are the **Twenty** different recipes of the remedies which are digestive (of the mucous accumulations) in cases of Áma-Atisára and should be administered (in the shape of powder) with *Dhányámla* (Kánjika), tepid water or wine, or their decoctions in luke-warm state should be used. This is a detailed list of the best remedies in cases of **Áma-Atisára**. 20.

A compound of *Haritaki*, *Ativishá*, *Hingu*, *Sauvarchala* and *Vachá* should be taken with tepid water in cases of Áma-Atisáras. Similarly a compound of *Patola*, *Yamáni*, *Vis'va*, *Vachá*,*Pippali*, *Nágara*, *Musta*, *Vidanga*, and *Kushtha*, or that of *S'unthi* and *Guduchi* should be taken with tepid water. 21-23.

The five following compounds separately composed (1) of all kinds of officinal salt, *Pippali*, *Vidanga* and *Haritaki*; or of (2) *Chitraka*, *S'ims'apá*, *Páthá*, *S'árngashtá*, and all kinds of officinal salt; or of (3) *Hingu*, *Vrikshaka*-seeds (Indra-yava) and all kinds of officinal salt taken in equal parts; or (4) of *Nága-danti* and *Pippali*, weighing two Tolás; or (5) of *Vachá* and *Guduchi*-stems, would be found beneficial, if taken with tepid water. Twenty *Musta*, should be boiled in a quantity of milk and thrice as much water. The milk which is left back after all the water is evaporated by boiling, should be used for the relief of the griping (Śula) due to the accumulation of mucus (Áma) in the intestines. 24-25.

Clarified butter mixed with *Saindhava*-salt and *Yava-kshára* should be given to a patient of weak digestive pcwer in a case in which the Váyu has not been restored to its normal condition in spite of the subsidence of the intestinal Śula (griping) and which is marked by scanty (but repeated) motions passed with pain. The Ghrita duly cooked with *Nágara*, *Chángeri* and *Kola* (Vadara) and with milk*, curd (Dadhi) and Amla (Kánjika), or simply the transparent part of clarified butter should be taken as a relief for Atisára attended with Śula (pain). In the alternative, clarified butter mixed with (an equal quantity of) oil and duly cooked with curd, together with a paste of *Tri-katu*, *Játi* (flower) and *Chitraka*, or with that of *Pippali-mula*, *Vilva*, *Dádima-bark* and *Kushtha* should be given. All these are the remedies to be employed in a type of Atisára due to the action of Váta or of Śleshmá ; and all the foregoing remedies with the exception of those of keen and heat-making potency, may be used in the Pittaja type of the disease. 26—27.

Fasting as already advised should be first observed and it should be broken with gruels (Yavágu) duly cooked with the two kinds *Valá*, or with *Ams's-mati*, or *S'vadamshtrá* and *Vrihati*, or *S'atávari* made cold and mixed with honey. The soup (Yusha) of *Mudga* duly cooked with the drugs of appetising virtue, or with mild and bitter drugs of appetising property would cure (the Dosha in) the acute stage (Ámá-dosha) of the stool. Decoctions of *Haridrá*, *Ativishá*, *Páthá*, *Vatsa*-seeds (Indra-yava) and *Rasánjana* ; or of *Rasánjana*, the two kinds of *Haridrá* and *Kutaja*-seeds (Indra-yava ; or of Páthá, *Guduchi*, *Bhu-nimba* and *Katu-rohini* would

* We have tha recipe of this Ghrita in Charaka Samhitá also. But there we find Kshárá in place of Kshira and that appears to be the better reading. See Chapter XIX,—under Chángeri Ghrita, Charaka Samhitá.

prove extremly useful in correcting (Páchana) the deranged **Pitta**. 28—29.

Six Yogas for Pittaja-Atisára :—Any one of the six decoctions respectively prepared with *Mustá*, *Kutaja*-seeds (Indra-yava.), *Bhu-nimba* and *Rasánjana* ; or with *Dárvi*, *Durálabhá*, *Vilva* and red *Chandana* ; or with *Chandana*, *Válaka*, *Mustá*, *Bhu-nimba*, *Durálavá* ; or with *Mrinála*, *Chandana*, *Rodhra*, *Nágara* and *Nilotpala* ; or with *Páthá*, *Musta*, the two kinds of *Haridrá*, *Pippali* and *Kutaja*-seeds ; or with the seeds and barks of *Vatsaka*, *S'ringavera* and *Vachá* mixed with clarified butter should be regarded as good remedies for the **Pittaja** type of Atisára. 30.

A case of **Pittaja**-Atisára in its acute (Áma) stage would yield to the use of a decoction of (unripe) *Vilva*, *Indra-yava*, *Ambhoda* (Mustá), *Válaka* and *Ativishá*. A decoction of *Yashti-madhu*, *Utpala*, *Vilva*, *Ámra*, *Hrivera*, *Us'ira* and *Nágara* mixed with honey proves curative in the case under discussion. 31—32.

Astringent or constipating (Samstambhana) remedies should be employed in a case of the chronic (Pakva) Atisára marked by dullness of the Grahani, *viz*, the digestive fire and by constant motions. Any of the four following medicinal compounds, *viz*., *Samangá*, *Dhátaki*-flower, *Manjisthá*, *Lodhra* and *Mustá* ; or of *S'álmali-veshtaka*, *Rodhra* and the bark of *Vrikshaka* (Kutaja) and of *Dádima* ; or of the stone of *Ámra*, *Lodhra*, the inner pulp of (unripe) *Vilva* and *Priyangu* ; or of *Yashti-madhu*, *S'ringavera* and the bark of *Dirgha-vrinta* (Śyonáka) should be taken with honey and the washings of rice in cases of chronic (**Pakva**) Atisára. 33—34.

The decoction of *Musta* alone should be taken with honey in the case under discussion, or a decoction of any of the nine Ganas, *viz.*, the *Lodhrádi*, *Amboshthádi*, or *Priyangvádi* groups, etc. (see Chapter XXXVIII, Sutra-Sthàna) should be employed. Similarly, the decoction of *Padmá*, *Samangá*, *Yashti-madhu* and dried *Vilva* and *Jambu* fruits should be taken with the washings of rice mixed with honey. A paste of the root of *Kachchhurá* weighing an *Udumvara* (two Tolás) should be similarly taken (with the same vehicles). A case of Pakvátisára marked by bloody stool or by emission of blood (from the intestines) would yield to the use of the decoction of *Payasyá*, *Chandana*, *Padmá* (Bhárgi), *Sitá* (sugar), *Mustá* and the polens of lotus. 35—38.

Application of Ghrita :—Clarified butter with *Yava-kshára* should be given to a patient with due regard to the state of his digestive power if, after being treated with fasting, etc., he be still found to be affected with Śula and dryness and if the stool would be found to be free from mucus i.e., in a case of Pakvátisára. The colic (in a case of Atisára) is relieved by taking (a potion of clarified butter duly cooked with) *Valá*, *Vrihati*, *Ams'u-mati* and *Kachchhurá*-roots mixed with a little honey and *Yashti-madhu* (as an after-throw). Clarified butter duly cooked with *Dárvi*, *Vilva*, *Kaná* (*Pippali*), *Drákshá*, *Katuka* and *Indra-yava* would prove curative in a case of Atisará due to the action of the Váta, Pittá and Kaphá (jointly or separately). A draught of milk, honey and clarified butter (in equal parts) mixed with sugar, *Ajamodá*, *Katvanga* and *Yashti-madhu* (as an after-throw) would relieve the griping (Śula) in the intestines (in a case of Atisára). 39—42.

Putapáka Preparations :—A case of long-standing (chronic) Atisára marked by stools of various colours and a keen digestion but unattended with any sort of pain or complication should be remedied with medicines prepared in the maner of **Puta-páka** preparation (described below). The barks of *Dirgha-vrinta* (*S'yonáka*), and polens of lotus should be pasted together and wrapped up in leaves of *Kás'mari* or of *Padma* (lotus) with their ends tied with string or thread (D. R.—Kus'a). The cover. should be then coated with a plaster of clay and duly scorched in the fire of (smokeless) charcoal (of *Khadira*). When well cooked, it should be taken out and the juice, squeezed out of its contents. This juice should be cooled and administered in combinaticn with honey in a case of Atisára. Similar preparations of the drugs known as *Jivanti* and *Mesha-s'ringi*, etc., may also be used in the same way. The skin of a *Tittira* bird should be peeled off and a paste of the drugs of the *Nyagrodhádi* group should be stuffed into its belly after it has been previously drawn. After this it should be duly stitched up and cooked (scorched) in the fire in the above manner. The juice should then be squeezed out therefrom and administered, when cool, with the admixture of honey and sugar in a case of Atisára. The drugs known as *Lodhra*, *Chandana*, *Yashti-madhu*, *Dárvi*, *Páthá*, *Sitá* (sugar), *Utpala* and the barks of *Dirgha-vrinta* pasted together with the washings of rice should be duly scorched in the fire in the above manner (of a Puta-páka). The juice pressed out of its contents and taken with honey, when cold, proves curative in cases of Atisára due to the action of the deranged Pitta and Kapha. Similar preparations may be made of the aerial roots of *Vata*, etc., and may be advantageously prescribed with the soup of the flesh of any Jángala bird (such as Tittira, Kapinjala, etc,). 43-47.

The *Kutaja*-bark taken with treacle would cure perforce the long-standing cases of Atisára attended with blood and marked by the diminished action of the bodily Váyu but a predominant action of the deranged Kapha. The drugs of the *Ambashtádi* group as well as those of the *Pippalyádi* group taken with honey would be similarly beneficial. 48-49

A **Peyá** duly prepared with the admixture of *Pris'niparni*, *Balá*, *Vilva* (D. R. Vis'va), *Bálaka*, *Utpala*, *Dhanyáka* and *Nágara*, should be taken by a patient suffering from Atisára. A case of Pakvátisára would yield to the curative efficacy of a light medicinal gruel (*Yavágu*) duly prepared with the admixture of the paste of *S'yonáka*-bark, *Priyangu*, *Yashti-madhu*, and tender sprouts of *Dádima* pasted together with curd. A case of Atisára attended with blood and colic (S'ula) would be readily cured by the use of *Rasánjana*, *Ativishá*, *Dhátaki*, *Nágara* and the bark and seeds of *Kutaja* taken with honey and the washings of rice. 50—52.

Yashti-madhu, (dried) green *Vilva*-fruit mixed with honey and sugar, or particles of *S'áli* and *Shashtika* rice (administered with the same drugs) would prove curative in a case of Atisára. *Badari*-roots pasted with honey should be given to be licked with the same result. Barks of *Badari*, *Arjuna*, *Jambu*, *Ámra*, *S'allaki* and *Vetasa* taken with honey and sugar would cure a case of Atisára. Gruels (Yavágu), Mandas (thick gruel squeezed through a piece of linen) and Yusha (soup) may also be duly prepared with the admixture of these drugs, and in a case marked by excessive **thirst**, the water for **drinking** should be prepared by duly boiling these drugs. The cold infusion of * *S'álmali*-stems kept in the open

* Powders of S'álmali stem should be kept immersed for whole

space for a whole night, may be given good with good results as a **drink** in combination with *Yasthi-madhu* and honey. 53—54.

Use of Milk in Atisára.:—Milk should be given in a case of Atisára marked by the suppression of stool and Váyu and attended with griping (Śula), constant scanty motions, symptoms of Rakta-pitta and thirst. Milk is ambrosia itself in such a case of Atisára (Dysentery), and in long-standing cases the milk to be taken should be duly boiled with thrice as much water. This would remove the remnant, if any, of the Dosha involved and is, therefore, considered as the best remedy in such cases. Oily purgatives and application of Pichchila-Vasti (slimy intestinal injections) as well as the medicated Ghrita duly prepared with the expressed juice of the barks of slimy trees, e. g., *S'yoná*, *S'álmali*, etc., are beneficial under the circumstances (in chronic or longstanding cases). 56.

Draughts of clarified butter duly prepared with the tender sprouts of the *Kshiri* trees and mixed with honey and sugar (as an after-throw) should be taken in a case of Atisára marked with a discharge of **blood** before or after the passing of the stool and with a cutting pain (in the region of the anus). Draughts of medicated clarified butter duly prepared with the barks of *Deva-dáru*, and with *Pippali*, *S'unthi*, *Lákshá*, *Indra-yava*, and *Bhadra-rohini* (Katuká) administered through the medium of any kind of *Peyá*, would prove highly efficacious in a case of **Tri-doshaja** Atisára of severe type. 57-58.

night in an equal quantity of water. In the morning the water should be passed through a piece of linen. Four-Pala-weight of this water mixed with a Karsha weight of Yashti-madhu and honey should be taken.

Exhibition of emetics or vomiting is an excellent remedy in a case of Atisára marked by heaviness (in the abdomen) and the predominance of the deranged bodily Kapha. A case attended with fever, burning sensation and suppression of stool and marked by an aggravation of Váyu should be treated as a case of Rakta-pitta. Intestinal injections with urine-purifying (Mutra-Śodhana) drugs should be speedily administered in the manner of an **Ásthápana** or **Anuvásana** Vasti, as the occasion might arise, in a case marked by an excessive accumulation of the deranged bodily Doshas in the affected locality as well as by the suppression (of stool) during the mature stage of the disease. 59-60.

Intestinal injections consisting of oil or clarified butter duly cooked and prepared with the drugs of sweet and acid tastes should be applied in the manner of an **Anuvásana** Vasti in a case marked by the protrusion of the bowel through violent and excessive straining and by painful obstruction of urine (Mutrágháta) and pain in the waist. Pitta-subduing **washes**, and **injections** prepared with the Pitta-subduing drugs and appiied in the manner of Anuvásana Vasti, are the remedies in a case marked by the suppuration of the anus due to the aggravation of **Pitta** in an injudicious or intemperate patient. **Anuvásana** Vasti charged with oil duly cooked with wine, *Vilva* and *Dadhi-manda* should be applied in a case of Atisára marked by the aggravation of the deranged bodily **Váyu**, and milk duly boiled and cooked with the admixture of *Kachchurá*-roots should be given to drink. 61-63.

Pichchhá-Vasti should be applied (into the rectum) in a case of Atisára marked by painful and frequent emission of blood, though in scanty quantities at a time, and by an entire suppression of Váyu (flatus). An atonic condition of the anus results from a long-standing attack of Atisára which should, therefore, be remedied by rubbing the part with oil. 64–65.

Diet :—The **diet** of the patient suffering from Atisára should be prepared with the admixture of *Kapittha*, *S'álmali*, *Phanji* (a kind of Páthá), *Vana-Kárpási* (D. R. Vata and Kárpási), *Dádima*, *Yuthiká*, *Kachchhurá*, *S'elu*, *S'ana*, *Chuchchu*, *Dadhi* (curd), *S'ála-parni*, *Pris'niparni*, *Vrihati*, *Kanta-káriká*, *Valá*, *S'vad-amstrá*, *Vilva*, *Páthá*, *Nágara* and *Dhanyáka* and may also consists of the pastes of sesamum and *Mudga* pulse or of *Mudga* soup. 66.

Causes and Symptoms of Raktáti-sára :—The bodily Pitta of a person already suffering from an attack of Pittaja-Atisára is further deranged and aggravated, if Pitta-generating eatables are taken, and ushers in the discharge of blood with stool accompanied by fever, burning sensation, thirst, gripings (Śula) and excessive suppuration (inflamation) of the anus (Guda). The above are the characteristies of the **Raktáti-sára**. 67.

Treatment :—Draughts of milk duly boiled and cooked with the leaves of *Vata*, etc. (those included within the Nyagrodhádi group) should be given with clarified butter, or with sugar and honey in a case marked by a discharge of **blood** before or after motions ; or the butter prepared by stirring the preceding preparation of milk should be taken ; and draught of the *Takra* (thus prepared) should be taken as an after-potion. The discharge of blood (in a case of Atisára) may be stopped by a potion consisting of the barks of *Piyála*, *S'álmali*, *Plaksha*, *S'allaki*, and of *Tinis'a* pasted together with milk and mixed with honey. The same result is obtained by administering the milk of a she-goat with a paste of *Yashti-madhu*, sugar, *Lodhra*, *Payasyá* (Arkapushpi) and *Dárvi* and mixed with honey, or with a paste (or powder) of *Manjishthá*, *S'arivá*, *Lodhra*, *Padmaka*, *Kumuda*, *Utpala* and *Padmá* (Bhárgi). 68-71.

Sugar, *Utpala*, *Lodhra*, *Samangá*, *Yashti-madhu* and *Tila*; or *Tila*, *Mocha-rasa* and *Lodhra*; or *Yashti-madhu* and *Utpala*; or *Kachchurá* and *Tila* are the ingredients of four recipes which, if taken with the she-goat's milk and honey, would remove the blood in the stool. Pastes of unripe *Vilva* fruits, treacle and honey taken before the meal would be a remedy in a case marked by watery motions mixed with blood. A case of blood-dysentry due to the deranged blood, and Pitta and attended with Śula yields to the use of a compound consisting of *Kos'akára* (a kind of sugar-cane) pulverised parched paddy fried in clarified butter and mixed with sugar and honey. A case of blood-dysentery due to the action of the deranged blood, and Pitta may be cured with a compound of the kernel of a (unripe) *Vilva*-fruit mixed with *Yashti-madhu* and taken with the washings of rice, honey and sugar. The remedies mentioned in connection with a case of Guda-páka (suppuration of anus) should also be employed in these cases. Application of **Pichchhá-Vasti** is recommended in the type where the pain begins to subside. A purgative consisting of the decoction of *Vidanga*, *Triphalá* and *Pippali* should be given to a patient with good appetite as soon as the stool would assume* the colour of blood. In the alternative, a purgative consisting only of milk cooked with *Eranda*-roots (castor plant) should be employed and the patient should be

* D. R.—When the stool would harden "सक्तविट्" ।

given *Yavágu* prepared with appetising and Váyu-subduing drugs. 72-78.

Treacle (Phánita) mixed with powdered *S'unthi*, curd, oil, milk and clarified butter should be given in a case marked by good appetite but by frothy motions devoid of all fœcal matter. *Badara*-fruits boiled with oil and treacle, or cakes prepared from them and dried unripe *Vilva*-fruits should be prescribed. Cakes prepared with boiled *Másha*-pulse should be prescribed to be taken with curd followed by a draught of *S'vetá* (cake-made) wine in the case marked by the absence of fecal matter in the stool. The blood-stained flesh of a hare cooked with *S amangá*, curd and clarified butter should be taken with well boiled rice. 79.

A decoction of *Másha*-pulse, *Kola* and barley duly cooked in equal parts of the oil and clarified butter and mixed with curd and the expressed juice of *Dádima* should be prescribed as **diet** in the case. The absence of any fecal matter in the stool (**Purisha-Kshaya**) would yield to the use of *Bit* (black salt), dried unripe *Vilva* fruit and *S'unthi* pasted with any acid juice and mixed with curd-cream and cooked in equal parts of oil and clarified butter. Clarified butter duly cooked with as- tringent and appetising drugs should be given in a case of Atisára attended with Śula where the patient feels a good appetite after the loss of fecal matter. 80—81.

Symptoms of Pravahiká :—The Váyu in the organism of a person addicted to the use of unwholesome food, is deranged and aggravated. It carries down the accumulations of Valása (mucus) into the lower part of the body, whence, mixed with stools, they are constantly passed off with tenesmus. The disease is called **Pravahiká** (mucous diarrhœa). The motions are attended with Śula (pain) in the **Vátaja** type of the disease, with burning sensation in the **Pittaja** one, with mucus in the **Kaphaja** one and with blood (blood-streaked mucus) in the **Raktaja** (blood-origined type). Excessive use of dry (Ruksha) or of fatty articles of food may be regaided as the exciting factor of these cases. The specific indications of Praváhiká as well as its **Áma** or acute and **Pakva** or mature stage are respectively identical with those of the several types of Atisára. 82-83.

Treatment :—In the event of fasting and other digestive (Páchana) compounds (of Praváhiká) producing no beneficial effect in serious cases they are found to readily yield to the use of boiled milk, oil, *Tila* (sesamum) or Pichchhila Vasti. The green stems of *S'álmali* well covered with green *Kus'a*-blades, should be scorched in the fire in the manner of Puta-páka. The juice should be squeezed out thereof and mixed with boiled milk, oil, clarified butter and powdered *Yashti-madhu*, and should be carefully injected into the rectum in the manner of Vasti application in cases of Praváhiká marked with the retention of stool and urine. Similar injections of a decoction of *Das'a-mula* duly cooked in milk and mixed with honey and applied in the manner of an **Ásthápana**-Vasti as well as the application of oil in the manner of an **Anuvásana** Vasti would prove highly efficacious in cases marked with painful tenesmus. 84—86.

Diet :—Oil duly cooked with the drugs of the Váyu-subduing (Vidári-gandhádi) group and with (the five officinal kinds of) salt should be used in (the preparation of) **food** and **drink**. A compound consisting of *Lodhra*, *Bit*-salt and dried unripe *Vilva*-fruit pasted with oil and mixed with *Tri-katu* should be given to be licked*. The food (boiled rice) of a diarrhœtic patient should be taken with honey and curd from which the cream has not been removed ; or with milk warmed by a piece of red-hot metal † (other than gold and silver) and mixed when cold with a profuse quantity of honey. The use of milk duly boiled and cooked with the admixture of *Tri-katu* and *Vidári-gandhá*, with the food would prove curative in a case attended with Śula. He should also be given soups (**Rasa**) prepared with the drugs of appetising, astringent (Gráhi) and Váyu-subduing virtues. Fish he may take and his soup should be prepared with oil and clarified butter with the admixture of Váyu-subduing drugs. The **diet** in this disease should consist of venison, mutton or goat's flesh cooked with the tender sprouts of a *Vata* tree or of blood of a fatty goat duly cooked with curd (Dadhi), oil and clarified butter. He may take his food with an unsalted soup (Yusha) of a peacock or of a Láva bird, or with well prepared curd. He may take (with benefit) well cooked *Másha-pulse* mixed with the transparent upper part of clarified butter (Ghrita-manda) and with curd, while chewing at intervals (with his teeth) the unpowdered *Maricha* (black pepper). 87—89.

A compound of milk, honey and clarified butter mixed with the decoction of *Yashti-madhu* and *Utpala* should be applied in the manner of Vasti-application in (a case of Praváhiká, marked by) excessive pain and painful micturation (Mutra-Krichchhra). The application of this Vasti would alleviate the burning sensation,

* According to some variants this compound should be taken thrice daily.

† In place of "कुप्य"—Kupya (any metal other than gold and silver) some read "कुर्प"—Kurpa which is explained to mean a kind of stone.

allay the the accompanying fever and remove the blood (in the stool). Injections of the decoction (of the drugs) of *Madhura* group (such as Kákoli, etc.) in the manner of an Anuvásana Vasti, should also be applied every day—at daytime or in the night, if the patient be feeling any pain. 90.

A Vasti applied with the admixture of oil would pacify the aggravated bodily Váyu and Praváhiká, would be removed with the pacification of the deranged bodily Váyu. The main treatment, therefore, in a case of Praváhiká is to restore the deranged local Váyu to its normal condition, (which is identical with a cure). 91.

Medical Treatment :—The drugs known as *Páthá*, *Ajamodá*, *Kutaja-seeds*, *S'unthi* and *Mága-dhiká* taken in equal parts, pasted together and dissolved in tepid water or milk duly boiled with the testicles of a goat and mixed with clarified butter would prove efficacious in a case of Praváhiká. Clarified butter mixed with oil and duly cooked with *S'unthi* and *Kshavaka* would give instantaneous relief, if licked. Yavágu duly prepared with the admixture of *Vilva* and the expressed juice of *Gajás'ana* (Śallaki), *Kum-bhiká* and *Dádima* and with curd, oil and clarified butter would prove highly beneficial. The use of milk just drawn would similarly prove beneficial in the case. 92.

A wise and experienced physician should employ the foregoing medicinal compounds and decotions in the complaints of the bowels and of the stomach (Udará-maya) as well as light, appetising and emulsive (Snigdha) articles of fare and other articles of food prescribed before as diet in the cases. 93.

Yavágu :—Yavágu (gruel) is always efficacious in cases of fever and Atisára in as much as it allays thirst, is light in digestion and appetising, and acts as a cleanser of the bladder (diuretic). 94.

General Principle of Treatment :— Drying (Ruksha) measures should be employed in a case due to the excessive use of any oily or emulsive food and emulsive (Snigdha) measures should be adopted in a case brought on through an excessive use of any dry (Ruksha) article. The cause of terror should be first removed in a case due to fright, while the mind should be calmed or consoled in the case due to any grief or bereavement. The treatment in cases (of Atisára) due to piles or worms (in the intestines) as well as in those due to the effect of poison (introduced into the system) consits in employing therapeutic agents which are simultaneously remedial both to the disease and to its exciting factors. Complications or distressing concomitants such as vomiting, thirst, fainting fits, etc., should be removed with drugs which are not incompatible with the main treatment of the disease, and which do not aggravate the exciting factors. In a case of fever or Atisára marked by the simultaneous aggravation of the deranged bodily Doshas, the deranged **Pitta** should be first remedied, while in all other affections, it is the deranged bodily **Váyu** which should be first curbed down or corrected. 95—96.

Indications of cure :—Non-emission of stool at the time of urination and the free emission of flatus (Váyu), as well as the rousing of the appetite, and the lightness of the abdominal cavity (Koshtha) are the **indications** of cure in a case of Udarámaya (Diarrhœa, etc.).* 97.

* The printed edition of Dallana's commentary says that these are the symptoms of cases of aggravated Atisára.

Static or Dynamic causes of Diseases and Treatment :—Some diseases are due to the dynamics of **Karmas** (deeds done by a man in the present or any prior existence), and some are due to the effects of deranged bodily **Doshas**, while there may be others which have their origin both in the dynamics of Karma and the necessary physiological (Doshaja) causes. Of these a Karma-origined disease may come on without any apparent exciting factor and it disappears with the extinction of its (Karma's) result effected by means of any remedial measure (e. g. penance, etc.) other than medical treatment, whereas as a **Dosha**-origined disease is conquered as soon as the involved deranged Doshas of the body are restored to their normal condition. Cases due to a slight derangement of the bodily Doshas but attended with a good deal of troubles as well as those due to the excessive aggravation of the Doshas but attended with only slight troubles should be attributed both to the physiological causes and to the dynamics of Karma, and these are cured only when both of these causes *viz.*, Karma and aggravated Doshas are removed. 98.

Grahani :—The **Grahani** (lit. the uppermost extremity or the receiving ducts of the intestines) is affected by the causes which produce dulness of appetite. The digestive fire of a patient is again deranged, even after * the subsidence of an attack of Atisára, if, with the dulness of appetite, he be still intemperate and injudicious in matters of food and drink. Hence the regimen of diet and conduct in a case of Atisára should be as laid down in connection with the

* The use of "अपि" in the text shows, say the commentators, that Grahani is possibie even without a previous attack of Atisára.

sequel of any purgative course (Virechana), until the deranged Doshas of the body would be completely restored to their normal condition, bringing in the natural health and strength in their train. The sixth Kalá which has been described as the Pitta-dhará Kalá (Pitta-containing sheath) is situated between Pakvás'aya and Ámás'aya (duodenum ?) is called **Grahani.** The strength of the organ of Grahani is dependent on the digestive fire (Agni) and the latter is situate in the former. Hence anything that impairs the digestive fire (Agni) necessarily affects the Grahani. 99-102.

The aggravation of one or all the bodily Doshas leads to the derangement of the Grahani into which the food taken is passed off in the shape of undigested fecal matter, or if it is digested, it sometimes produces constipation of the bowels and sometimes liquid motions accompained (in both cases) by pain and fetid smell. The disease is called **Grahani** (chronic diarrhœa ?) by experienced Physicians. 103.

Premonitory Symptoms :—Incomplete digestion, lassitude or a sense of physical langour, laziness, thirst, a sense of exhaustion, weakness, aversion to food, cough, ringing in the ears (Karna-Kheda) and rumbling sound in the intestines are the symptoms which mark the **premonitory** stage of the disease. 104.

Symptoms :—Swelling or œdema of the hands and of the feet, emaciation, pain at the joints, greediness, thirst, vomiting, fever, aversion to food, burning sensation, eructations of bitter, acid or fermented taste, or of those smelling of blood or smoke, water-brash, bad taste in the mouth and non-relish for food, as well an attack of Tamaka-S'vása (variety of asthma) are the indications of the developed stage of the disease (Grahani). 105.

Specific Symptoms of Grahani :—A case of the **Vátaja** type is accompained by a severe aching pain at the anus, thorax (Hridaya), sides, abdomen and the head. A case of the **Pittaja** type is marked by a burning sensation in the body, while the one of **Kaphaja** origin is characterised by a sense of heaviness in the limbs. A case of **Tri-Doshaja Grahani** exhibits symptoms belonging to all the symptoms of the three cases (Vátaja, Pittaja and Kaphaja types). The deranged bodily Dosha involved in a case imparts its characteristic colour to the finger-nails, eyes, face and excreta (stool and urine) of the patient. Thus it furnishes a **satisfactory** clue to the diagnosis of the disease, which, if neglected or unchecked at the outset, may usher in an attack of Hrid-roga (disease of the heart), Pándu (chlorosis), Udara (ascites, etc), Gulma, piles and enlargement of spleen. 106.

Treatment and Diet :—Appropriate emetics and purgatives should be exhibted (for cleansing the upper and lower parts of the body) in accordance with the aggravation of the Dosha or Doshas involved, and Peyás (gruels) and other articles of diet duly prepared with appetising drugs should then he prescribed in their due order. Therapeutic agents possessed of digestive, astringent and appetising virtue should then be employed through the vehicles of *Surá*, *Arishta* (wine), *Sneha* (oil or clarified butter), cow's urine, tepid water, or *Takra*. The use of Takra in the morning is in itself an excellent cure for the disease (Grahani). Remedies mentioned in connection with the treatment of worms in the intestines, Gulma, ascites or piles may also be adopted with benefit in the disease uuder discussion. The compound known as the *Hingvádi-churna*, or the medicated clarified butter described as remedial in a case of enlarged spleen, or the one duly cooked with the expressed juice of *Chángeri* and with the drugs of the *Mágadhádi* (Pippalyádi) group as Kalka may be likewise prescribed with beneficial results. Clarified butter duly cooked with four times as much curd (Dadhi) may also be used with benefit. Whatever is appetising (medicines, drugs and diet, etc.) would be beneficial in cases of Grahani. Complications (Upadrava) such as fever, etc. should be subdued with drugs not incomptible with the main treatment of nor in any way aggravative of the main disease. 107

Thus ends the fortieth chapter of the Uttara-Tantra in the Sus'ruta Samhitá which deals with the (symptoms) and medical treatment of Atisára.

CHAPTER XLI.

Now we shall discourse on the (symptoms and) medical treatment of Phthisis (**Śosha-Pratishedha**). 1.

Nomenclature :—Wasting or a general emaciation of the frame marks the sequel of and comes in as a premonitory symptom of an organic disease. Any cachectic condition of the body accompanied by a low lingering fever is called Kshaya. A correct diagnosis and a radical cure of the disease under discussion has baffled many a skilful physician. The disease is nameds **Śosha** from the fact of its consuming or drying up (Śosha—withering) the vital principles of the body such as Rasa—serum, etc. It is called **Kshaya** (wasting) since a wasting process is found to accompany all the functional activities of the body during its attack. Since the Moon-god, the king of the Bráhmanas, was the first to fall a victim to its attack, it is also called **Rája-yakshmá** (king's disease) † by some authorities. 2.

Some say that the disease is produced by the separate action of the three fundamental Doshas of the body. It being usually found to be attended with all

* The mythological origin of **Śosha** (Phthisis) is :—

The Moon-god married 27 daughters of Daksha of whom he was attached to Rohini in the extreme. Thereupon the personated wrath of his father-in-law, Daksha entered the Moon-god in the shape of Phthisis, whereby the body of the Moon-god began to emaciate. The Moon-god became penitent and the wrath of his father-in-law having been subdued at the intervention of the other gods, he managed to send down the personated Phthisis to earth to take possession of men indulging in any kind of excess and more particularly—**sexual excess**. The moon-god was then medically treated and radically cured by the celestial physicians, the twin As'wins.

† Cf. Scrofula which is now known as the "King's disease."

the eleven distressing symptoms which are manifested simultaneously with the ushering in of the disease, and being the only instance in the science of therapeutics in which the treatment does not vary according to the variation of symptoms. This disease, **Śosha**, is more properly said to originate in the simultaneous aggravation of all the three Doshas, and it is the symptoms of the most predominant Dosha only that are manifested. 3.

Ætiology and general symptoms:—The process of any wasting disease in the system, repression of any physical urging or propulsion, over-fatiguing physical exercise and irregular diet are the causes which, by aggravating the bodily Doshas and propelling them all over the organism, give rise to the disease. The aggravated Doshas with Kapha as the most predominant factor having obstructed the lymphatic channels, or the semen of a person having been exhausted by sexual excesses consequently produce a loss of the other Doshas or the principal elements of the organism, thereby producing a cachectic condition of the body, and the following symptoms, *viz*, aversion to food, fever, asthma, cough, emission of blood, loss of voice, numbering six in all are found in cases of Rája-yakshmá. 4—6.

Specific Symptoms:—The symptoms which mark the action of the deranged bodily **Váyu** in the disease are loss of voice (hoarseness), aching pain (in the chest), contraction of the sides and stoop at the shoulders (Amśa), while those which are exhibited through the action of the deranged **Pitta** are fever, burning sensation, Atisára and expectoration of blood, and the features which indicate the action of the deranged **Kapha** in the disease are a sense of fullness in the head, aversion to food, cough and a sense of the presence of a lump or plug in the throat (as if something is rising up). 7.

Prognosis :—A physician having an eye to his professional reputation or good name should not take in hand the treatment of a case of Śosha (Phthisis) whether marked by all the preceding eleven kinds of symptoms or attended with six of them *viz.* cough, Atisára, pain at the sides, loss of voice, aversion to food and fever, or accompanied by only three symptoms, *viz.* fever, cough and blood-spitting. 8.

Other causes of Śosha and their symptoms :—Sexual excess, grief, old age, over-fatiguing physical exercise, toils of journey, fasting, ulcers and ulceration of the Urah (lungs) are included by certain authorities within the exciting factors of this disease, Śosha. A case of Śosha due to sexual excess is attended with all the symptoms due to loss of semen and is marked by palour or yellowness of the complexion, the vital organic principles beginning with semen being wasted up in succession in their inverse order of enumeration. Constant brooding over the departed person, looseness of the limbs and all the symptoms of sexual excess other than the actual discharge of semen mark a case due to grief. A general cachectic condition of the body accompanied by imbecility of the mind, diminution of bodily strength, impaired functions of the sense-organs, laboured or difficult breathing (D. R. shivering of the limbs), aversion to food, a gong-like voice, expectorations marked by the absence of mucus (A. R. heaviness of the limbs), a general apathy to the concerns of life and (constant mucus) secretions from the ears, nose, eyes and mouth are the symptoms which indicate the origin of the disease in the natural and spontaneous waste of an extreme **old age**. 9–12.

A case due to the toils of journey or travel develops such symptoms as looseness of the limbs, flabbiness of the muscles, scorched or burntness of complexion, a haggard and cadaverous look, a gone-feeling in the limbs, the absence of natural gloss of the body and dryness of the mouth, throat and of the Kloma. These symptoms in addition to those of the ulcerated lungs (Urah-Kshata) without actual ulceration, characterise the type due to over-fatiguing physical exercise. 13–14

If a case of ulcer is attended by loss of blood, pain and difficulty in eating, it is turned to a case of Śosha and is pre-eminently the most uncurable type of the desease. Rupture or ulceration in the lungs (Urah-kshata) is caused by physical exercises, lifting up heavy loads, excessive and loud reading, a hurt or a blow, or excessive sexual congress and such other acts as require the active co-operation and entail excessive straining of the chest (Urah). They ultimately discharge blood and pusy secretions. Yellowish, black or purple coloured blood is expectorated or hawked out by coughing. A burning sensation is felt inside the region of the chest. A fetid smell is felt in the mouth and in the breath. The complexion of the body and the tone of the voice is changed and the patient becomes senseless from the excessive pain he suffers from. In certain cases the symptoms vary according to the varied natures of their exciting factors, and all the specific symptoms are not fully exhibited. Nevertheless these diseases also go under the denomination of Kshaya (consumption) owing to the fundamental vital principles of the body being equally consumed or withered up in them, and the specific mode of their treatment has already been explained before (Chapter XV, Sutra-Stháná). 15-17.

Premonitory Symptoms:—Laboured or difficult breathing, a gone-feeling in the limbs and a sense of physical lassitude, secretion of mucus, dryness of the palate, vomiting, dulness of appetite, vertigo or fainting fits, nasal catarrh, cough, somnolence, whiteness of the eyes, desire for meat, and increased sexual propensities are the symptoms which mark the advent of the dreadful disease—**Śosha**. The patient dreams that he has been borne on the wings of a crow or a parrot or a vulture or a pea-cock or has been riding a porcupine or a lizard or a monkey or sees in dreams river-beds dried up and trees dried up or fanned by gales of wind or surrounded by flames or fumes of fire. 18.

Prognosis:—A gradual wasting of the body inspite of sufficient food, presence of Atisára (diarrhœa) and swelling of the abdomen and scrotum are the symptoms of a comsumptive patient who should be given up. The treatment, however, of a patient temperate in his habits and strictly conforming to the instructions of the physician and possessed of a good digestive fire and not much reduced in body may be taken in hand provided the disease be an acute one. 19-20.

Treatment:—The patient should be made first to use the medicated clarified butter prepared from the milk of a ewe or a she-goat and duly cooked with the drugs of the *Sthirádi* (Vidári-gandhádi) group and then mild emetics and purgatives. Intestinal injections after the manner of an Ásthápana Vasti should follow the preceding medicinal measures and head-purgative (Śiro-vireka) should be applied. The diet should then be given consisting of (cooked) wheat, barley *S'áli-rice* together with meat-essence. Constructive tonics or tissue-builders (Vrimhana) should be given to a patient with a good digestion and relieved of all distressing symptoms or concomitants. Complications peculiar to the action of the deranged bodily Váyu generally mark a case due to sexual excess, wherein constructive tonics and remedial agents of Váyu-subduing virtue would be found to be extremely efficacious. 21—22.

Diet—meat, etc. :—The flesh of a crow or an owl or a mungoose or a cat or a *Gandupada* (earthworm) or a cormorant or a beast of prey (Vyála) or of any animal of the Vilesaya or Jángala class mixed with *Saindhava* salt and fried in mustard oil, should be prescribed in various ways for a patient laid up with Phthisis. The diet may also consist of *Mudga*-soup or of *Ádhaki*-soup or of the flesh of an ass, camel, elephant, mule or horse variously prepared and well cooked. Meat in combination with any Arishta as well as wine mixed with *Mádhvika* may also be given. 23.

Various articles of food made of barley-grains previously soaked in the alkaline water duly prepared with *Arka* and *Amritá* may likewise be prescribed. Clarified butter skimmed off from the milk of a ewe or a she-goat, may be given with gruel at the meal-time to an extremely emaciated patient. A compound consisting of *Tri-katu*, *Chavya* and *Vidanga* made into a paste with honey and clarified butter should be given to be licked up by a patient suffering from Phthisis. The use of a medicated clarified butter duly cooked with the essence of the flesh of any carnivorous animal and mixed with *Pippali* and honey as an after-throw proves remedial in a case of Phthisis. A lambative consisting of *Drákshá*, sugar and *Mágadhiká* pasted together with honey and oil proves efficacious as a cure for Phthisis A case of Phthisis would yield to the use of a lambative consisting of *Tila*, *Másha*-pulse and *As'vgandhá* ground to a fine paste with the addition of honey and clarified butter skimmed out of the milk of a she-goat, or of sugar, *As'vagandhá* and *Pippali* pounded together and made into a fine paste with the addition of honey and clarified butter. Milk duly cooked with the admixture of *As'vagandhá* may be prescribed as a constructive tonic. Butter skimmed out of the preceding preparation of milk and mixed with copious quantity of sugar should be taken, as an alternative, every morning and this should be then followed by a draught of milk. 24.

As'vagandhá, *Punarnavá* and *Yava* should be used in rubbing (Utsádana) the body of the patient. Clarified butter duly cooked with (the decoction of) the whole of a *Vásaka* tree (*viz.*, its roots, leaves, branches and barks) and with its flower (as Kalka) and mixed with an adequate quantity of honey* should be taken by a consumptive patient strictly conforming to the regimen of diet. Thus a virulent attack of Phthisis accompanied with cough, asthma and chlorosis would be speedily conquered. 25–26.

A wise physician should take equal parts of clarified butter, milk, decoctions of *Murvá*, *Haridrá* and of *Khadira* and the expressed liquid of the dungs of a cow, a horse, an elephant, a she-goat and a ewe. Ten equal parts of the above ten articles should be duly boiled and cooked together with the Kalka of powdered *Tri-katu*, *Tri-phalá*, *Devadáru* and the drugs of the sweet (Kákolyádi) group. This medicated clarified butter would be found highly beneficial in the cure of Phthisis (Yakshmá). 27.

Six Pátra measures of the duly prepared decoction of *Das'a-mula*, *Varuna*, *Karanja*, *Bhallátaka*, *Vilva*, the two

* This preparation is also found in the Charaka Samhitá though in different language under the treatment of Rakta-pitta.

kinds of *Punarnavá*, *Yava*, *Kulattha*, *Badara*, *Bhárgi*, *Páthá*, *Chitraka* and *Mahi-Kadamba* should be cooked with a Pátra measure of clarified butter and with (the Kalka of) *Vyosha* (Tri-katu), the milk of *Mahá-vriksha* (Snuhi), *Abhayá*, *Chavya*, *Devadáru* and *Saindhava* salt (D. R. Pippali). The medicated clarified butter thus prepared proves efficacious in cases of Phthisis, Ascites and Vátaja-Prameha. Clarified butter duly cooked with the milk, blood, meat-essence and the expressed liquid of the dungs of a cow, a mare, a ewe, a she-goat, a cow-elephant, a hind, a she-ass and a she-camel and with the Kalka of *Drákshá*, *As'vagandhá*, *Magadhá* and sugar proves extremely beneficial in cases of Phthisis. 28-29.

Eládi-mantha :—A Prastha measure of clarified butter should be duly cooked with the decoction of *Elá*, *Ajamodá*, *Ámalaka*, *Abhayá*, *Aksha*, *Gáyatri*, *Arishta*, *Asana*, *S'álasára*, *Vidanga*, *Bhallátaka*, *Chitraka*, *Ugrá**, *Tri-katu*, *Ambhoda* and *Suráshtrajá*-earth. When duly cooked it should be taken down from the oven and thirty Pala weight of candied sugar, six-Pala-weight of *Tugá-kshira* (Vams'a-lochana) and two-Prastha-measure of honey should be added to it and stirred with a laddle. A Pala weight of this preparation followed by a draught of milk should be given to be licked every morning to a Phthisical patient. The present elixir is possessed of ambrosial sanctity. The extent of its therapeutic application embraces such diseases of the body as Phthisis, chlorosis, fistula-in-ano, asthma, loss of voice, cough, troubles of the heart, enlarged spleen, Gulma and chronic diarrhea or indigestion. It imparts longevity to a person using it, leads to the expansion of his intellectual faculties and

* Chakradatta does not read Ugrá in the list.

tends to invigorate his eye-sight. It is the best of all rejuvenating preparations of our pharmacopea and no strict regimen of diet and conduct is required to be followed while it is used. 30.

The medicated clarified butter mentioned under the treatment of Plihodara (dropsy of the abdomen owing to the enlargement of spleen—Chapter XIII, Chikitsita-sthána) as well as the three others mentioned in that connection may be also used with advantage in the disease under discussion. The accompanying symptoms or complications such as hoarseness of voice, etc. should be remedied with appropriate medicines presented for those diseases in the S'ástras. The patient should be made to use regularly the milk, butter, urine, blood, meat and the (expressed liquid of the) dung of a goat as his bath or in any other way possible (e.g., in drinking) and to live in a goat-shed (in the company of goats) whereby he would be cured of his Phthisis in a month. A Phthisical patient should likewise be made to take *Rasona* (garlic) or *Nága-valá* or *Mágadhiká* or *S'iláјatu* with milk, in the prescribed manner (laid down in connection with the medical treatment of Mahá-váta-Vyádhi). 31-34.

Rules of conduct :—He should not allow any grief, anger or jealousy to disturb the equilibrium of his mind, should lead a life of strict continence, deal in the discussion of sublime subjects and conform to the injunctions of his medical advisers or physicians. He should pay respects to the gods, superiors and Bráhmanas and listen to the discussions of the spiritual truths from the lips of Bráhmans. 35.

Thus ends the forty-first chapter of the Uttara Tantra in the Sus'ruta Samhitá which deals with the (symptoms and) treatment of Phthisis.

CHAPTER XLII.

Now we shall discourse on the chapter which deals with the (symptoms and) medical treatment of Gulma **(Gulma-Pratisheda).** 1.

Definition and number of Gulmas :— The fundamental principles of the body, deranged and aggravated by their respective or specific exciting causes and factors tend to accumulate in the cavity of the abdomen (Koshtha) and help the formations of ball-like tumours or Gulmas (internal tumours inculsive of those known as the phantom tumours) somewhere inside the body lying between the extreme confine of the regions of the heart and of the bladder (Vasti). The Gulma is of **five** kinds and found to be round or spheroid in shape and may be either fixed or mobile (lit. shifting) in their character and subject to variations in their mass and size. 2.

Localisation and nomenclature :— They have **five locations** inside the abdominal cavity, *viz.* the two sides, the region of the heart, the bladder (Vasti) and the region of the umbilicus). The Gulmas are so named because their root or base cannot be exactly localised as well as their cause cannot be exactly ascertained owing to the fact of their having their origin in the aggravated condition of the local bodily Váyu, or because of their being but a agglomeration of the deranged bodily Doshas in the affected locality and the shrub-like large converse outline of the surface (Gulma-shrub). Since a Gulma, like a bubble of water, is a self-contained agglomeration of the deranged bodily Doshas and freely moves about in the cavity of its growth, it is not marked by the advent of any suppurative process in its mass or body. The Gulmas are the products of either the several or concerted actions of the three Doshas, while in females a separate class of tumours (such as the ovarian or uterine tumours) intimately connected with the deranged or vitiated condition of the **blood** (catamenial fluid, etc) is also recognised. 3—5.

Primonitory Symptoms :—A sense of lassitude, dulness of appetite, pain and rumbling in the intestines, suppression of stool, urine and flatus, incapacity to take food to the full, aversion to food, and an upward coursing of the internal Váyu are the indications whieh may be set down as the **premonitory** symptoms of Gulma. 6.

Specific Symptoms :—Pain (Śula) in the region of the heart and the belly (Kukshi), dryness of the throat and of the mouth, suppression of Váyu (flatus), irregularity of digestion and all other symptoms which specifically indicate the deranged condition of the bodily Váyu are the characteristics of the **Vátaja-Gulma**. Fever, perspiration, defective digestion, burning sensation, thirst, redness of the body (Anga-rága), bitter taste in the mouth and all other specific symptoms of the deranged Pitta mark the **Pittaja** type of the disease. A sensation of wetness all over the body, an aversion to food, lassitude, vomiting, water-brash, sweet taste in the mouth and all other specific indications of the deranged Kapha are exhibited in the **Kaphaja** type of the disease. The **Tri-doshaja** type exhibits the symptoms specifically belonging to each of the preceding ones and should be regarded as incurable. 7—9.

Symptoms of Raktaja-Gulma :—The symptoms of Raktaja-Gulma are mentioned below. The bodily Váyu of a woman newly delivered of a child as well as that of a woman who has recently miscarried, or of a woman in her courses is deranged by the use of unwholesome or injudicious food (and regimen of conduct), and by supressing the discharge of the blood (lochia) it gives rise to Gulma attended with pain and burning sensation. A Gulma of this type is easily mistaken for a case of conception, which exhibits all the symptoms of pregnancy as well as those which are peculiar to the state of the Pittaja type, with the exception that the abdomen does not enlarge and there is no movement (in the womb). The medical treatment of a Gulma of the present type should be taken in hand after the lapse of the natural term of gestation and this is known as the **Raktaja-Gulma** * by the experienced physician. 10.

General Treatment :—A person suffering from an attack of **Vátaja** Gulma should be duly treated with a Sneha, purged with any fatty purgative and then treated in the proper time with Nirudha and Anuvásana Vastis. In a case of **Pittaja** type of the disease, the patient should be treated (rubbed) with clarified butter duly prepared and cooked with the drugs of the *Kákolyádi* group and then being properly purged with the compounds of sweet drugs (of the Áragvadhádi group) he should be treated with Nirudha Vastis. In a case of the **Kaphaja** type, the patient should be first anointed with a medicated Ghrita duly cooked and prepared with the drugs of the *Pippalyádi* group, then purged with a strong (Tikshna) purgative and then treated with Nirudha Vastis of the same

* This Raktaja Gulma is peculiar to the females only. But some authorities are of opinion that a kind of Raktaja (blood-origined) Gulma due to the vitiated blood of the organism may be possible both in the males and females.

character. In a **Tri-doshaja** type, measures held to be remedial for each of the Doshas should be adopted or employed. Measures laid down in connection with the Pittaja type of the disease should be as well employed in cases of **Raktaja** (blood-origined) Gulma in female patients. Now hear me describe the recipes of the medicines which would particularly lead to the disintegration of the blood (in cases of Raktaja Gulma). Clarified butter duly cooked and prepared with the alkaline preparation of *Palás'a* wood (water charged with the burnt ashas of Palás'a) should be internally administered, and the medicated clarified butter known as the Pippalyádi Ghrita should be employed after the manner of an **Uttara-vasti.** In the alternative, the discharge (of blood) should be induced with the help of the drugs of heat-making (Ushna) potency (*e.g*, Pippalyádi group) and measures laid down in connection with menorrhagia (Asrigdara) should be adopted after the flow has fairly set in. 11.

Anuvásana :—The use of curd, clarified butter, oil, lard (Vasá) and marrow of Ánupa (such as boar buffalo, etc.) and Audaka (aquatic) animals, boiled together and applied after the manner of an **Ánuvásana-vasti,** proves beneficial in a case of **Vátaja**-Gulma. The application of similar Vastis charged with a solution of clarified butter and the lard of animals of the Jángala and Eka-s'apha groups proves efficacious in the **Pittaja** type of the disease, while the application of these containing solutions of oil and the marrow of any Jángala animal will prove beneficial in a case of the **Kpahaja** type*. 12-15.

* Dallana recommends the use of Váyu subduing, Pitta-subduing and Kapha-subduing drugs as Kalka in the preparation of these three Vastis respectively.

In a case of the **Vátaja** type of Gulma, the patient should be made to use the medicated Ghrita duly cooked with the expressed juice of *Ámalaka* and with the Kalka of the six drugs * and with the admixture of sugar and *Saindhava* (as an after-throw). 15.

Chitraka Ghrita :—Clarified butter duly cooked with curd, fermented rice-boilings (Kánjika) as well as with the decoction of *Vadara* and the expressed juice of *Mulaka* and with the Kalka of *Chitraka*, *Tri-katu*, *Saindhava*, *Prithviká*, *Chavya*, *Dádima*, *Dipyaka*, *Granthika*, *Ajáji*, *Habushá* and *Dhanyáka* taken in equal parts, proves curative in cases of **Vátaja** Gulma, Śula (colic), distention of the abdomen and dulness of appetite. 16.

Hingvádi Ghrita :—Clarified butter duly cooked with *Hingu*, *Sauvarchala-salt*, *Ajáji*, *Vit-salt*, *Dádima*, *Dipyaka*, *Pushkara*, *Vyosha*, *Dhanyáka*, *Amla-vetasa*, *Yava-kshára*, *Chitraka*, *S'athi*, *Vachá*, *Ájagandhá*, *Elá* and *Surasa* as Kalka and with the admixture of curd (Dadhi) as liquid, proves efficacious in a case of Vátaja Gulma, colic-pain and suppression of stool and urine. 17.

Dádhika Ghrita :—Clarified butter duly cooked with *Vit-salt*, *Dádima*, *Saindhava*, *Chitraka*, *Vyosha*, *Jiraka*, *Hingu*, *Sauvarchala-salt*, *Yava-Kshára*, *Kushtha*, *S'unthi*, *Vrikshámla* (turmerie) and *Amla-vetasa* as Kalka and with the expressed juice of *Vija-pura* and with curd weighing four times as much as of Ghrita, proves curative in cases of Gulma, enlargement of spleen and Śula. The clarified butter thus prepared is called **Dádhika-Ghrita**. 18.

Rasona Ghrita :—Clarified butter duly cooked with the admixture of the expressed juice of *Rasona*

* The six drugs to be used as Kalka are Pippali, Pippali-mula, Chavya, Chitraka, Nâgara and Yava-kshâra taken one Pala of each.

and with the decoction of (major) *Pancha-mula* as well as with wine (Surá), Áranála (fermented rice-boilings), curd, and the expressed juice of *Mulaka*, with the Kalka of *Vyosha*, *Dádima*, *Vrikshámla*, *Yamáni*, *Chavya*, *Saindhava*, *Hingu*, *Amla-vetasa*, *Ajáji* and *Dipyaka* (Ajamodá) taken in equal parts, includes within the range of its curative efficacy such diseases of the body as Gulma, Grahani (chronic diarrhœa), piles, asthma, insanity, consumption, fever, cough, epilepsy (Apasmára), dulness of appetite, enlargement of spleen, colic, and the derangements of the bodily Váyu. 19.

An Ádhaka measure each of curd, *Sauviraka* (a kind of Kánjika), clarified butter and the decoctions of *Mudga* and *Kulattha* pulse should be cooked with the admixture of two Pala weight of each of the following drugs, *viz.*, *Sauvarchala*, *Sarjiká*, *Devadáru* and *Saindhava*. The medicated Ghrita thus prepared proves curative in cases of Vátaja Gulma and acts as a good appetiser. 20.

Ghritas in Pittaja and Raktaja Gulmas :—Clarified butter duly cooked with the Kalka of the drugs or the *Jivaniya* (Kákolyádi) group and with the decoction of the component members of the *Trina-pancha-mula*, or of the *Nyagrodhádi* or of the *Utpaládi* group, would undoubtedly prove curative in cases of **Pittaja** and **Raktaja** Gulma. 21.

Ghritas in Kaphaja Gulma :—A Gulma of the Kaphaja type would surely yield to the use of medicated Ghritas duly cocked with the drugs of the *Dipaniya* (Pippalyádi) group as Kalka with the admixture (as liquid) of the decoction of the component members of either the Áragvadhádi group, the alkaline (Mushkakádi) group or the *Áragvadhádi* Gana, or with the officinal group of (animal) urines. 22.

A Gulma of the **Sánnipátika** type (due to the concerted action of all the three fundamental Doshas of the body) should be treated according to the predominance of any specific deranged bodily Dosha involved therein. The patient should be made to take at the proper time (*i.e*, as soon as the disease sets in) the pulverised compound known as the *Hingvádi-churna* or the medicated Ghrita known as *Tilvaka-Sarpih* or the one (*viz*. Shatpalaka Ghrita) which has been described as curative of the enlargement of the spleen, as these would prove curative in a case of Gulma. 23—24.

Internal use of Kshára :—Alkaline preparation should be duly made with the following drugs, *viz*., the ashes of (dried stems of) *Tila*, *Ikshuraka*, *Sarshapa* and *Yava* and of (the barks of) *Palás'a* and of *Mulaka* with the urines (weighing four times as much) of a cow, she-goat, ewe, she-ass and she-buffalo. This alkaline preparation should then be cooked in an iron vessel and on a slow fire with one Pala weight of each of the following pulverised drugs, *viz*, *Kushtha*, *Saindhava*, *Yashti-madhu*, *Nágara*, *Vidanga* and *Ajamodá* and with ten Pala weight of *Sámudra-salt* thereto added and, should be taken in the form of a lambative with one or the other of clarified butter, curd, wine, fermented rice-boilings (Dhányámla), warm water or the soup of *Kulattha*. The alkaline compound, thus prepared, undoubtedly proves curative in cases of Gulma and in the derangements of the bodily Váyu. Compounds consisting of *Sarjiká-Kshára*, *Kushtha* and the ashes of *Ketaki* taken with oil*, or of *Sarjiká-Kshára*, *Kushtha*

* According to Dallana, Sarjiká-Kshára, Kushtha and Yava-Kshára with oil would form the 1st compound and the Ketaká-Kshára with oil would form a separate compound.

and *Saidhava* taken with tepid water, would subdue an attack of the deranged bodily Váyu. 25–26.

Vris'chirárishta :—The drugs known as *Vris'chira*, *Uruvuka*, *Varshábhu*, the two kinds of *Vrihati* and *Chitraka* should be duly boiled together with a Drona-measure of water and taken down from the oven after three-fourths of the water are evaporated by boiling. It should then be poured into an earthen pitcher of which the interior has been previously coated with pastes of *Mágadhi*, *Chitraka* and honey. One Seer of powdered *Pathyá* and four Seers of honey shonld be subsequently added to its contents and the pitcher should be then kept buried in a heap of husks for ten days, after which it should be taken out and its contents should be given to the patient after the digestion of his daily food. The **Arishta** (fermented wine) thus prepared proves curative in cases of Gulma, indigestion and aversion to food. 27.

Powders of *Páthá*, *Nikumbha*, *Rajani*, *Tri-katu*, *Triphalá*, *Agnika* (*Chitraka*), *Saindhava*-salt and *Vriksha-vija* (Indra-yava) in equal parts should be taken with matured treacle of their combin d weight ; or the powders of the above drugs with pulverised *Pathyá* (weighing a fourth part only of the other powders taken together) should be cooked with cow's urine (weighing four times) to a thick consistency and made into pills which should be taken in an empty stomach (by the patient). These medicines would radically cure the cases of Gulma, enlarged spleen, indigestion, heart-disease, chronic diarrhæa and violent forms of chlorosis. 28.

Blood-letting :—Blood-letting by the application of leeches or by venesection should be effected in a case of elevated and immobile (unshifting) Gulma characterised by Śula, burning sensation, inflamation and piercing pain. 29

Diet and Sveda :—Drinks composed of the meat-essence of an animal of the Jángala group, profusely salted with *Saindhava* and mixed with clarified butter and *Tri-katu* and taken lukewarm are good for Gulma-patients **Peyás** prepared with the Váyu-subduing drugs and the soup of *Kulattha*-pulse cooked with a *Sneha* as well as the **Khada-yusha** prepared with *Pancha-mula* also are likewise efficacious as **Diet**. Draughts of milk with *Árdraka* should be prescribed in a case of Gulma attended with the suppression of stool and flatus. **Fomentation** (Sveda) after the manner of Kumbhika, Pinda and Ishtaka (see Chapter XXXII) Chikitsita Sthána) are also efficacious 30—32.

Purgatives preceded by the application of fomentation should be exhibited to a Gulma-patient, since it is extremely difficult to purge him. Vilepana (massage of the Gulma), application of unguents and poultices, Samdahana (cauterisation) as well as tepid fomentation after the manner of Śálvana-Sveda and the like are likewise applicable. Medicated Ghritas, powders and Vartis mentioned in connection with the treatment of Udara as well as medicated salts mentioned under the head Udarámaya* are likewise applicable in the present disease. 33—34.

Medicated **Plugs** or Vartis made of *Sámudra* †,

* Udarámaya may mean either indigestion or ascites. Anilámaya (Váta-vyádhi) is a variant addopted by Dallana and is undoubtedly preferable since there are several medicated salts *e. g.*, Patra-Lavana, Kánda-Lavana, in the treatment of Váta-Vyádhi. See Chap. IV, Chikitsita Sthána.

† According to some 'Sámudra' means Sámudra-salt and others, it means Samudra-Phena.

Árdraka, *Sarshapa* (mustard) and a profuse quantity of *Maricha* pasted together should be inserted into the rectum in suppression of stool and flatus in a case of Gulma. Arishtas made with *Danti* -roots, *Chitraka*-roots, or with theVáyu-subduing drugs according to the manner laid down in the Sutra-sthána should be prescribed, or the patient should be made to use the duly fried tender sprouts of *Putika* and *Nripa-Vriksha*. A Gulma patient with the upward coursing of his bodily Váyu should not be treated with Nirudha-Vasti. 35—37.

Compounds of *Trivit* and *S'unthi* or of treacle and powdered *Haritaki** as well as of *Guggulu*, *Trivit*, *Danti*, *Dravanti*, *Saindhava* and *Vacha* should be administered through milk, wine or the expressed juice of grapes, according to the strength (of the disease and of the patient). *Pilu* made into a paste and salted with the addition of *Saindhava* should also be similarly taken. Wine surcharged with *Pippali*, *Pippali*-roots, *Chavya*, *Chitraka* and *Saindhava* and taken at an opportune moment (*i. e.*, when attended with tympanities, etc.) would prove readily curative in a case of Gulma. A Gulma-patient afflicted with a suppression of stool and of flatus should take barley with milk or *Kulmásha* (Másha-cakes) profusely saturated with salt and clarified butter. 38–39.

Supervening Symptoms :—If S'ula which is its supervening symptom anyhow appears whereupon the patient suffers a kind of digging and piercing pain resembling that arising from the piercing of a dart, there will also appear the following distressing concomitants according to the Dosha or Doshas involved,

* According to some commentators the first two compounds should be taken with water.

viz., supression of stool and urine, difficult respiration, and numbness or stiffness of the limbs (in cases of aggravated **Váyu**), thirst, burning sensation, vertigo, ill-digestion of food, and excess of the colic pain (in cases of aggravated **Pitta**), and goose-flesh, aversion to food, vomiting, increase of pain after the taking of food and a sense of lassitude in the limbs (in cases of aggravated **Kapha**). The course of medical treatment in such cases should be determined by the nature and number of the deranged bodily Doshas specifically lying at the root and should be as follows. 40.

The following three compounds, *viz.*, (1) *Pathyá*, the three kinds of salt (Saindhava, Sauvarchala and Vit) *Yava-Kshára*, *Hingu*, *Tumburu*, *Pushkara*, *Yamáni*, *Haridrá*, *Vidanga* and *Amla-vetasa* ; (2) *Vidári*, *Triphalá*, *Satávari*, *S'ringáta*, *Guda-s'arkará* (Gángeri-phala), *Kás'mari-phala*, *Yashthi-madhu*, *Parushaka*, *Hima* (sandal wood) and (3) *Shad-granthá* (Vacha), *Ativishá*, *Deva-dáru*, *Pathyá*, *Maricha*, *Vrikshaka*, *Pippali-mula*, *Chavya*, *Nágara*, *Kshára* (Yava-kshára) and *Chitraka* should be respectively given in the Vátaja, Pittaja and Kaphaja types of the disease. The medium through which these compounds should be given would be tepid *Amla-Kánjika*, luke-warm milk and tepid water respectively. The preceding three compounds should be jointly administered in sets of two or three when two or three Doshas are involved in any case. 41.

Sprinkling (of water), baths, plaster (Pradeha) unguents and dietetic treatment should be similarly applied in Vátaja cases. Contacts with vessels filled with cold water should be applied in Pittaja cases, while the use of emetics, rubbing, fomentation (Sveda), fasting and other Kapha-subduing remedies should be recommended in Kaphaja types. Applications of Sneha and such-like remedial measures are specifically recommended in the disease, according to the Dosha or Doshas involved in each case. 42.

Prohibited articles :—A person suffering from Gulma, should refrain from taking Vallura (dried meat), *Mulaka* (radish), fish, dried pot-herbs, any preparation of pease, *Áluka*, (potato of any kind) and any kind of sweet fruit. 43.

Causes and symptoms of Śula :—Now I shall deal with the causes, the characteristic symptoms and the treatment of **Śula** occurring in any specific locality of a Gulma even without its actual presence or formation therein. A voluntary retention of flatus (Váta), stool or urine, over-eating, indigestion, eating before the digestion of previous food, over-exertion, use of articles of food which are incompatible in their combination, drinking water when hungry, use of germinated grains, dry food or cakes of dry meat, as well as the use of other such-like articles of fare, derange and aggravate the bodily Váyu, which produces a violent cutting and spasmodic pain (Śula) in the main cavity of the trunk (Koshtha). The patient complains of as if being pierced with a Śamku (spear) in the inside and of a feeling of suffocation under the influence of that excruciating pain, which fact has determined the nomenclature of **Śula** (lit.—a spear). 44—45.

Vátaja Śula :—The patient experiences a violent colic whenever in an empty stomach and he feels a difficulty of respiration. The limbs seem to be numbed or stuffed and the flatus, stool and urine are evacuated with the greatest difficulty—these are the symptoms which mark the **Vátaja** type of the disease. 46.

Pittaja Śula :—Thirst and a burning sensation in the body attended with an excruciating pain, giddiness, loss of consciousness, desire for cold things and amelioration on application of cooling measures, are the specific features of the **Pittaja** type. 47.

Kaphaja and Sánnipátika Śulas :—An agonising pain attended with nausea, excessive fullness of the stomach and a sense of heaviness in the limbs are the indications which distinguish the **Kaphaja** type of the disease. The type due to the concerted action of the three simultaneously deranged Doshas of the body (**Sánnipátika Śula**) exhibits all the series of symptoms which respectively mark the preceding types, and hence it is said to be incurable. 48–49.

General treatment :—The symptoms have been described. Now hear me describe the mode of medical treatment (to be generally pursued in curing a case of Śula) Since the deranged bodily Váyu (which is the principal and immediately exciting factor, is very active in its operation, hence it should be speedily subdued. Fomentations with *Páyasa*, *Kris'ará* or cooked meat saturated with any Sneha (clarified butter, etc.) should be resorted to. Fomentation naturally gives relief to a patient suffering from Śula. The patient should take cooked *Trivrit*-leaves (as pot-herbs) with his meals cooked with a Sneha (clarified butter) and served hot ; or he should eat the tender sprouts of *Chiravilva* fried with oil, or drink the meat-essence of the flesh of any birds of the Jángala group charged with a Sneha, or take the meat of any animal of the Viles'aya group. 50.

Treatment of Vátaja Śula :—*Surá*, *Sauviraka* (fermented rice boilings), *S'ukta*, the cream of curd and *Udas'vit* (half-diluted Takra) saturated with *Kála-salt* *, should be taken in a case of **Vátaja** Śula. The

* Kála Lavana generally means 'Vit-salt', but here, according to Dallana, it means 'Sauvarchala-salt'.

soup of *Kuluttha* with an adequate quantity of the acid articles (e. g. pomegranate, etc.) and cooked with the soup of *Láva* bird salted with *Saindhava* and seasoned with pepper, exercise a curative efficacy in a case of the Váyu-origined type. The compound of *Vidanga*, *S'igru*, *Kampilla*, *Pathyá*, *S'yáma*, *Amla-vetasa*, *Surasá*, *As'va-karna* and *Sauvarchala* should be taken with wine in an attack of the Vayu-origined type of Śula. 51—52.

A pulverised compound consisting of *Prithviká*, *Ajáji*, *Chaviká*, *Yaváni*, *Vyosha*, *Chitraka*, *Pippali*, *Pippala-mula* and *Saindhava* pounded together should be taken with milk or *Kámbalika* or *Madhvásava* (wine of honey) or *Chukra* or *Surá* (wine) or with *Sauviraka* (fermented rice-boilings) as alternatives. The above pulverised compound should be soaked in the expressed juice of *Mátulunga* and with the decoction of *Badara* several times after the manner of Bhávaná saturation, and the compound should be taken with a profuse quantity of *Hingu*, and with sugar. A Varti made of the same powders and pulverised (pith of) *Dádima* wood mixed together should be licked with treacle or honey or taken with wine in cases of Vátaja Śula as giving an instantaneous relief. 53.

In a case of Śula due to hunger, light and sparing diet should be given with lukewarm milk, *Yavágu* or meat-soup charged with clarified butter. Emulsive diet should be given in a case of Vátaja Śula to a patient of dry or parched organism, use of well seasoned Ghrita-puras being specially recommended. The patient should also take Váruni wine wherefrom he will get relief. 54—55.

Treatment of Pittaja Śula :—The treatment of Vátaja Śula has been described above. Now I shall narrate the therapeutic agents and remedies in respect of **Pittaja-S'ula**. A person afflicted with an attack of the present type of the disease, should be made to vomit without any violent effort by drinking (a stomachful of) cold water. He should have recourse to cooling measures and avoid all heat-making ones. Vessels of copper, silver, or precious stones and cooling gems and filled up to the brim with water, should be placed upon the seat of affection (S'ula) in his body. Treacle, barley, *S'a'li* rice, milk, (draughts of, clarified butter, purgatives, the flesh of any Jángala animals—these should be prescribed in cases of Pittaja S'ula. All Pitta-generating articles should be avoided and those which soothe the Pitta should be used. The soup of the meat of Jángala animals may be taken with sugar as an alternative. *Parushaka*, grapes, dates and aquatic fruits such as *S'ringa'taka*, etc., should also be taken with sugar as they tend to relieve Pittaja S'ula. 56.

Treatment of Kaphaja S'ula :—A fit of S'ula due to the action of the deranged Kapha is aggravated just after eating. Vomiting should be induced in such a case with draughts of the decoction of *Pippali**. Dry fomentations and other heating measures should be likewise resorted to and the patient should be made to take *Pippali* and *S'unthi* (in any shape) in cases of Kaphaja S'ula. *Páthá*, *Vachá*, *Tri-katu*, and *Katuka-rohini* should be used with the decoction of *Chitraka*, or the soup (of any S'ula-subduing article) should be taken with an equal part of *Arjaka*. 57–58.

Seeds and roots of *Eranda*, *Gokshura*-roots, *S'ála-parni*, *Pris'ni-parni*, *Brihati*, *Kantakári*, *S'rigála-vinná* (a kind of Prisni-parni), *Sahadevá*, *Mahásahá* (Máshaparni),

* Some commentators, according to Dallana, take Pippali to mean seeds of Madana-phala.

Kshudra-sahá (Mudga-parni) and Ikshuraka-roots should be duly boiled with a Drona measure (sixty-four seers) of water and should be boiled till reduced to a quarter part. This decoction should be used with the admixture of *Yava-kshára* *. By this compound attacks of Vátaja, Pittaja, Kaphaja and **Tri-doshaja** types of Śula would be thrown off just as the floating clouds are shattered and driven by the wind. *Pippali*, *Yava*, *Chitraka*, *Us'ira* and *Sarjiká-kshára* should be burnt together and reduced to ashes. Taken with tepid water, this compound proves curative in an attack of Kaphaja Śula. 59-60.

Symptoms of Párs'va-Śula :—The deranged Kapha in the regions of the Párśva (sides) arrests the course of local Váyu which thus irritated causes an immediate distention of the abdomen and a rumbling in the intestines. A pricking pain is felt in the affected part, which seems as if being pierced with needles, and the patient complains of insomnia and has no relish for food and his respiration becomes painful and difficult. The disease is named **Párśva-Śula** (side-colic) and is brought on by the action of the deranged Váyu and Kapha. 61.

Treatment of Párs'va-Śula :—A pulverised compound of *Pushkara*-roots, *Hingu*, *Sauvarchala*, *Vit-salt*, *Saindhava*, *Tumburu* and *Pathyá* should be taken with a decoction of barley in a case of (colic) pain at the sides, at the region of the heart and at the region of the bladder. The medicated Ghrita mentioned in connection with abdominal dropsy due to the en-

* The total weight of the drugs should be 8 seers, according to Dallana. According to others, however, it should be 12 seers. The preparation should be used in any shape both internally and externally *e. g.* a bath, washings, etc.

larged spleen, or clarified butter mixed with *Hingu* should be as well administered in such cases. *Vija-puraka-Sára** duly cooked in milk as well as draughts of castor oil mixed with wine, *Mastu*, milk or meat-soup (whichever of these may be conducive to the health of the patient) should be taken and the diet should be taken with milk or with the meat-soup of Jángala animals. 62.

Symptoms of Kukshi-Śula :—The deranged and aggravated bodily Váyu, affecting the fire of digestion and incarcerated in the region of the Kukshi (loins) interferes with the digestion of the food previously taken which remains stiff and undigested in consequence. The patient breathes heavily owing to the accumulation of undigested (fecal) matter and tosses about in agony of pain, finding no relief in any posture whatever, whether sitting or lying. The disease is called **Kukshi-Śula**, and is due to indigestion incidental to the action of the deranged bodily Váyu. 63.

Treatment of Kukshi-Śula :—Vomiting should be induced and fasting should be prescribed in the case according to the strength of the patient. Acid and appetising drugs should be employed for the alleviation of the Doshas (Váyu and Áma). A decoction of *Nágara*, *Dipyaka*, *Chavya*, *Hingu*, *Sauvarchala*, *Vit*, † and the seeds of *Mátulunga*, *S'yámá*, *Uruvuka*, *Brihati* and of *Kantakári*, should be taken for the relief of the pain (Śula). *Vachá*, *Sauvarchala*, *Hingu*, *Kushtha* *Ativishá*, *Abhayá* and *Kutaja*-seeds taken together would instantaneously relieve Śula. Purgatives should be administered, and Sneha-Vastis and Nirudha-Vastis should be applied for the amelioration of the deranged

* Vijapuraka-sára, according to Dallana, means the fruit of Vijapuraka. Vijaka-sára (the pith of Vijaka) is, however, a variant.

† Hingu, Souvarchala and Vit salt should be used as an after-throw.

Doshas according to their nature and intensity. Sneha-Sveda and poultices should be applied and *Dhányámla* (fermented paddy-boilings) should be employed as washes. 64–66.

Symptoms and treatment of Hrich-chhula :—The deranged bodily Váyu aggravated by the vitiated Rasa (chyle) and incarcerated in the region of the heart through the action of the deranged Pitta and Kapha, produces Śula (pain) in the heart and gives rise to difficulty of respiration. This disease which is called **Hrich-chhula** (cardiac colic) is ushered in through the action of the deranged Váyu and Rasa of the body. Remedial measures mentioned in connection with the treatment of the diseases of the heart should be as well employed in the present malady. 67–68.

Symptoms of Vasti-Śula and Mutra-Śula :—The local Váyu aggravated by the suppression of stool and urine is incarcerated in the region of the Vasti (bladder) and gives rise to a pain in the bladder, in the groins and about the umbilicus causing a further suppression of the stool, urine and flatus. The disease is called **Vasti-Śula** (bladder colic) and is due to the action of the deranged bodily **Váyu**. A cutting pain experienced in the genital, the intestines and the loins as well as at the sides and in the inguinal regions and about the umbilicus and causing a complete suppression of urine, is called **Mutra-Śula**. The disease should be likewise attributed to the action of the deranged bodily Váyu 69–70.

Symptoms of Vit-Śula :—The bodily Váyu deranged and aggravated by the use of dry food, etc., affects or impairs the digestive fire and obstructs the evacuation of feces accumulated in the bowels and gives rise to an excruciating pain in the locality by stuffing or choking the channels of the intestines. The pain is first experienced in the region of the right or left Kukshi (loin), but it soon extends over the whole abdomen with rumbling sounds therein. Thirst becomes unquenchable and vertigo and epileptic fits follow in its train, and the patient finds no relief even after the evacuation of the bladder and of the bowels. This disease is called **Vit-Śula** and is a very violent one. *71.*

Treatment :—An experienced physician should instantly employ (in such cases) the medicinal remedies which have the virtue of eliminating the deranged Doshas from the system. Fomentations, emetics as well as Sneha-Vastis and Nirudha-Vastis should be applied, and the bowel-cleansing compounds dealt with before should be administered. Medicinal measures mentioned in connection with the treatment of Udávarta should be likewise employed with advantage. *72.*

Symptoms of Annaja Śula :—A voracious eating in an impaired state of digestive fire, aggravate the local Váyu which makes the food taken remain stiffed in the Koshtha. The food thus undigested in the Koshtha causes an intolerable colic, which brings on a distension of the abdomen, epileptic fits, eructation, nausea and an attack of Vilambiká. The patient shivers, vomits, or passes stool, and even loses consciousness. Anti-colic (pain-killing) pills, powders and medicinal Ksháras are recommended in the case. All the medical remedies applicable in cases of Gulma should likewise be applied in cases of Śula. *73—74.*

Thus ends the forty-second chapter of the Uttara-Tantra in the Sus'ruta Samhitá which deals with the medical treatment of Gulma.

CHAPTER XLIII.

Now we shall discourse on the chapter which deals with the (symptoms and) medical treatment of the disease of the heart **(Hridroga-Pratishedha).** 1.

Etiology and Nomenclature :—The deranged Doshas of the body, aggravated by such causes as voluntary repression of any natural urging (of stool, urine, etc.), external blow or hurt, use of extremely dry (Ruksha) and heat-making articles of fare in inordinate quantities or of such articles as are indigestable or are incompatible in combination or are uncongenial to the system as well as taking food before digestion, contaminate the bodily Rasa (lymph chyle) and find lodgement in the heart, producing the characteristic pain in the organ, which is known as **Hridroga** (the disease of the heart). The disease may be divided into **five** distinct types, of which four are Dosha-origined, (*viz.*—Vátaja, Pittaja, Kaphaja, Sánnipátika) and the fifth is due to the presence of worms (Krimi). The different symptoms should be first described and then the medical treatment thereof. 2-3.

Specific symptoms :—In the **Vátaja** type, a pain is felt in the region of the heart which seems as if being drawn and crushed, pierced and cracked, pricked and split. Thirst with a burning sensation, a gone-feeling and a sucking pain in the heart, epileptic fit, perspiration, fumy eructation and dryness of the mouth, are the symptoms which characterise the **Pittaja** type. A sense of heaviness in the chest, secretion of mucus (from the nose and the mouth), an aversion to food, feeling of numness (in the body), dulness of appetite and

34

a sweet taste in the mouth are the features which mark the **Kaphaja** type of the heart-disease. 4-6.

Krimija Hridroga:—Nausea, salivation (spitting), piercing and cutting pain (in the heart), dark vision, an aversion to food, a dull yellow hue of the eyes, as well as emaciation of the body (D. R. swelling) are the indications which point to the presence of worms (**Krimija Hridroga**) as the exciting factor of the disease 7.

Supervening symptoms:—Vertigo and a sense of exhaustion attended with a feeling of physical lassitude and emaciation of the body exhibit themselves as the distressing concomitants in all the cases, while the supervening symptoms of Kaphaja worms exhibit themselves in case of Krimija Hridroga also. 8.

Medical treatment of the Vátaja type:—In a case of the **Vátaja** type, the patient should be first treated with a Sneha and then made to vomit (out the contents of his stomach) with a draught of the decoction of *Dasá-mula* mixed with salt and a Sneha. After being purged he should be made to take a pulverised compound consisting of *Pippali*, *Elá*, *Vachá*, *Hingu*, *Yava-kshára*, *Saindhava*-salt, *Sauvarchala*, *S'uthin* and *Ajamodá* through the medium of the juice of (acid) fruits, fermented rice-boilings, decoction of *Kulattha*, curd, wine, Ásava or with any kind of Sneha. The patient should be made to have his meal of matured *S'áli* rice, with the soup of any Jángala meat cooked with clarified butter. Oil duly cooked with the Váyu-subduing drugs should be applied as a Vasti in an adequate quantity in the case. 9.

Treatment of Pittaja type:—In a case of **Pittaja-Hridroga**, vomiting should be induced with the decoction of *S'ri-pari*-fruit, *Yashti-madhu* and *Utpala* (D. R.—treacle) mixed with honey and sugar. Clarified butter duly cooked with the drugs of the *Madhura* group, as well as the decoction efficacious in Pittaja-fever, should be internally administered. The food of the patient should be prescribed with the soup of the flesh of the principal animals of the *Jángala* group cooked with clarified butter, and he should then be treated with a Vasti, charged with honey and oil duly cooked with *Yashti-madhu*. 10.

Treatment of Kaphaja type :—In the **Kaphaja** type of the disease, vomiting should be induced with the decoction of *Vachá* or of *Nimba* and the pulverised medicinal compound prescribed for the Vátaja type, should be adminstered. The patient should also be advised to take clarified butter with his food. A decoction of *Tri-phalá* or of the drugs of the *Phaládi* (Madana-phaládi—Sutra, Ch. XXXIX) or the *Mustádi* (Sutra, Ch. XXXVIII) group, should be prescribed for internal use, or the patient should be purged with clarified butter mixed with powdered *S'yámá* (Vriddha-dáraka) and *Trivrit*. A physician skilled in the art of applying Vasti should prescribe a Vasti charged with Valá-oil under the circumstances. 11.

Treatment of Krimija type :—In the type (**Krimija**) characterised by the persence of worms, the patient should be first treated with a Sneha. A meat-diet with curd or (fried and) powdered sesamun should then be given to the patient for three days in succession after which he should be purged with the compound of *Ajáji* and sugar mixed with the salt-predominating* purgative preparation (see—Sutra,

* Some read "Su-pala-lair-jogaih" in place of 'Salava-nair-jogaih'. It would mean that the compound should be mixed with fried and powdered sesamum.

XLIV.) and mixed with the scented drugs (mentioned in the Sutra-sthána, Ch. XLIV). An adequate quantity of fermented-rice boilings (Dhányámla) with a profuse quantity of *Vidanga* should then be internally administered, whereby the worms would be dislodged from the hearts (and expelled through the lower orfices of the body). A dlet consisting of cooked barley grains saturated with powdered *Vidanga* should then be given to the patient. 12.

Thus ends the forty-third chapter of the Uttara Tantra in the Sus'ruta Samhitá which treats of the (symptoms and) treatment of Hridroga.

CHAPTER XLIV.

Now we shall discourse on the chapter which deals with the (symptoms and) medical treatment of Jaundice, etc. (**Pándu-roga Pratishedha**). 1.

Etiology and Nomenclature:—The deranged bodily Doshas of a person addicted to sexual excesses* or to eating clay or salts or articles of keen potency and of acid or saline taste or to strong liquors in excessive quantities or to sleeping in the day, contaminate the blood and produce a yellowish (Pándu) colour of the skin. This is known as Pándu-roga and is divided into **four** distinct types † according as they are severally originated through the action of the deranged Váta, Pitta, or Kapha, the fourth being the one incidental to their concerted action. The disease has got the name of **Pándu-roga** from the fact that a deep yellow (Pándu) colour is imparted to the skin of the patient suffering therefrom. 2

Premonitory symptoms:—Cracking of the skin, salivation (spitting) a sense of lassitude in the limbs, (desire for) eating clay, swelling of the eyelids, yellow colour of stool and urine, and indigestion are the premonitory symptoms which usher in an attack of Pándu-roga. The diseases known as Kámalá-Pálaki-Pándu (popularly called Kámalá), Kumbha-Kámalá,

* Mádhava in his Nidána reads "Vyáyáma" (physical exercise) in the place of "Vyaváya" "sexual enjoyment." Charaka, however, includes both "Vyaváyá" and Vyáyáma" in the long list of the causes of Pándu-roga.

† A variant reads that Pándu-roga is of **eight** kinds. In that case the four different varieties of Pándu, separately mentioned below should be added to the four kinds mentioned here. Charaka says that Pándu-roga is of five different types:—by separating and adding the one due to the eating of clay to the four kinds enumerated here.

Lágharaka and Alasa (otherwise known as Halimaka) are all included within Jaundice (Pámdu-roga), the characteristic symptoms of which are fully enumerated in succession below. 3-4.

Specific Symptoms:—A black colour of the eyes and of the skin marked by the prominent appearance of black-coloured vein (on the surface), black colour of the stool and of the urine, blackness of the face and of the finger-nails as well as other symptoms characteristic of the deranged bodily Váyu are manifested in the **Vátaja** type of Pándu. Yellowness of the eyes and of the skin marked by the appearance of veins (Śirá) of the same colour (on its surface), yellowness of the stool and of the urine, yellowness of the face and finger-nails and other specific symptoms of the deranged Pitta, mark the **Pittaja** type of the disease. Whiteness of the eyes and of the skin, marked by the appearance of veins of the same colour (on its surface), whiteness of the stool and urine, whiteness of the face and of the finger-nails and other specific symptoms of the deranged Kapha mark a case of the **Kaphaja** type of the disease. All the preceding symptoms are exhibited in a case of the **Sánnipáta** type. Now I shall describe the symptoms which mark the disease known as Kámalá. 5-8.

The Pitta of a patient suffering from any disease not radically cured gets deranged by the use of any acid, or unwholesome food or drink, and imparts a (deep) yellow tint to his complexion and produces physical weakness as well as all the specific symptoms (of Pándu-roga) described above. This disease is known as **Kámalá**. When it is accompanied by a general swelling (edema) of the body and a crushing pain in the joints, is called **Kumbha-Kámalá**, which, when it developes in its course such symptoms as fever, aching pain in the limbs, vertigo, physical langour, drowsiness and emaciation comes to be known as **Lágharaka**. This, in its turn, when marked by an excessive preponderance of the deranged Váyu and Pitta is called **Alasa**, otherwise known as **Halimaka**, by those who are conversant with its nature. 9-12.

Supervening Symptoms :—Aversion to food, thirst, vomiting, fever, headache, dulness of appetite, swelling about the neck, weakness, epileptic fits, exhaustion and a pain in the region of the heart are included their distressing concomitants. 13.

General Treatment :—Having ascertained the curable nature of an attack of Pándu-roga, the patient should be treated with clarified butter *. He should then be purged and vomited with the compounds containing powdered *Haritaki* mixed with a copious quantity of honey and clarified butter. Clarified butter duly cooked with turmeric or the one known as Traiphala-Ghriita † as well as the one known as Tailvaka-Ghrita ‡ may also be used for the purpose. Drugs possessed of purgative properties should also be taken in combination with clarified butter (or clarified butter duly cooked with purgative drugs should be prescribed). Half a Pala (four Tolás) of *Nikumbha* duly cooked in an adequate quantity (eight Palas) of the urine of a she-buffalo should be daily used. Similarly half a Kudava measure of treacle mixed (D. R. duly cooked)

* Some say that the Sneha used should be the Kalyánaka-Ghrita (Ch. LXII.). Others says that simply matured clarified butter should be used.

† Traiphala-Ghrita may mean either the Ghrita duly cooked with Tri-phalá or the one known as Traiphala-Ghrita mentioned in.

‡ Similarly Tailvaka-Ghrita may mean the Ghrita of that name mentioned in Chap. V. Chikitsita-sthána or the one duly cooked with Tilvaka.

with pulverised *Haritaki* should be taken by the patient. A decoction of the drugs of the *Áragvadhádi* group, may be likewise prescribed for internal use. Powdered (dead) iron mixed with pulverised *Vyosha* and *Vidanga*, or powdered *Haridrá** and *Tri-phalá* should be licked up with honey and clarified butter.† Any other medicinal compound mentioned anywhere as remedial to Gulma should also be administered. 14.

The aggravated Doshas should be gradually eliminated from the system in as much as an quick and excessive elimination of the Doshas under the circumstances might produce swelling in the patient. Either the expresed juice of *Dhátri* or of sugar-cane, or a *Mantha*‡ should be taken with honey by a patient and he should take wholesome diet. 15-16.

Clarified butter duly cooked with the Kalka and decoction of the two kinds of *Vrihati*, *Rajani*, *S'ukákhyá* (*S'uka-s'imbi*), *Kákádani*, *Kákamáchi*, *Ádári-vimbi* and *Kadamba-pushpi* (*Bhumi-Kadamba*) should be taken as a remedy for **Pándu-roga**. *Pippali*-powder dissolved in milk should also be taken according to the condition of the appetite. The use of a decoction of *Yashti-madhu*, or of powdered *Yashti-madhu* mixed with honey would likewise prove efficacious. Powdered

* Here we have followed Dallana in the text. Some take Haridrá to mean Dáru-Haridrá.

† According to Charaka's recipe, however, we find that the two compounds here have been combined into one and there we find the definite mention of Dárvi (Dáru-haridrá). In our practice also we follow Charaka in this case.

‡ **Mantha** is prepared by mixing powdered grains of barley with clarified butter and a copious quantity of water. Some commentators, however, on the authority of other medical works, are of opinion that in cases of Pándu (jaundice) the word "Mantha" is technically used for the preparation of the powdered grains of barley mixed with the expressed juice of A'malaki and of sugar-cane and with honey.

leaves of *Tri-phalá* and powdered (dead) iron should be frequently taken as an electuary in combination with cow's urine. A compound composed of powdered coral, pearl, antimony and conch-shell, or powdered *Giri-mrittiká* (ferrugnious earth) should be similarly used by the patient. 17–18.

A compound consisting of half a seer of powdered goat's dung together with a Pala weight of each of the drugs known as *Vit*-salt, *Haridrá* and *Saindhava*-salt, should be licked with honey by a patient living on wholesome diet. A compound of *Mandure* (iron-rust), *Agni* (Chitraka), *Vidanga*, *Pathyá*, *Tri-katu* all taken in equal parts with *Tápya* (Svarna-mákshika) equal to their combined weight should be duly soaked in cow's urine and formed into a lambative with the addition of honey, the same being prescribed for an immediate cure of a serious type of Pándu-roga. 19–20.

Vibhitaka, *Mandura* (iron-rust), *Nágara* and *Tila* should be pounded together and made into a paste with the addition of a profuse quantity of treacle. Pills prepaied from this compound should be administered through the medium of *Takra* whereby a violent attack of jaundice would be defeated. Pills of the Kaláya weight of each of *Sauvarchala*, *Hingu* and *Kiráta-tikta* pasted together, should be taken wlth tepid water. As an alternative, a lambative compound of *Murvá*, *Haridrá* and *Ámalaka* pounded together and alternately dried and soaked in cow's urine for a week, should be given to be licked by the patient. 21–22.

A patient suffering from Pándu-roga should observe a proper regimen of diet and take two-Tolá-weight of the compound of the powders of *Valá* and *Chitraka* (with cow's urine or tepid water). The compound of *Saindhava* salt and powdered *S'igru*-seeds taken in equal parts should be taken with tepid water, followed by a meal of cooked rice with milk. The decoction of the drugs of the *Nyagrodhádi* group should be taken, when cold, with honey and sugar followed by a proper regimen of diet. Powders of the drugs included within the *S'ála-sárádi* group or of *Ámalaka* should be formed into a lambative with the addition of honey and given to be licked by the patient. 23-26.

The pulverised compound of *Vidanga*, *Musta*, *Triphalá*, *Ajamodá*, *Parushaka*, *Vyosha* and *Chitraka* as well as clarified butter, honey, sugar and treacle should be duly cooked in the decoction of the drugs of the *S'ála-sárádi* group till reduced to the consistency of a lambative. It should then be taken down and preserved inside a covered vessel prepared of Mokshaka (Mushkaka). This lambative proves curative in cases of Pándu attended with a general edema as well as in cases of the violent types of Kámalá. 27.

Treatment of Kámalá, etc :—*Tribhandi* (Trivrit) taken with sugar as well as *Gavákshi* or *S'unthi* taken with treacle, is beneficial to a patient suffering from an attack of Kámalá. Clarified butter duly cooked with *Káleya*-wood and mixed with turmeric as an after-throw is also efficacious. In the alternative the patient should take *Srotánjana* and *S'ilájatu* with cow's urine in a case of **Kumbha-Kámalá**. *Mandura* (rust of iron) kept immerged in cow's urine should be likewise taken with *Saindhava*-salt continually for a month. *Mandura* should be burnt in the fire of *Vibhitaka*-wood and cooled with cow's urine. The process should be repeated eight times in succession. The iron-rust thus tempered should be subsequently reduced to powders. Licked with honey it would act as a speedy cure in cases of Kumbha-Kámalá. 28-30.

Saindhava-salt once made red-hot by heating (in the fire of *Vibhitaka*-wood) should be cooled in cow's urine. Iron-rust (Mandura) should be successively heated in fire and cooled with cow's urine as directed above, the process being repeated many times. The two substances (Saindhava and iron-rust) thus prepared, (taken in equal parts) and made into a paste with (five times of) cow's urine, should be cooked on an oven, care being taken to guard against their ignition. When dried, the compound should be reduced to powder and taken with *Udas'vit* (a kind of Takra). The medicine acts as a good appetiser and proves curative in cases of Pándu. The patient using it should take his diet with *Takra* after the assimilation of the medicine. Clarified butter duly cooked with the expressed juice of *Drákshá*, *Guduchi* and *Ámalaki* proves curative in cases of **Lágharaka** 31.

Articles of Diet :—*Arishtas* and *Ásavas* prepared with treacle or with honey or with sugar or with cow's urine or with *Kshára* (alkali) as well as the essence of meat of any Jángala animal saturated with clarified butter and mixed with the expressed juice of *Ámalaka* or of *Kola* should be prescribed and meals of cooked barley grains or of *S'ali* rice and the preparations prescribed in cases of swelling (Śopha) should be daily taken by a patient suffering from an attack of Pándu-roga. 32.

Treatment of supervening Symptoms :—The supervening symptoms such as difficulty of breathing, diarrhœa, aversion to food, cough, epileptic fits, thirst, vomiting, colic pain, fever, swelling (Śopha), burning sensation in the body, indigestion, hoarseness, lassitude, etc. should be remedied on the principles laid down in the Śástras with due regard to the nature and intensity of the deranged bodily Doshas, severally lying at their roots. 33.

Prognosis :—If a patient afflicted with Pándu have an edematious swelling of the extremities with an emaciation of the abdominal region and *vice versa* or if he have a swelling of the scrotum or of the genitals or about the anus or if he be suffering from fever or diarrhæa or be lying in a sub-comatose state, he should be given up and should not be attended by a physician caring anything for his fame. 34.

Thus ends the forty-fourth chapter of the Uttara-Tantra in the Sus'ruta Samhitá which deals with the (symptoms and) medical treatment of Pándu-roga.

CHAPTER XLV.

Now we shall discourse on the Chapter which deals with the symptoms and) medical treatment of Hemorrhage **(Rakta-Pitta-Pratishedha).** 1.

Cause and Pathology :—Excessive indulgence in grief, fright or anger, excessive physical labour, exposure to the sun and fire, constant use of pungent, acid, saline and alkaline food, or, of articles of fare which are keen or heat-making in potency, or incompatible in their combination, or are followed by deficient gastric or intestinal digestion are the factors which tend to aggravate the Rasa (chyle), which, in its turn, aggravates the Pitta. The aggravated Pitta thus imperfectly assimilated affects or invades in virtue of its own essence the blood (lit. leads to its imperfect digestion) which finds an outlet through the upper or the lower channels of the body or through the both. The deranged blood accumulated in the Ámás'aya (stomach) finds out an upward outlet, while it flows out through the lower orifices in the event of its continuing in a similar state in the Pakvás'aya (intestines), and it escapes through both the upward and downward orifices in the event of its being deranged and accumulated in both the Ámás'aya and the Pakvás'aya. According to several authorities, the ejected blood in the disease comes from the spleen and the liver. 2.

Prognosis : - A case of Rakta-pitta in which the blood finds outlet through an upward channel of the body is amenable, while palliation is all that is possible in a case in which it fiowes out through a downward orifice of the body. A case marked by the emission of blood through both these outlets, upward and downward, should be regarded as incurable 3.

Premonitory Symptoms :—A sense of lassitude in the limbs, desire for cooling things, a sense as if fumes are rising in the throat, vomiting and fetor of blood in the breath are the symtoms which usher in an attack of Rakta-pitta. The number of the cases of Rakta-pitta as well as the aggravation of the different Doshas involved in each case should be ascertained from the colour and nature of the ejected blood (as described before in Chap. XIV-Sutra-sthána). 4-5.

Supervening Symptoms :—Weakness, laboured breathing, cough, fever, vomiting, mental aberration (lit : a state like intoxication), yellowness of complexion, burning sensation in the body, epileptic fits, acidity of the stomach,restlessness, extreme pain in the region of the heart, thirst, loss of voice (D. R. loose stool), heat in the head, fetid expectoration, aversion to food, indigestion and absence of sexual desire (D. R. bending of the body after sexual act) are the usual **complications** in a case of Rakta-pitta. 6.

Symptoms of Incurable Types :—In a case of Rakta-pitta the emitted matter resembling the washings of meat or drug-decoction, or turbid water or fat or pus, or being liver-coloured or dark-black or blood-red in colour or looking like a ripe *Jambu*-fruit or blackish blue or variously coloured like a rain-bow or having a very fetid smell as well as the presence of the above mentioned supervening symptoms—these are the indications which show that the case should be given up as incurable. 7.

General Principles of Treatment :—It is improper to arrest the emission of blood immediately at the outset of the disease if the patient be a sufficiently strong man, in as much as such a procedure may bring on an attack of * Pándu-roga, Grahani, Kushtha (cutaneous diseases), Gulma, or fever or enlargement of the spleen. An attack in which the blood makes a downward course should be arrested with **emetic** medicines, while **purgatives** should be exhibited in a case in which the blood finds an upward course. But weak patient, under the circumstances, should be treated in both cases with **soothing** remedies. Fasting should be first enjoined in the case of an **excessive** emission † of blood in respect of a strong patient with an unimpaired digestion and an unemaciated frame. A Peyá prepared with a small quantity of rice should be given to the patient after fasting ‡. Tarpana measures, decoctions of digestive drugs, as well as a variety of medicinal lambatives and Ghritas should be the proper applications in the disease under discussion. Purgation should be induced with the compound of *Drákshá*, *Yashti-madhu*, *Kás'marya* and sugar, while vomiting should be induced with an emetic compound consisting of *Yashti-madhu* mixed with honey. 8—11.

Articles of Fare:—The use of milk, the drugs of cold-producing potency (e g. the drugs of the Utpaládi group), essence of the meat of an animal of the Jángala group, soup of *Satina* (cerials), *S'áli*-rice, *Shashtika*-grains, leaves of *Patola*, *S'elu*, *Sunishanna*, *Yuthiká*

* Both Chakrapáni and Vrinda read "हृत्पाण्डुग्रहणी etc." *i.e.*, they say that it may bring on an attack of heart-disease also.

† Both Chakrapáni and Vrinda read "ऊर्द्धं प्रवृत्तदोषस्य" i.e. in cases of upward emission. There is also another variant "ऊर्द्धं प्रवृद्धदोषस्य" i.e. in cases of excessive upward emission or in cases where a good deal of the vitiated Doshas takes an upward course.

‡ Additional Text :—Meat-essence (Rasa) and soup (Yusha) seasoned with clarified butter prepared from cow's milk.

and *Sindhuvára* (Nirgundi) as well as the tender sprouts of *Vata* and *Atimuktá* (Tinduka) as pot-herbs and cooked with clarified butter are recommended as diets. Soup of the meat of pigeons, *S'amkha* (conch) and tortoise as well as the gruels mentioned before mixed with the expressed juice of *Dhátri* and pomegranate and with a profuse quantity of clarified butter should be given to the patient as diet. Milk should be duly cooked in combination with the drugs of the *Utpalâdi* group, and the cream therefrom should be likewise prescribed with a copious quantity of honey and sugar. Cold Pradehas, honey, sugar, and clarified butter are said to be beneficial in cases of Rakta-pitta. 12—13.

An experienced physician should prescribe any one of the four lambatives composed of the powders of the flowers of *Madhuka*, *S'obhánjana*, *Kovidára* or of *Priyangu*, mixed with honey to be licked up by a patient suffering from Rakta-pitta. Similarly lambatives of *Durbá*, or the tender leaves of *Vata*, or of white *Karnika* pasted together with the honey should be given to be licked up by the patient*. Dates and other friuts of the same therapeutic virtue, taken with honey, would prove efficacious in the disease. 14—15.

Medicinal compounds mentioned in connection with the treatment of Raktâtisára (blood-dysentery) may be as well employed with advantage in the present instance. A piece of sugar-cane devoid of its skin and crushed should be kept immersed in cold water contained in a new earthen pitcher. The picther with its lid off should be kept in an open place for a night. Its contents duly strained in the morning should be given with powdered *Utpala* and honey to a patient suffering from

* Dallana takes only Durbá and Vata under one *recipe*. Some commentators would prescribe all these together under one *recipe*.

Rakta-pitta. A cold infusion of *Jámbu, Ámra* and *Arjuna* should be taken with honey. As an alternative, the expressed juice of *Udumbara* fruit should be taken (with honey). 16—A.

The best six Yogas :—A paste (Kalka) of *Trapusi*-roots in combination with honey and washings of rice or two Tolás of the pasted *Yashti-madhu* should be taken (with the same vehicles). A compound consisting of *Chandana, Yashti-madhu,* and *Rodhra* taken in equal parts or *Karanja*-seeds made into a paste with sugar and honey should be similarly used In a similar way, the pith of *Ingudi* together with *Yashti-madhu* should be taken. As an alternative, salt (Saindhava) and *Karanja*-seeds turned into a paste with curd-cream should be taken lukeworm for three days in succession by a person suffering from an attack of Rakta-pitta. The six preceding medicinal compounds act as excellent cures for the disease under discussicn. 16.

Pathyá should be employed as an errhine after the manner of Avapida-Nasya in the event of the blood passing through the nostrils. In case of excessive hæmorrhage (in the disease) the patient should drink blood in combination with honey, or eat a goat's raw liver with the bile. 17.

Clarified butter duly cooked with the admixture of an adequate quantity of the expressed juice of (the bark of) *Palás'a* trees should be taken, when cool, in combination with honey, or clarified butter prepared by churning the milk duly cooked with the expressed juice of (the bark of) the *Vanaspati*-trees (Vata, etc.) should be used with sugar. A Pala weight of each of *Drákshá, Us'ira, Padmaka* and sugar should be kept immersed in cold water during the (whole) night. This cold infusion would cure a case of Rakta-pitta. A draught of milk with an equal quantity of water is also recommended for a patient comforming to a proper regimen of diet and conduct. 18.

The watery secretion of the dung of a horse or a bull should be taken with honey and sugar. In the alternative, powders of the seeds of *Vástuka* or (of the roots, of *Tanduliyaka*-plants should be licked with honey. A lambative formed of Lája (parched paddy) and *Anjana* * mixed with honey, or powdered *Tugá-kshiri* mixed with honey and sugar should be licked. A patient suffering from an attack of Rakta-pitta should take a compound of *Drákshá*, *Tikta-rohini*, *Yashti-madhu* and sugar with cold water, or lick a compound of pulverised *Pathyá*, *Ahinsrá* and *Rajani* with clarified butter. 19.

The compound of (blue), *Utpala Sourásthra mrithiká* (red earth), *Priyangu*, *Lodhara*, polens of lotus and sugar mixed together and taken with honey and a decoction of *Vásaka* would speedily stop the emission in a virulant type of Rakta-pitta. Similarly a compound consisting of flowers of *Khadira*, *Jambu*, *Arjuna*, (red) *Kovidára*, *S'irisha*, *Lodhra*, *Asana*, *S'álmali* and *S'igru*, pounded together and mixed with honey should be licked by the patient in a case of Rakta-pitta. 20—21.

The alkaline water prepared with the ashes of *Indivara* and taken with honey, powdered *Karanja*-seeds taken with honey and clarified butter and the decoction of *Jambu*, *Arjuna* and *Ámra*—these three compounds prove curative in cases of Rakta-pitta. A paste made of the roots and flowers of *Mátulunga* should also be taken with the washings of rice. 22—23.

* Kálánjana is a variant, in place of Lája and Anjana. For Kálánjana Dallana reads Souviránjana. This should be the proper reading because there is a word in the receipe which shows that there will be only one thing and not two.

A solution of milk or water saturated with sugar should be applied into the nostrils in the event of bleeding from the nose. The expressed juice of grapes, clarified butter prepared by churning milk or the expressed juice of sugar-cane should be taken cold (through the nostrils) in combination with sugar *. All cooling measures and sweet-drugs should be employed in the present disease 24—25.

Ásthápana and Anuvásna :—The application of an Ásthápana-Vasti charged with milk duly cooked with the drugs of the *Vidári-gandhádi* group and mixed with honey, clarified butter, sugar and *Drákshá*, proves extremely efficacious in the disease under discussion. The application of an Anuvásna-Vasti charged with clarified butter * would be attended-ded with equal benefit. The drugs known as *Priyangu, Lodhra; Souviránjana, Gairika, Utpala, Suvarna-gairika, Káliyaka,* conch-shell, *Chandana,* sugar, *As'va-gandhá, Ambuda, Yashti-madhu, Mrinála* and *Sougan-dhika,* taken in equal parts, should be pounded together and mixed with copious quantities of milk, honey and clarified butter. This solution should be injected into the rectum after the manner of Nirudha-Vasti. The patient should be sprinkled with cold water and given his diet with milk after which clarified butter duly cooked with *Yashti-madhu* should be injected into the rectum of the patient after the manner of Anuvásana-Vasti. This measure proves extremely beneficial in cases of **down-coursing** Rakta-pitta and violent types of blood-dysentery. In the case of an excessive discharge of

* S'rikantha Datta, the commentator of Vrinda, would mix sugar with the juice of sugar-cane only and not with the other two. All these should be applied into the nostrils.

blood, if the patient be strong enough, vomiting should be induced after the cessation of the blood-discharge. 26-27.

Urethral-injections composed of the aforesaid drugs should be applied (after the manner of **Uttara-vasti**) in the event of bleeding from the bladder. Measures laid down in connection with the treatment of Rakta-pitta should be resorted to in cases of bleeding-piles. In cases of menorrhagia as well as in cases of excessive bleeding incidental to any surgical operation, the above measures (of the medical treatment) should be adopted by an experienced physician. The subsequent treatment of the cases should be determined by the nature and intensity of the deranged bodily Doshas as well as of the blood involved therein. 28–29.

Thus ends the forty-fifth chapter of the Uttara-Tantra in the Sus'ruta Samhitá which deals with (the symptoms and) the medical treatment of Rakta-pitta.

CHAPTER XLVI.

Now we shall discourse on the chapter which deals with (the symptoms and) the medical treatment of fainting fits **(Murchchhá-Pratishedha).** 1.

Defination :—The deranged and aggravated Doshas of the body of a person who is emaciated or accustomed to the use of incompatible articles of food or who has become very weak on account of a sudden suppression of his natural urgings or of any external blows or injury give rise to fainting fits. The deranged bodily Váyu, etc. choking up the sense-carrying nerves of the body, produces that giddy state in a patient in which the world seems to vanish from the eyes of the afflicted person and the perception of the pleasure or pain is suspended for the time being. The patient, in consequence of this suspension of the sense-perception drops down insensible as a log of wood and this disease is called **Murchchhá** or **Moha**·(fainting). It admits of being divided into **six** kinds or types according as an attack is due to the action of the deranged **Doshas** separately or to that of **blood, wine** or **poison**, but a predominance of the deranged **Pitta** may be detected in all forms of the diseases due to any cause whatever. 2.

Premonitory Symptoms :—Pain or oppression of the heart, yawning, lassitude, loss of consciousness and of strength are the symptoms which usher in an attack of the disease (Murchchhá) according to the nature of the deranged bodily Dosha lying at its root. 3.

The natural elements, water (Ap) and earth (Kshiti) abound with the attribute of Tamas (insensibility). A smell of blood also contains the same attribute, Tamas.

It is therefore that persons generally lose their consciousness at the smell of blood. Several authorities hold that the loss of consciousness in these instances happens in virtue of the natural properties of the thing itself, *viz.*, blood, wine and poison which also possess these properties in a greater degree and it is therefore that an use of either of these substances suspends animation and produces Moha (fainting). 4-5.

Symptoms:—A case of Murchchhá (fit of unconsciousness) due to the effects of (deranged) **blood** is characterised by stiffened condition of the limbs and by the fixedness of the eyes (Drishti) and by deep breathing. Delirious talks, mental aberration and the state of the patient convulsively lying flat on the earth until the wine is perfectly assimilated into the system are the symptoms of a case of Murchchhá due to the effects of **wine**; while shivering, drowsiness, thirst and numbness of the body) attended with the specific symptoms of poisoning form the general characterstics of the type due to the effect of **poison**. 6.

General Treatment:—Constant sprinkling of water over the body (water-spray) plunge-bath in cold water, contact of cold gems and garlands of flowers, cold plasters and compresses, (cold) breeze and fanning, cold and perfumed drinks and cooling measures in general are efficacious in all cases of the desease under discussion. Cordials prepared with the expressed juice of *Ikshu*, *Piyála* and *Drákshá* and with sugar or with the expressed juice of *Drákshá* and *Madhuka* (Maula) or those prepared by boiling *Kás'marya* and *Kharjura* or clarified butter duly cooked with the drugs of the *Jivaniya* group with the d-ugs of the *Madhura* group, or the essence of Jángala meat in combination with the expressed juice of pomegranate should be taken in a case of Murchchhá. The diet should consist of cooked red *S'áli*-rice or barley grains or *Satina*-pulse.* 7—8.

Specific Treatment :—A compound consisting of *Nága-kes'ara, Maricha, Us'ira,* the kernal of *Kola* as well as *Visa* (lotus stock) and *Mrinála* (lotus-stem) taken in equal parts should be taken with the decoction of *Satina* (D. R.—with cold water). *Pippali* with honey or *Pathyá* with sugar should also be taken. The mouth and the nostrils should be pressed close during a fit and the breast-milk should be given to the patient to be drunk. 9.

Strong medicinal errhine should be administered and strong emetics should be as well employed in cases of repeated attacks of the fit. Clarified butter duly cooked and prepared with the decoction of *Haritaki* or with expressed juice of *Ámalaki* should be prescribed. The decoction remedial to Pittaja-fever should be given in a cold state, mixed with *Drákshá,* sugar, parched paddy, *Nilotpala* and *Padma* and well perfumed with any good-smelling scent. 10.

Sannyása :—The case of a patient lying in a comatous state and incapable of being roused up or brought to under the circumstances owing to the aggravated nature of the delusion (unconsciousness) due to an extensive preponderance of the deranged bodily Dosha (involved therein) should be looked upon by an intelligent physicion as extremely hard to cure. This is said to be a case of **Sannyása** (Epilepsy ?). Just as a lump of clay, when thrown into water, should be instantaneously taken up before it is being finally desolved therein, so a patient lying unconscious under an attack of suspended

* Chakrapáni and Vrinda both read Mudga also in the list of the diet.

animation (Sannyása) should be speedily restored to consciousness with the help of medecinal remedies before the process of final dissolution (lit.—death) sets in his body. 11—12.

Treatment :—The patient should be tried to be roused up with the application of strong eye-salves (Anjana), unguents and inhalation of smoke (Dhuma) or by pricking needles into his finger-nails or by discoursing sweet words and music in his hearing or by shaking his limbs roughly or by rubbing his skin with the fruits of *Átma-gupta* creepers. An attack of the present disease not amenable to the above remedies but attended with, salivation, laboured breathing, retention of stool and urine and distension of the abdomen should be given up as **irremediable**. Strong emetics and purgatives should be exhibited after the return of consciousness and **diet** should consist of light articles of fare. *S'ilájatu** mixed with *Tri-phalá*, *Chitraka*, *S'unthi*, etc. should be employed in combination with sugar and continued for a month. Matured clarified butter should be used in particular. Medicinal compounds remedial to any case of fever originated by the Dosha in the case may be as well prescribed in any case of Murchchhá ; and a case due to the action of **poisom** should be remedied with the antitoxine remedies (mentioned in the Kalpa Sthána). 13—14.

Thus ends the forty-sixth chapter of the Uttara-Tantra in the Sus'ruta Samhitá which deals with the (symptoms and) treatment of Murchchhá.

* According to Dallana S'ilájatu should be prepared with the said drugs after the manner of Bhávaná saturation and then be applied with sugar.

CHAPTER XLVII.

Now shall discourse on the (symptoms and) medical treatment of alcoholism and its kindred maladies **(Pánátyáya-Pratishedha).** 1.

Properties and actions of Wine :— Wine is heat-making in its potency, keen or sharp in its properties, subtile in its essence, acts as a soaker or cleanser of moisture and albuminous matter (Vis'ada), is dry, and instantaneous in its action (Ás'ukara), stimulating or exhilarating in its effect (Vyaváyi) and is diffusive (Vikás'i). It destroy cold and shivering by virtue of its heat-making potency. It suspends all cognitive process (lit.-intellectual motions) on account of its keenness or sharpness, enters into every limb and member of the body by reason of its subtlety (Sukshmatva), destroys Kapha (phlegm) and semen in virtue of its Vais'adya, enrages or aggravates the bodily Váyu on account of its dryness (Rukshmtva), and is instantaneous in its action by reason of its Ás'ukáritva. It is exhilarating on account of its Vyaváyitva and diffusive (coursing swiftly all through the body) for its Vikás'itva. Wine is acid in its taste, is light and appetising, and produces fresh relish for food. Others assume the presence of all the tastes except the saline one in it. 3—4.

Wine taken in combination with cooked meat and boiled rice, or any other articles of food profusely saturated with a Sneha (clarified butter, etc.) adds to the longevity, muscular strength and corpulency of a person (using it in moderate quantities) and to the exhilarated state of mind accompanied with beauty, fortitude, vigour and valour and these benefits one may derive from the **proper** use of wine. This fiery liquid in combination with the aggravated bodily fire (Káya-Agni) produces the symptoms of intoxication and unconciousness, etc. (**Mada**) in a foolish person taking it without food or in an empty stomach and in an inordinate quantity. 5.

Evil effects of Drinking :—Excessive drinking produces incidental nescience which gradually creeps into and clouds the sense-perceptions, destroying all power of self control (control over the sense-organs) and giving publicity to the innermost thoughts (in the mind) of the intoxicated person. 6.

Three stages of Alcoholic Intoxication :—There are three stages of intoxication—*viz.*, the first, the second or intermidate and the third or last. The **first** or preliminary stage (of intoxication) is marked by an exhilarated state of mind with increased valour, and conviviality as well as satisfaction and talkativeness, etc. The **second** or intermediate stage is indicated by incoherent speech, exhilaration and the performance of proper and improper acts. In the **third** or last stage the man lies down unconscious, bereft of all powers of action, of memory and of judging the ethic effects of his acts. 7.

A man who is in the habit of taking fatty food or in whom Śleshmá predominates, or in whose constitution, there is only a little of Pitta, is not so easily affected by the action of wine, which, however, proves distressing in a person of contrary nature. Wine, if taken daily without food by a man in an empty stomach, gives rise to many distressing and dangerous diseases in his organism and leads to the ultimate dissolution of his body. 8–9.

Cases where wine is prohibited :—Wine should not be taken by a person under the influence of anger, grief, fright, thirst or hunger. The use of wine is prohibited immediately after a fatiguing journey, physical exercise or an act of load-carrying, or after the repressing of any physical urging, or after the use of excessively acid food, (D. R. excessive water and food) to the full, or before the proper digestion of food or by a weak person, or by one suffering from the effects of heat. In the above cases, wine undoubtedly proves a source of a host of bodily derangements such as Pánátyaya, Paramada, Pánájirna and the violent Pána-vibhrama the characterstic symptoms of which I shall presently describe. 10.

Specific symptoms of Pánátyaya :—The **Vátaja** type of **Pánátyaya** is marked by such symptoms as numbness and aching pain in the limbs, palpitation, a catching and pricking pain in the region of the heart and headache. Perspiration, delirium, dryness of the mouth, burning sensation and fainting fits (loss of consciousness) and yellowness of the face and eyes are the features which distinguish the **Pittaja** type (of Pánátyaya). Vomiting, shivering and water-brash are the indications which mark the **Kaphaja** type. The symptoms of all the three preceeding types being exhibited in the one due to the concerted action of the three deranged bodily Doshas—**Tri-Doshaja** type of Pánátyaya. 11.

Symptoms of Para-mada :—Heat and a sense of heaviness in the body, bad taste in the mouth, excessive accumulation of Śleshmá in the body, an aversion to food, supression of stool and urine, thirst, headache and a crushing pain in the joints are the symptoms which the learned physicion sets down to **Para-mada** (reactionary effects of the abuse of wine). 12.

Pánájirna and Pána-Vibhrama :—Distension of the abdomen (tympanites), acid or sour taste (in the mouth), vomiting, deficient gastric digestion are the symptoms which are exhibited in a **Pánájirna** type (alcoholic indigestion). Aggravation of the deranged Pitta should be regarded by a physicion as the exciting factor of the disease. The malady which exhibits such symptoms as piercing pain in the heart and limbs, vomiting, fever, a sensation of the rising of fumes into the throat, salivation, epileptic fits, headache, a burning sensation in the throat and an aversion to all sorts of food and wine (in connection with an abuse of wine) is called **Pána-Vibhrama**. 13-14.

Prognosis:—A patient suffering from the effects of excessive drinking and exhibiting such symptoms as protuded upper lip, excessive shivering or burning sensation and clamminess of the face, black or blue colour of the tongue, lips or teeth and yellowness or blood-colour of the eyes should be givin up as **incurable**. Hiccough, fever, vomiting, shivering, tremor, cramp of the sides, cough and vertigo are the supervening symptoms (**Upadrava**) which are found in all forms of Pánátyaya (alcoholism). 15.

Treatment of Vátaja type:—Now hear me describe the medicinal remedies for all the above said maladies. Wine saturated with the mixture of pulverised *Chukra*, *Maricha*, *Ádraka*, *Dipya* (Yamáni), *Kushtha* and *Souvarchala* should be given for the relief of the **Vátaja** type of Pánátyaya, or one mixed with *Prithviká*, *Dipyaka*, *Mahoushadhi* and *Hingu*, or with *Souvarchala* should be taken for comfort. Shádavas or cordials made of *Ámrátaka*, *Ámra-fruits*, *Dádima* and *Mátulunga* should be given for relief. In the alternative, the cooked flesh of an animal of *Ánupa* group *i.i.* tortoise, etc. should be seasoned with the expressed juice of above fruits and be taken. 16.

Treatment of Pittaja type:—In the **Pittaja-type** of Pánátyaya, wine mixed with the decoction of the drugs of the *Madhura* group and saturated and flavoured with the admixture of sugar and scented drugs should be taken, or wine profusely mixed with the expressed juice of sugar-cane should be taken and fully vomited out, a short while thereafter. Meat-juice (Rasa) of *Láva*, *Ena* and *Tittira* unmixed with any acid, or *Mudga* soup should be taken with sugar and clarified butter. 17.

Treatment of Kaphaja and Tri-Doshaja type, etc.:—In the **Kaphaja** type of Pánátyaya, the mucus should be eliminated by taking a potion of wine mixed with the expressed juice or decoction of *Vimibi* and *Vidula* (Vetasa). Meat-juice of any fatty *Jángala* animal mixed with bitter and and pungent articles as also the *Mudga*-soup made bitter and pungent should be taken as beneficial to the patient. The **diet** should consist of preparations of barley, flesh of *Jángala* animals and also the Kapha-subduing articles, as well as those calculated as remedial to the present type of Pánátyaya. The above kinds of medicines and diet should be combinedly applied in the one due to the concerted action of the three Doshas of the body (**Tri-Doshaja type**), while in the **Dvi-Doshaja** types, the treatment should be according to the nature of the predominant Doshas. 18—19.

Now I shall describe the medicinal compounds which tend to relieve the delirious state of mind and may be employed for the relief of all forms of Pánátyaya in general. The fine powder of *Nága-pushpa*, *Mágadhiká*, *Elá*, *Madhuka*, *Dhánya*, *Ajáji* and *Maricha* taken in equal parts mixed copiously with the expressed juice of *Kapittha*, water and *Parushaka* should be duly taken in all forms of Pánátyaya after the mixture is strained through a piece of cloth. The body of the patient should be anointed with a paste of *Haridrá*, *Padma*, *Paripelava*, *Karavira*, *Padmaka*, drugs of the *Sárivádi* group and acquatic flower pasted togather, and clear and cold water should be sprinkled over the body of the patient in a case of Madátyaya. 20–21.

Pánaks :—A **Pának** prepared with *Tvak*, *Patra*, *Chocha*, *Maricha*, *Elá*, *Nága-pushpa* and flowers of *S'leshmátaka* ground together into a paste and mixed with treacle and *Drákshá*, should be filtered and perfumed and given to a person suffering from an attack of Pánátyaya. The patient would find relief by the frequent use of a **Pánaka** (draughts) composed of *Yashti-madhu*, *Katurohini*, *Drákshá* and *Trapusha*-roots, or of *Kárpása*-roots, *Nága-valá* and *Suvarchalá* (Surjávarta) all taken in equal parts. 22—23.

Treatment of Para-mada :—A **Pánaka** (cordial) made of the fruits of *Káshmarya*, *Dáru*, *Dádima*, *Vit*, *Pippali*, *Drákshá* pasted together and disolved in water and taken in combination with the expressed juice of *Vijapuraka*, instantly gives relief in discomforts due to an abuse of wine (**Para-mada**). Pánakas made of sugar, *Drákshá*, *Madhuka*, *Jiraka*, *Dhánya*, *Krishná* (Pippali) and *Trivrit*, or of *Souvarchala*, the meat-soup (Rasa) of any fatty *Jángala* animal and *Phalámla* should be taken. Cold infusion of *Bhárgi* would be found beneficial in **sprinkling**. 24—25.

Treatment of Pánájirna :—Vomiting should be induced with an Anjali measure of milk duly cooked with the admixture of *Ikshváku*, *Dhámárgava*, *Brikshaka* and two kinds of *Udumvariká* after which the patient should be advised to take wine in the evening in a case of indigestion due to an abuse of wine (**Pánájirna**). *Phalámla* in combination with *Tvak*, *Pippali*, *Nága-pushpa*, *Vid*, *Hingu*, *Maricha* and *Elá*, or a compouud consisting of *Saindhava*, *vid*, *Tvak*, *Chabya*, *Elá*, *Hingu*, *Pippali*, *Pippali-roots* and *S'unthi* pounded and desolved in warm water should be taken. The food of the patient should be made palatable with the admixture of Khada-jusha * in the present instance. 27.

Treatment of Pána-vibhrama:—A Pánaka composed of *Drákshá*, *Kapittha*, *Phala* (Mátulunga, etc.) and *Dádima* sweetened with profuse quantity of sugar and honey, as well as the one made with the expressed juice of *Kola* and *Ámrátaka* sweetened in the same manner would prove curative in a case of **Pána-vibhrama**. A compound consisting of *Kharjura*, *Vetra*, *Karira*, *Parushaka*, *Drákshá* and *Trivrit* pounded together and disolved in cold water should be taken, sweetened with sugar, or the same should be taken in combination with *S'ri-parni*. In the alternative, the tender sprouts of *Kshiri*-trees, *Visa* (Mrinála), *Jiraka*, *Nágapushpa*, *Patra*, *Elaválu*, *Sita-sárivá*, *Padmaka*, *Ámrátaka*, *Bhavya*, *Karamarda*, *Kapittha*, *Kola*, *Vrikshámla*, *Vetra*-fruits, *Jiraka*, *Dádima*, *Yashti-madhu* and *Utpala*, all pounded together and mixed with the cold infusion of such drugs as *Maricha*, *Jiraka*, *Nága-pushpa*, *Tvak*, *Patra*, *Vis'va*, *Chaviká* and *Elá* filtered through a piece of thin linen duly perfumed with the addition of scented drugs would be found curative in the seven types of distempers which have their origin in drinking excesses. 28.

Objects which are pleasing to the five sense-organs of man and gratifying to the mind and heart, as well as

* Dallana in his commentatory says that some read "मद्यै:" in place of "हृद्यै:" and others read "फलै:" in place of "खडै:".

light wine should be always prescribed in a case of **Panátayaya** and the patient should be enlivened with the embrace of handsome and youthful damsels exceedingly attached to the gratification of the senses with splendid hips and thighs with their slender waists drooping under the weight of the exuberance of their breasts. 29.

Potions prepared with powders of *Nága-pushpa, Ajáji, Krishná* and *Maricha* taken in equal parts mixed with sugar, *Madhuka* and *Tri-sugandhi* and then disolved in the expressed juice of *Kushmánda* fruits, should be taken. The drugs known as *Varshábhu, Yashtyáhva, Madhuka, Lákshá, Tvak,* tender sprouts of *Karvudara, Jiraka, Drákshá, Krishná* and *Kes'ara* should be given mixed with tepid milk. 30—31.

A person afflicted with diseases due to the excess of Surá, Ásava, etc. should be treated with the same wines (Surá, Ásava, etc.) duly administered otherwise he will be ruined, in the same manner as a person who has incurred the king's displeasure, should be saved by courting the royal favour. An inveterate drunkard giving up his habit of drinking is afflicted with the symptoms of Pánátyaya if he suddenly revert to his former pernicious habit. 32—33.

The Ágneya and Váyaviya virtues of wine tend to produce a dryness in the water carrying channels of the body, hence **thirst** is experienced by a drunkard person. A cold infusion of *Patola*, flowers and bulbs of *Utpala*, and *Mudga-parni* mixed with *Mágadhika'* should be taken under the circumstances (reactionary thirst), or oil, clarifiied butter, Vasá (lard) and marrow (D. R.—milk) should be duly cooked with curd (four times), expressed juice of *Bhringa-ra'ja* (four times), and the decoction of *Vilva* and *Yava* (four times) with the Kalkas of the drugs known as the *Sarva-gandhá* should be applied as an **Abhyanga**. The body should be sprinkled (Seka) with the cold decoction*. Palatable foods and cold, pleasing and scented cordials should be prescribed according to the nature and intensity of the deranged bodily Doshas underlying the disease. 34-35.

The heat generated by drinking being aggravated by bodily Pitta and blood of an intoxicated person, escapes through the surface of the skin and causes a feeling of intense burning (**Dáha**) which should be remedied with measures and therapeutic agents prescribed in connection with the aggravation of Pitta. 36.

Remedies for Dáha :—Now I shall describe the cooling measures which should be employed for alleviating the burning sensation (**Dáha**) in the case of a rich patient. The body of such a patient under the circumstances should be smeared at the outest with *Chandana* (white sandal wood) pastes made cooler by the contact of cold beams of the moon, pearl-necklaces and the water produced from melted ice. He should be laid down in a bed of full-blown lotus flowers sparkling with dew drops or of lotus-leaves sprinkled with spray of translucent water, and youthful damsels decked with necklace and bangles of lotus-stems cooler even than cold water, should be asked to touch him. He should try to alleviate the burning feeling by strolling on the banks of a tank in a garden in the soft, cool and sweet breeze bearing on its wings the soft perfume of *Kalhára* (red) lotus and water-moss dancing in the adjoining tank. Water cooled and charged with *Us'ira*, *Válaka* and (white) sandal paste should be sprinkled over his body, or he should be made to sport in a cleansed tank filled with freshly collected water em-

* Decoction of the drugs of Madhura-gana and of the drugs of cold virtues.

balmed with full-blown red and blue lotus-flowers and scents (*e. g.* sandal pastes) after being smeared with sandal paste and with the hairs of his body standing on their roots with the magnetic touch of beloved female hands. Here he should take his bath with young, gay and beautiful damsels skilful in aquatic sports refreshing him with the lotus-like touch of their cold hands, thighs and mouth and hard (*i.e.*, full-grown) breasts and with their sweet words. 37-A.

He should lie down, when tired, in a cool chamber cooled with watery breeze, fitted with fountains and made dusky with the misty jets (vapours, of water. The floor of the chamber should be sprinkled over with scented water and flowers and the walls thickly coated with pastes of sandal wood, *Teja-patra* and *Válaka*. The chamber should be scented and decorated with *Mánsi*, *Tamála*, *Musta*, *Kumkuma*, *Padma*-leaves, *Játi*-flower, *Utpala* (blue-lotus), *Priyangu*, *Kes'ara* (Bakula), and *Pundarika* (red-lotus), *Punnága*, *Nága-Kes'ara*, and *Karavira* and there in the room with garlands of flowers gently swinging in the sweet and lazy wind, the patient should lie down and listen to the sweet discourses about the Hemanta, the Vindhya, the Malaya or the Himálaya mountains as well as about cold water, leaves of *Kadali* or of any other evergreen tree or plant and about the receptacles of full-blown blue or red lotus, as well as about topics of moon-rise, or any other subject which may be calculated to be agreeable to his mind under the circumstances. Young and beautiful damsels with their full and thick-set breasts and thighs anointed with sandal pastes, being clad in wet clothes (adhering to and advantageously showing the splendid contours of their limbs, etc.,) and with their necklaces and girdles loosely sliding down their bosoms and slender waists should lie there with him in their firm embrace. These damsels should refresh him with their secret charms in that lonely chamber and by means of their bodily coolness would be able to alleviate the burning sensation of aggravated Pitta due to **over-drinking**. 37.

These are the measures in general which should be employed also in the cases of burning sensation due to the aggravated condition of **blood, Pitta** and **thirst**. Now hear me discourse on the measures which are to be specifically employed in the case of a burning sensation in the body under different circumstances. 38 A.

Symptoms of Raktaja Dáha :—The blood coursing through the whole body when aggravated by any cause whatsoever becomes heated and imparts a copper colour to the skin, complexion and the eye-balls of the patient. It produces a bloody smell in the mouth and the body, and the patient feels a burning and contracting sensation as if he is surrounded by fire. 38.

Treatment :—Fasting should be prescribed at the outset in such a case and then the diet should be regulated conformably to the nature and intensity of the deranged bodily Dosha involved therein. If such burning sensation (in the body) be still unrelieved, the patient should be treated with a diet largely composed of the soup of *Jángala* flesh and venesection in the extremeties should then be resorted to duly in conformity with the rules (prescribed in Chapter VIII—S'árira Sthána). Cases of burning sensation due to the aggravation of **Pitta** would produce the symptoms of Pittaja fever and remedies for Pittaja fever should in such cases be resorted to. 39.

Symptoms and treatment of Dáha due to thirst :—The watery part is dried up in the event of an unslaked thirst, thus generating a heat in the organism. This produces an extreme dryness of the lip, throat and palate and a burning sensation (**Dáha**) both in the skin and inside the organism of the patient followed by the coming out of the tongue and the trembling of the whole body. The medical treatment under such circumstances consists in alleviating the heat and adding to the watery component of the body. A large draught of cold water or cooled milk saturated with a copious quantity of sugar, or of the expressed juice of sugar-cane or of *Mantha* should be given to the patient to his satiety under the circumstances. 40-41.

An intense burning sensation in the body is caused by the presence of accumulated **blood** in the abdomen (Koshtha), the symptoms and therapeutics of which are those mentioned in the chapter on Sadyo-vrana (Chap. II—Chikitsita-Sthána) A burning sensation of the body incidental to the waste (**Kshaya**) of any of its fundamental organic principles (Dhátus) brings on thirst, fainting fits, feebleness of voice, suspension of physical and mental faculties or functions, weakness and lassitude in its train which should be remedied with measures laid down under Rakta-pitta. Emulsive and Váyu-subduing remedies are likewise applicable therein. 42-43.

A severe internal burning sensation in the body may also be produced by (the aggravation of) **blood** due to (the breach of the rules of) diet and to grief of any kind. The symptoms in such cases are thirst, fainting fits and delirium The remedy should consist in giving the patient the wished-for objects, and the diet under the circumstances should largely consist of milk and meat-essence to be partaken of in company with friends in the manner described before. A burning sensation in the body incidental to a **hurt** or to a **blow** on any of its vulnerable or tender parts (Marma) is the seventh of its kind and should be deemed as incurable. All kinds of burning sensation in the body with a coolness of its surface are incurable. Emetics and purgatives should be exhibited according to the Dosha involved even after the subsidence of the supervening symptoms of excess in wine. 44–46.

Wine mixed with half its quantity of water and scented with *Jiraka*, *Sauvarchala*, *Árdraka* and *S'unthi* becomes palatable and immediately allays thirst. Wine, taken with meal and with cooked meat by a person besmeared with sandal paste and wearing wet clothes and garlands of flowers, does not produce any of its bad after-effects nor brings on intoxication which in its turn would throw the mind and mental faculties off their balance. 47–48.

Thus ends the forty-seventh chapter of the Uttara-Tantra in the Sus'ruta Samhitá which deals with the (symptoms and) medical treatment of alcoholism.

CHAPTER XLVIII.

Now we shall discourse on the chapter which deals with the (symptoms and) medical treatment of thirst **(Trishná-Pratishedha Adhyáya).** 1.

He who is not satisfied even with the constant drinking of water but craves for more and more water should be regarded as afflicted with the disease known as thirst (morbid desire for water). 2.

Etiology :—The Pitta and Váyu of the body become extremely aggravated by such factors as (excessive) exercise, grief (or any violent mental agitation), fatigue, drinking, use of any extremely dry, acid, hot or pungent fares, or of those which cause a parched condition in the organism, or waste of any vital organic principle (Dhátu), of the body, fasting or exposure to the sun, and combinedly affect the water-carrying channels of the body (diminish the liquid portion of the bodily lymph-chyle). The water-carrying channels thus affected give rise to violent **thirst.** The disease is divided into **seven** types. 3.

Classification :—The first three are due to the action of the deranged Doshas (Váyu, Pitta and Kapha). The fourth and fifth are respectively incidental to any ulcer and to the waste of any of its fundamental organic principles. The sixth is due to the presence of undigested fecal matter in the intestines (lit. mucus) and the seventh is due to errors in diet. Now hear me describe their specific symptoms and the therapeutic agents to be employed in curing them. 4.

Premonitory Symptoms :—An extreme dryness of and a burning sensation in the palate, throat, lips and mouth, external heat, vertigo, loss of consciousness, and delirium are the general **premonitory** symtoms which usher in an attack of the disease. The specific symptoms are given below. 5.

Symptoms of Vátaja, Pittaja and Kaphaja Thirst :—Dryness of the mouth with a tingling sensation in the regions of the temples, and the head (D. R.—throat), obstruction of the (water-carrying) channels of the body and a bad taste in the mouth, are the symptoms which specifically mark a case of the **Vátaja** type in which the drinking of cold water leads to a distinct aggravation of the disease (thirst). Loss of consciousness (epileptic fits), delirium, an aversion to food, dryness of the mouth, yellowness of the eyes, extreme burning sensation in the whole body, desire for coldness, a bitter taste in the mouth and a fumid sensation (in the throat) are the features which specifically mark the **Pittaja** type of the disease. The vapours produced by the fire of digestion being enveloped and obstructed in their course by the layer of accumulated Kapha, the heat (pent up in the body tends to dry up the moisture of its water-carrying channels and) produces a kind of thirst which is characterised by somnolence, a sense of heaviness in the limbs, a sweet taste in the mouth, extreme emaciation, cold-fever, vomiting, an aversion to food and suppuration in the skin are the symptoms of **Kaphaja** type. And where such symptoms are present, the patient has no excessive desire for drinking water. 6—8.

Kshataja and Kshayaja Thirsts :—A case of thirst which is engendered in consequence of pain in or discharge of blood from, any cut in the body is the fourth type and is known as **Kshataja** thirst. The days of the patient in such a case pass with great uneasiness even if he drinks water. In the type due to the waste of the fundamental organic fluid (Rasa) which is known as **Kshayaja** thirst, the patient constantly drinks water in large quantity both in the day and in the night but still finds no relief. This type is attributed by several authorities to the concerted action of the three deranged Doshas and all the specifice symptoms due to the waste of the vital organic principle (Rasa) described before are expected there. 9—10.

Ámaja and Annaja Thirst:—The symptoms of all the three (aggravated) Doshas in addition to pain in the heart, spitting and a sense of lassitude in the limbs are present in the type which is due to indigestion (**Ámaja**). The case of thirst which is produced by using extremely fatty and saline articles of fare, as well as those which are hard to digest is due to errors in diet (and is known as **Annaja** thirst). 11—12.

Prognosis:—A patient who has become extremely weak and deaf in consequence of thirst and who suffers from a mental stupour and lies with his tongue protruded and hung down should not be taken charge of (by a physician) for treatment. 13.

General Treatment:—Vomiting should be induced with a solution of powdered *Pippali* in a case of thirst in which the stomach of the patient becomes fully loaded (with water). A plaster composed of *Dádima*, *Ámrátaka* and *Mátulunga* is also beneficial. Drugs which are cooling in their virtue and potency should be applied in the three cases of thirst (due to the three Doshas). A gargle composed of a solution of powdered *Ámalaka* with any acid drug (Mátulunga, etc.) should be retained in the mouth for removing the bad taste in the mouth under the circumstances. Water made hot by immersing bits of heated gold, silver, etc, as well as pieces of heated stone or baked clay in it and taken in a tepid state, or cold water charged with sugar and honey, is possessed of the efficacy of allaying thirst. 14—16.

Specific Treatment :—A patient suffering from **Vátaja** thirst would find relief by taking lukewarm and in a little quantity at a time the water boiled with the drugs of any of * the five *Pancha-mula* groups or with the drugs of the first group (Vidári-gandhádi-gana). A decoction of the drugs of the Pitta-subduing groups † subsequently cooled and taken with the addition of honey and sugar, or milk duly boiled with the admixture of the drugs of the *Jivaniya* group (Kákolyádi Gana) would allay a case of **Pittaja** thirst. Water duly boiled with *Vilva*, *Ádhaki*, the drugs of the *Kantaka-Pancha-mula* ‡ and *Darbha* allays a case of **Kaphaja** thirst. Vomiting induced with the help of a draught of the infusion of tender *Nimba*-leaves taken lukewarm would likewise prove curative in such a case. 17—19.

The Pitta-subduing remedies and measures should, in the alternative, be applied in all types of thirst which cannot otherwise be allayed. The expressed juice or a decoction of ripe *Udumvara* should be taken with

* The five Pancha-mula groups are (1) The major pancha-mula, (2) The minor Pancha-mula, (3) The Valli Pancha-mula, (4) The Kantaka-Pancha-mula, (5) The Trina-Pancha-mula. See Chap. XXXVIII, Sutra sthána.

† The Pitta-subduing groups are Utpaládi, Sárivádi and Kákolyádi groups.

‡ In place of "कण्टकपञ्चमूली, etc.", some read "कण्टकपञ्चकोल" etc., *i.e.* Kantaka (Gokshura) and the drugs included in the group known as "पञ्चकोल," viz. Pippali, Pippali-mula, Chavya, Chitraka and Nágara. The commentator Kártika Kundu supports this:—Dallana. For Kantaka—Pancha-mula, see Chap. XXXVIII—Sutra-Sthána.

sugar under the circumstances. A thirst-afflicted patient should likewise drink the water duly boiled with the drugs of the *Sárivádi* group sufficiently cooled down for the purpose. 20—21.

Water duly boiled with *Kas'eru*, *S'ringátaka*, *Padma*, *Mocha* (plantain-flower) and *Vis'a* is efficacious in allaying thirst incidental to hurt (**Kshataja**). Water containing *Nilotpala*, *Us'ira* and red *Chandana* should be kept in an open space during the night and a physician should give this well-scented water mixed with sugar and honey and with a large quantity of *Drákshá* to the thirst-afflicted patients on the following morning for their benefit. Cold infusions of the drugs of any of the *Trina-pancha-mula*, *Utpalâdi* and *Madhura* (D. R. the first group *i.e.*, Vidárigandhádi) groups mixed with the drugs of the *Sárivádi* group as well as that of the drugs of the *Madhuka-pushpádi* groups should be prepared in the preceding manner and prescribed. The six kinds of cordials (Pánaka) separately prepared (in the preceding manner) with the (four kinds of) *Rájádana*, *Kshiri* or *Kapitana* are also beneficial in such cases. Fruits of *Tundikeri* (wild Kárpása) and of *Kárpása* pasted together (and dissolved in water) and taken internally would prove beneficial. A case of thirst incidental to any ulcer (Kshataja) is allayed with the stoppage or removal of the pain or by taking meat-soup or the blood (of deer, goat, etc.). 22—26.

A case of thirst due to the waste (**Ksháyaja**) of any fundamental organic fluid (Rasa) is removed by taking draughts of clarified butter churned from milk,*

* In places of "क्षीरघृतं" "मांसोदकं" and "मधुकोदकं" some read "क्षीरजलं" (milk mixed with water), "माषोदकं" (soup of Másha pulse) and मधूदकं (honey mixed with water) respectively.

as well as those of meat-soup and infusion of *Yashti-madhu.* Thirst which is incidental to the presence of mucus and undigested fecal matter in the intestines (**Ámaja**) should be remedied with the decoction of *Vilva, Vachá* and the drugs of the *Dipaniya* (Pippalyádi) group or with the decoction of the drugs of the *Dipaniya* group mixed with *Ámrátaka, Bhallátaka* and *Valá.* The type which has its origin in the use of heavy and indigestible fares or due to errors in diet as well as all other types of thirst with the exception of the one which is incidental to the waste of any fundamental organic principle should be cured by inducing vomiting. 27—28.

Solution of common treacle or *Mantha* or meat-soup is efficacious in allaying thirst which is due to physical fatigue. Warm *Yavágus* or cold *Manthas* * would alleviate a thirst caused by the obstruction of the participated meal. A man should drink warm water in cases of thirst due to an excessive taking of any fatty substance (Sneha). The thirst of a habitual drunkard which is due to the reactionary effects of wine is allayed by draughts of half-diluted wine. Thirst due to heat, may be allayed with draughts of cold water surcharged with sugar or with the expressed juice of suger-cane. 29—33.

General Treatment :—Vomiting should be induced in these cases with the decoction of such drugs as are remedial to the deranged bodily Doshas involved in each case and the digestive (Páchana) remedies as prescribed in cases of fever should also be prescribed in these cases. Use of cooling plasters and of cold

* Warm Yavágu should be prescribed in cases where Váyu preponderates and cold Mantha in cases where Pitta preponderates.

baths and spray, residence in cold chambers, exhibition of emetics and purgatives, use of milk, meat-essence, clarified butter and sweet and cooling lambatives would be likewise prescribed in all cases of thirst. 34—35.

Thus ends the forty-eighth chapter of the Uttara-Tantra in the Sus'ruta Samhitá which deals with the (symptoms and) treatment of thirst.

CHAPTER XLIX.

Now we shall discourse on the chapter which deals with the (symptoms and) medical treatment of vomiting **(Chhardi-Pratishedha).**

Causes and Nomenclature :—The bodily Doshas are deranged and aggravated per force by the use of extremely liquid, emollient, unpalatable or oversalted food or of one taken at an improper time or in an inordinate quantity or which is incongenial to the physical temperament of its user, as well as by over-fatiguing physical exercise, fear, mental agitation, indigestion, presence of worms (in the intestines), or quick eating or owing to pregnancy or any disgusting or loathsome causes. Thus deranged, the Doshas rush up to the mouth and after covering the whole of it come out with great force and with an aching pain in the limbs. This is, therefore, called **Vomiting** (Chhardi). 2.

The vital Váyu known as the Udána-Váyu coming in combination with the one known as the Vyána-Váyu in a man addicted to incompatible food and drink leads to the derangement of the bodily Doshas and rushes up to the upper part of his body (which causes vomiting). 3.

Premonitory Symptoms :—Nausea, suppression of eructations, thin and saline water-brash and an aversion to food and drink are the premonitory symptoms of vomiting. 4.

Specific Symptoms :—Scanty ejections of frothy matter of strong astringent taste accompanied with a loud sound and cramps at the back and the sides produce a sense of exhaustion or fatigue and increase after the digestion of a meal and this should be ascribed to the action of the deranged bodily **Váyu**. Vomiting of yellow, greenish or blood-streaked matter with an excessively acid, pungent or bitter taste in the mouth and attended with such complications as fever, dryness of mouth, fainting fits and burning and sucking (Chosha) sensations in the body, should be ascribed to the action of the deranged **Pitta**. Excessively cold, white, sweet, thick and mucous vomiting attended with horripilation, an aversion to food, heaviness of the limbs and lassitude should be ascribed to the **Kaphaja** type of vomiting. The specific features of all the three preceding types are present in the type due to the concerted action of all the **three Doshas**. 5—8.

Traumatic Cases :—The five cases of vomiting due to any disgusting or loathsome cause or to pregnancy, indigestion, presence of worms (in the bowels) or the taking of uncongenial food and drink, should be duly classified according to the Dosha aggravated in each case. The stomach is irritated in all types of vomiting. Fasting should, therefore, be the first remedy in these cases. Violent cramps and nausea as well as the symptoms of Krimija-Hridroga are the special characteristics of a case of vomiting due to the presence of worms in the bowels. 9—10.

Prognosis :—A skilful physician shall not take in hand the medical treatment of a patient afflicted with vomiting, where the patient is emaciated and is distressed with the supervening symptoms,* and in which the ejected matter is mixed with pus and

* The **supervening** symptoms are :—Cough, asthma, fever, hiccough, thirst, mental dejection, heart-disease and Tamaka-S'vása.

blood, and resembles the variegated colour of a peacock's plume and where vomiting is almost constant. 11.

General Treatment :—In a case of vomiting marked by an excessive preponderance of any Dosha (or by the presence of all the three Doshas), emetics or purgatives should be administered with a due regard to the nature and intensity of the Dosha or Doshas involved. In cases due to the concerted action of any two of the deranged bodily Doshas the medical treatment should be determined according to their relative order of preponderance. **Diet** in these cases should consist of dry and light articles and what the patient is accustomed to. Febrifuge decoctions should be administered according to the nature and intensity of the deranged bodily Doshas involved in each case. 12.

Treatment of Vátaja Type :—Draught of clarified butter churned from milk,* or the soup of *Mudga* and *Ámalaka* taken with clarified butter and *Saindhava*-salt, or gruels (*Yavágu*) prepared with the drugs of *Pancha-mula* and taken with honey, would prove curative in the **Vátaja** type of vomiting. The use of the essence of any bird of the *Vishkira* group (*e.g.* chicken, etc.) taken with a little quantity of salt and juice of acid-fruits would likewise prove efficacious. Lukewarm oily purgtives mixed with salt are also recommended in such cases 13.

Pittaja Type :—Cold drinks and decoctions of Pitta-subduing virtue would relieve vomiting due to the derangement of **Pitta**. Emetics or purgatives composed of the drugs of the *Madhura*-drugs and mixed

* "चीरघृतं" has been explained by some commentators as milk mixed with clarified butter. Chakradatta reads "चीरोदकं" milk and water in place of "चीरघृतं",

with the expressed juice of *Drákshá* may likewise be employed in the present type. In violent attacks of vomiting the medicated clarified butter known as Tailvaka-ghrita should also be prescribed. 14.

Treatment of Kaphaja Type:—A decoction of the drugs of the *Áragvadhádi*-group or of *Das'a-mula* should be given with honey in a case of vomiting due to the aggravation of **Kapha**. A cold infusion (Hima-Kasháya) of *Guduchi* mixed with honey would prove an excellent remedy in all the three preceding types of vomiting. 15—16.

Vomiting due to (the use or sight of) any disgusting or loathsome thing should be treated with agreeable things, while that peculiar to **pregnancy** should be relieved by giving to the *enceinte* the things she longs for.

Traumatic Types:—Vomiting due to the use of any unaccustomed or incongenial food should be relieved with fasting, vomiting or with the administration of habituated or congenial food. Vomiting due to the presence of worms in the bowels (**Krimija**) should be treated with remedies applicable in a case of Krimija Hrid-roga (heart-disease of parasitic origin). The measures and remedies prescribed before should be employed with a due regard to the nature and intensity of the deranged bodily Dosha or Doshas involved in each case. 17.

General Treatment:—Vomiting is relieved by frequently licking a lambative made of *Pippali*, honey and the expressed juice of *Kapittha*-fruit. *Madhurasá* * with the washings of rice and with honey may be likewise taken for the purpose. Tarpana (soothing) measure with the admixture of honey would be bene-

* "Madhurasá" may mean (1) Drak'shá (2) Gámbhári fruit (3) Murvá or (4) Yashti-madhu. The practice is to prescribe Drákshá.

ficial in all the three cases (due to the aggravation of the Doshas). A potion composed of powdered *Átma-gupta*-seeds and *Yashti-madhu* mixed with a copious quantity of rice-washing and with honey as well as gruels prepared with the admixture of *Karanja*-leaves should be administered. *Kustumburu* pasted and mixed with salt and acid would also be benificial. *Kapittha* should also be taken with *Tri-k tu* and rice-washing. 18—A.

The excreta of flies should be licked with sugar, honey and sandal paste. A lizard should be immersed in hot milk and this milk, when cooled, should be given to the patient to drink. Powdered fried paddy mixed with honey and clarified butter should be given to drink or pulverised *Pippali* mixed with honey, sugar and clarified butter should be licked. Sandal-paste * with the expressed juice of *Ámalaka* or the decoction of the leaves of *Mudga* † as well as a lambative composed of the marrow of *Kola* and *Ámalaka* spiced with the *Tri-sugandhi* drugs (*viz.*, Elá, Patra and Tvak) powdered together should be prescribed. Gruels of fried *S'áli* paddy mixed with honey should also be prescribed. The use of perfumes which are agreeable both to the mind and to the organ of smell, is also recomended. 18-B.

Diet :—The meat of any Jángala animal and palatable cordials and victuals of various plates should be likewise taken with care in all cases. 18.

Thus ends the forty-ninth chapter of the Uttara-Tantra in the Sus'ruta Samhitá which deals with the (symptoms and) treatment of Vomiting.

* The practice is to take white Sandal in this case.

† Vágbhata prescribes the decoction alone as a separate remedy.

CHAPTER L.

Now we shall discourse on the chapter which deals with the (symptoms and) medical treatment of hiccough **(Hiccá-Pratishedha).** 1.

Causes :—Hiccough, cough and asthma are the result of using those articles of fare which are heavy, dry, or secreting (Abhishyandi) or which are followed by an acid reaction or which remain long in an undigested state (in the stomach) as well as of cold drinks, residence in cold places, exposure to cold or dust or smoke or fire or wind, over-fatiguing physical exercises, physical exertion, load-carrying, toils of journey, voluntary repression of (physical urgings), fasting (Apatarpana), accumulation of Áma-dosha (mucus in the intestines), blow or hurt, emaciation (weakness) due to sexual excesse, concomitant distress or agony of any existing or continuing physical ailment, irregular diet, eating before the digestion of a previous meal or of a wrong application of Samśamana remedies. 2.

Derivation :—The Váyu (wind) constantly belches out of the mouth with a report shaking, as it were, the spleen, the liver and the intestines. The physicians have bestowed the name **Hiccá** on the disease owing to fact of its speedily extinguishing the vital spark in man (from Sanskrit root—Hins to kill). 3.

Classification :—Hiccá is divided into **five** kinds which are styled Annajá, Yamalá, Kshudrá Gambhirá and Mahati, all of which are the effects of the derangement of the bodily Váyu acting in unison with the deranged Kapha. 4.

Premonitory Symptoms :—An astrigent

taste in the mouth, an aversion to all sorts of pursuits, heaviness about the throat and cardiac region and a rumbling sound in the abdomen (Jathara) are the premonitory symptoms which usher in a fit of hiccough. 5.

Symptoms :—The bodily Váyu being suddenly deranged by taking too much food and drink, is pushed upward and belched out in gusts which are known as **Annajá Hiccá**. The hiccough which occurs in double strokes and at long intervals shaking the head and the neck is called **Yamalá**. The hic-cough which rises with a mild force and at long intervals from the root* of the clavicles (Jatru) is called **Kshudriká**. The violent hiccough which rises from the region of the umbilicus accompained by a deep sound and interfering with free respiration, causing dryness of the lips, throat, tongue and of the mouth and producing pain at the sides and complicated with many other distressing symptoms, is called **Gambhirá** The hiccough which produces a feeling of crushing pain as it were, at the vulnerable parts (Marmans) and stretches out the body in full, shaking all the limbs and which occurs frequently and with a considerable force accompained by a report, and produces a severe thirst is called **Mahá-Hiccá**. 6—10.

Prognosis :—A hiccough-patient whose body is stretched out in full during a fit, with his eyes turned upward and fixed in a gaze as well as the one suffering from weakness, frequent sneezing (D. R.—cough) or an aversion to food as well as those suffering from the last two cases of Hiccá *viz.*, Gambhirá and Mahati should be given up as incurable. 11.

* By the word "Mula" (*i. e.*, root) of the Jatru (clavicles) Gayadás'a understands the regions of the heart, Kloma, throat, etc.—Dallana.

Treatment:—Practice of Pránáyáma (control of breath-wind), tickling, frightening and producing confusion by pricking with needles may be effectively resorted to in a case of (simple) hiccough. *Yashti-madhu* mixed with honey, or *Pippali* mixed with sugar, or a lukewarm compound of milk, clarified butter and the expressed juice of sugar-cane* should be employed after the manner of an Avapida-Nasya. Vomiting and purging may be induced in a patient not extremely weak. Red sandal-wood made into a paste with the breast-milk, or lukewarm clarified butter mixed with *Saindhava* salt, or powdered *Saindhava* dissolved in water is beneficial, if administered as a medicinal snuff. 12.

Gummy exudation of *S'ála* trees, *Manah-s'ilá*, or cow's horn, or cow's hairs and skin, charged with clarified butter, should be used in fumigation (Dhupana). As an alternative, the seats of hiccough (*viz.*, umbilical region, etc) should be duly fomented. The patient should be advised to use a lambative composed of *Svarna-Gairika* or the ashes of the bones of any domestic animal pasted with honey. Hairs of Śvávidh †, a sheep, a cow or of Śallaki should be burnt in a covered pot and given to be licked with honey. Plumes of a peacock or the fruit of *Udumvara* or (the bark of) *Lodhra* should be similarly burnt and the ashes thus prepared should be licked by the patient in combination with honey and clarified butter. *Sarjiká-kshára* licked with the expressed juice of *Vijapura* and with honey

* Tepid milk, tepid clarified butter and expressed juice of sugar-cane are also separately used as snuff.

† S'vávidh and S'allaki are the two different kinds of porcupine.

would also give instataneous relief in a paraxysm of hiccough. 13.

Lukewarm gruels (Yavágu) saturated with clarified butter as well as lukewarm Páyasa prove curative in a case of hiccough. The milk of a she-goat duly cooked with *S'unthi* and water * (in the manner of Kshira-páka) and mixed with sugar could be as well taken with benefit. The urine of a she-goat and of a ewe taken to satiety would readily cure a fit of hiccough. Similarly the smell of *Puti-keeta* † duly soaked in the infusion of radish, *Vachá* and *Hingu* ‡ after the manner of Bhávaná saturation would have the same result. 14.

Nága-kes'ara mixed with sugar and honey should be taken with a copious quantity of) the expressed juice of sugar-cane and of *Madhuka* flowers. A Pala weight of *Saindhava* salt should be used with two-Pala weight of clarified butter. *Haritaki* should be first taken and then a draught of tepid water. Clarified butter should be taken with milk and honey. A Pichu (two Tolás) weight of the expressed juice of *Kapittha* should be taken with honey and powdered *Pippali* for the relief (of hiccough). A lambative prepared with *Pippali*, *A'malaka*, *S'unthi*, sugar and honey, or one prepared with *Anjana* (Souviránjana), powdered fried paddy, and the kernel (of the stone of) *Vadara*-fruit should be licked as a remedy for an attack of Hiccá. 15.

The four different liquid compounds ‖ prepared

* Some render शुण्ठीतोय as the decoction of S'unthi.

† Puti-keeta is a kind of bad-smelling worm appearing generally during the rainy season.

‡ Some read 'हिङ्गुब्ज' (Hingu and lotus) in place of 'हिङ्गुस्तु'। In both cases, however, 'भावित' means simply 'mixed'.

‖ According to Vrinda and Chakrapáni lambatives should be prepared with these drugs. According to some, the decoction should be used.

with the drugs mentioned in the four quarts of the present verse, *viz.*, (1) The fruit and flower of *Pátalá*, (2) *Gairika* and *Katu-rohini* (3) the kernel (inner pulp) of *Kharjura* and *Pippali* and (4) *Kásisa* (sulphate of iron) and *Kapittha* (D. R.—Dadhi), should be mixed with honey and administered by an experienced physician in cases of Hiccá. 16.

Meat as diet :—The soup prepared with the meat of *S'allaka* (porcupine), *S'vadamshtrá*, *Godhá*, *Vrisha-dams'a* (wild cat), *Rishya* (D. R. Riksha—a bear) and *Mriga* (different kinds of deer; as well as of *Kapota* and *Párávata* (different kinds of pigeon), *Láva* and other birds should be taken lukewarm with the expressed juice of acid fruits and with *Saindhava* and a Sneha (clarified butter, etc.). 17.

Purgatives as well as potions of tepid clarified butter mixed with *Saindhava*-salt and sugar should be regarded as highly beneficial in an up-coursing of the bodily Váyu in cases of Hiccá. Some authorities are of opinion that the application of an Anuvásana-vasti would be also beneficial in such cases. 18.

Thus ends the fiftieth chapter in the Uttara-Tantra of the Sus'ruta Samhitá which deals with the (symptoms and) treatment of hiccough.

CHAPTER LI.

Now we shall discourse on the chapter which deals with the (symptoms and) medical treatment of Asthma **(Śváśa-Pratishedha).** I.

Ætiology :—To the same group of exciting factors which bring in an attack of hiccough should be attributed the origin of that voilent disease which is known as Śvása (asthma). The vital Váyu known as the Prána-Váyu foregoing its normal function rises upward in unison with the deranged Kapha of the body and produces that gasping and laboured breathing which is called **Śváśa** (asthma). This dreadful disease though virtually one in its nature and origin is divided into five spicific types, *viz.*, Kshudra-Śvása, Tamaka-Śvása, Chhinna-Śvása, Mahá-Śvása and Urddhva-Śvása. 2 4.

Premonitory Symptoms :—Pain in the region of the heart and at the sides, aversion to food as well as to all other pursuits, suppression of stool and urine and a bad taste in the mouth, may be regarded as the premonitory symptoms of the disease. 5.

Specific Symptoms :—The type in which the least movement or exertion brings on an aggravation of the disease, and a distinct amelioration or relief is restored in a sitting posture, is called **Kshudra-Śváśa** The type which is accompained by such symptoms as thirst, perspiration, vomiting and a rattling sound in the throat and finds aggravation specially in foul weather is called **Tamaka-Śvasa**. In a case of Tamaka-Śvása the patient is weak and has a loud (wheezing) sound in the throat, as also cough, the symptoms of (bronchial) catarrh and an aversion to food. He is oppressed with difficult breathing even in sleep which abates only when the cough subsides and is aggravated when the patient sleeps. If a case of Tamaka-Śvása be attended with fever and fainting fits, it is then called **Pratamaka.** 6—9.

The case wherein the patient pants for breath and has tympanites and a burning sensation in the bladder, and wherein the breaths are painful, detached and intermittent, is known as **Chhinna-Śvása.** The case wherein the patient breathes heavily lying unconscious and with a loud rattling sound in his throat and with cramps at his sides, the lips and the throat being parched and the eyes riveted in a fixed gaze or stare, is known as **Mahá-Śvása.** The case wherein a patient breathes hurriedly, lies unconscious with choked voice and upturned eyes and with his Marmans stretching out fully with each stroke of breath is called **Urddhva-Śvása.** 10—12.

Prognosis :—Of these (five) types the one known a Kshudra-Śvása is easily curable, while the one known as Tamaka-Śvása is hard to cure, and the three remaining ones, as well as Tamaka, ocurring in a weak or enfeebled patient are regarded as incurable. 13.

General Treatment :—Several authorities aver that mild emetics and purgatives (lit. upward and downward cleansing—Śodhana—of the system) with the exception of the application of Sneha-vasti would be the chief remedies in cases of asthma, if the patient possesses sufficient vitality. Old and matured clarified butter duly cooked with *Abhayá*, *Vit*-salt and *Hingu* or with *Souvarchala*, *Abhayá* and *Vilva* would be beneficial in cases of cough, asthma, hiccough and heart-disease. Similarly old and matured clarified butter duly cooked with the pulverised drugs of the *Pippalyádi* group as Kalka and with (the decoction of) the drugs of the first *i.e.* the *Vidárigandhádi* group and with the five officinal kinds of salt added to it by way of an after-throw, relieves both cough and asthma. 14—15.

Himsrádi Ghrita :—Clarified butter should be duly cooked with a Kola (D. R. Karsha) weight each of * *Himsrá*, *Vidanga*, *Putika*, *Tri-phalá*, *Vyosha* and *Chitraka*, and with milk twice as much and water four times as much as clarified butter. A draught of this mediated Ghrita relieves both cough and asthma and proves curative in cases of piles, aversion to food, Gulma, diarrhœa and consumption (Kshaya). 16.

A quantity of clarified butter, duly cooked with four times as much of the decoction of all the parts (viz.—leaves, branches, barks, flowers and roots) of *Vásaka* and with its roots and flowers as Kalka, should be used with honey when cold (in cases of asthma). 17.

Śringyádi-Ghrita,—A Prastha measure of clarified butter duly cooked with *S'ringi*, *Madhuriká*, *Bhárgi*, *S'unthi*, *Rasánjana*, sugar, *Ambuda*, *Haridrá* and *Yashti-madhu* all taken in equal parts and as Kalka and with four times of water, would cure cases of cough, asthma and hiccough. 18.

Suvahádi Ghrita :—A Prastha measure of clarified butter should be duly cooked with twice as much of water and with a Kola (one Tolá. D. R.—Karsha) weight each of *Suvahá*, *Kaliká*, *Bhárgi*, *S'ukandsá*, *fruits of Nichula*, *Kákádani*, *S'ringavera*, *Varshábhu* and the two kinds of *Vrihati*. Taken hot after being made pungent (by the addition of some pungent drug *e. g.*, Pippali), it would cure all forms of asthma. 19.

Calrified butter duly cooked with the admixture of *Souvarchala*, *Yava-kshára*, *Katuka*, *Vyosha*, *Chitraka*, *Vachá*, *Abhayá*, *and Vidanga*, proves curative in a case

* Some prescribe the Kalkas to be taken in the ordinary way and say that the dose would be one Kola weight.

41

of asthma. Similarly clarified butter duly cooked with the decoction of *Gopa-valli* (Sárivá) weighing twice as much as the clarified butter is also prescribed. Physicians prescribe these **five** medicated Ghritas in cases of asthma and cough.* 20-21

Tálisádi-Ghrita :—Clarified butter mixed with *Hingu* weighing a quarter part of its own weight and duly cooked in combination with four times as much of water and with *Tális'a*, *Támalaki* and *Ugrá*, *Jivanti*, *Kushtha*, *Saindhava*, *Bilva*, *Pushkara*, *Putika*, *Souvarchala*, *Kaná* (*Pippali*), *Agni* (*Chitraka*), *Pathyá*, (Haritaki) and *Tejovati* as Kalka proves curative in all forms of asthma. The medicated Ghrita known as **Vásá-Ghrita** † and **Shatpala-Ghrita** ‡ would likewise prove beneficial. 22.

The proper use of oil duly cooked in combination with the expressed juice of *Bhringa-rája* weighing ten times as much, would relieve cough and asthma. 23.

Meat as Diet :—Essence of any bird of the Vishkira species (e.g. chicken, Láva, etc.) charged with the juice of any acid fruit (e.g. pomegranate, Vijapura, etc.) and with clarified butter and salted with a profuse quantity of *Saindhava*, or the soup of *Kulattha* cereals, properly cooked with the heads of Ena deer, etc., as well as milk duly cooked with (Anti-asthmatic and Váyu-subduing) drugs (e.g. Pancha-mula) would destroy cough and asthma. 24.

The five Lambatives :—A lambative com-

* Some editors add this sentence after the next (Tálisádi) Ghrita.

† **Vásá-Ghrita** is mentioned in the treatment of Rakta-pitta (Ch. XLV, 20, Uttara-Tantra). It should be prescribed in cases of asthma when **Pitta** predominates.

‡ **Shatpala-Ghrita** is mentioned in the treatment of Váta-Vyádhi. It should be prescribed if **Váyu** prevail.

posed of any of the following five groups of drugs mentioned in a hemistich each, *viz*, *Tinis'a*-seeds, *Karkata-S'ringi* and *S'uvarchiká* (*Jatuka-creeper*), or *Durá-labhá*, *Pippali*, *Katuka* and *Haritaki*,; or porcupine's hair, peocock's feather, *Kola'* (Chavya) *Mágadhiká*, and *Kana'*,* or *Bhárgi*, *Tvak*, (cardamom), *S'ringavera*, *S'arkara'* (sugar) and *S'allaka*-bark, or the well-pounded seeds of *Tri-kantaka* alone, should be licked with honey and clarified butter by a patient suffering from cough and asthma. 25.

Powders of *sapta-chchhada*-flowers and *Pippali* should be taken with curd-cream (Mastu) or powders of fried barley grains (?) previously soaked for several times in the expressed juice of tender *Arka*-twigs together with honey should be taken. As an alternative, a patient suffering from asthma wou'd drink the *Tarpana* (cordial) prepared with the above-mentioned barley-powder (by mixing it with a copious quantity of water and) with honey. 26.

A potion prepared with the flowers of *S'irisha*, *Kadali* and of *Kunda* and with *Mágadhiká* and dissolved in the washings of rice would completely cure all forms of asthma. The pith or inner pulp of *Kola*-stone, roots of *Tála* (palm) tree (D. R.—Tála-muli) and the burnt skin † of a deer of the Rishya species, should be taken with honey ; or *Bhárgi* with honey and clarified butter, or *Kadamba*-seeds and *Nimba* in combination with honey and the washings of rice. 27—28.

Drákshá, *Haritaki*, *Krishná*, *Karkata-s'ringi* and

* Maghadhiká and Kaná are synonyms and mean Pippali. Some, therefore, prescribe two parts of Pippali in the compound. Others prescribe one part of Pippali, and one of Gaja-pippali.

† The skin of the deer should be burnt in a covered earthen pitcher and the black contents should be used.

Durálabhá in combination with honey and clarified butter, should be licked by a patient whereby he would get rid even of a violent attack of asthma. A lambative composed of the equal parts of *Haridrá Maricha, Drákshá*, treacle, *Rásná, Kaná* and *S'athi*, should be given to be licked with oil by an asthma-patient, conforming to the regimen of wholesome diet. 29—30.

The expressed liquid of cow-dung and horse-dung should be licked by the patient with honey and powdered *Pippali* in cases of cough and asthma. The medicinal remedies or compounds mentioned in connection with Pándu-roga, and edema (Śotha) or cough, may be employed with efficacy both in cough and asthma. A compound made of *Bhárgi, Tvak, Tryushana*, oil, *Haridrá, Katurohini, Pippali, Maricha, Chandá* and the expressed liquid of cow-dung should be given (to be licked). **Utkáriká** should be prepared with *Tala-keeta-vija**. Taken internally, it instantaneously subdues even a violent attack of asthma. 31—34.

Articles recommended :—Matured clarified butter, *Pippali*, soups of *Kulattha*, or of the flesh of any Jángala animal, Surá, Souviraka (fermented rice-boilings), *Hingu*, the expressed juice of *Mátulunga*, honey, *Drákshá, Ámalaki* and *Bilva* are recommended (as diet) in cases of asthma and hiccough. 35.

Application of Sveda :—Oily fomentation (**Snigdha-Sveda**) with the help of oil and salt should be applied to the patient suffering from asthma and hiccough, whereby the hardened Kapha (accumulated in the channels) would be liquefied and the deranged bodily Váyu pacified. If the Váyu and Kapha be not thereby

* We do not know what 'Tala-keeta' is. Some printed editions read "Talpa-keeta" which would evidently mean a "bug". Dallana is silent on the point.

pacified, the patient should be first treated with Sneha and then with a diet consisting of boiled rice cooked with meat-soup. Application of Dhuma-inhalation should then be resorted to. 36A.

Application of Dhuma :—The stick (**Varti**) to be used in the process should be duly made of *Manah-s'ilá*, *Deva-dáru*, *Haridrá*, *Patra*, *Guggulu*, *Lákshá* and *Eranda*-roots made into a paste. Compounds made of clarified butter, fresh wax and resin ; or of cow's horn, hairs, hoof, tendon and skin ; or of *Turashka* (Śilá-rasa), *S'allaki* (Mocha-rasa), *Guggulu* and *Padmaka*, should be pounded together (and made into sticks) with the addition of clarified butter. An intelligent physician should use these (sticks) for the purpose of smoke-inhalation in the disease. 36.

Purging and vomiting should be induced in a patient overwhelmed with the action of the deranged Kapha, while Tarpana measures with the administration of a potion of the well-cooked soup of mutton or of the flesh of any Jángala or Ánupa animal, should be prescribed in the case of a weak or enfeebled patient, or in respect of one suffering from an internal parched condition of the body. 37.

A lambative should be prepared with *Nidigdhiká* paste of the weight of an *Ámalaka*, mixed with half as much of powdered *Hingu* and with a copious quantity of honey. Duly taken, it would per force conquer a paroxysm of asthma within three days. 38.

Irresistible is an attack of asthma like that of a fire fed with heaps of fuel (D. R. fauned by the wind) or like that of the thunderbolt hurled by the wrathful Indra, the king of the gods. 39.

Thus ends the fifty-first chapter in the Uttara-Tantra of the Sus'ruta-Samhitá which deals with the (symptoms and) treatment of asthma.

CHAPTER LII.

Now we shall discourse on the chapter which deals with the (symptoms and) medical treatment of cough. **(Kása-Pratishedha).** 1.

Cause and Etiology :—Cough has its origin in the same sets of causes, which excite or usher in an attack of hiccough or asthma. The vital Váyu of the body known as the Prána-Váyu combined with other Doshas (Pitta and Kapha) is deranged by such causes as the entrance of smcke or of particles of dust (into the larynx and nostrils), over-fatiguing physical exercise, inordinate use of any dry or parched (Ruksha) food, any food going wrong way, voluntary repression of sneezing or of any natural propulsion of the body. Thus deranged, it is suddenly pressed upward and emitted through the mouth in unison with the deranged Udána-Váyu (situated in the trachea) producing a peculiar sound resembling that of broken Indian bell-metal. This is called **Kása** (cough) by the learned. 2—3.

Classification :—This disease is divided into **five** types according as it is originated through the action of the deranged Váyu, or Pitta or Kapha of the body, or is due to the presence of any ulcer (Kshata) or to any wasting process (Kshayaja) in the organism. These five types of cough are recognised by the physicians (in practice), which, when fully developed, (*i.e.*, if neglected) would tend to produce phthisis (Yakshmá). 4.

Premonitory Symptoms :—Itching in the throat, a sense of obstruction in eating (difficulty of deglutition), a sticky feeling in the throat and in the palate, changed voice, aversion to food, and dulness of the digestive fire are the symptoms which usher in an attack of cough. 5.

Specific Symptoms:—A person affected with a cough of the **Vátaja** type, complains of an aching pain in the region of his heart, in his temples, head, stomach and the sides and has dry and frequent coughs (unattended with mucous expectorations), with a pale face, a weak and hoarse voice and diminished strength and vigour (Ojas). A burning feeling in the region of the heart, fever, sense of dryness, and a bitter taste in the mouth, thirst, yellow and pungent expectoration, paleness of complexion and a burning sensation in the body, are the indications of the **Pittaja** type of Kása. A sticky sense in the mouth, a sense of physical lassitude, headache, aversion to food, a sense of heaviness in the body, itching, frequent fits of cough and thick mucous expectorations are the features which distinguish the **Kaphaja** type. 6—8.

Symptoms of Kshataja Kása:—Ulceration in the Vakshas (chest ?) caused by loud reading, over-fatiguing physical exercise or carrying loads of excessive weight, or incidental to any blow or hurt dealt thereon, affects the locality and gives rise constant fits of cough accompained by blood-spitting. The disease is called **Kshatja Kása** or cough of ulcerated chest. 9.

Sexual excess, carrying heavy loads, excessive toils of journey, over-exertion in battle, forcible controlling of horses and elephants and such other fatiguing feats tend to produce parchedness of the system and ulcers in the Uras (chest) whereby the bodily Váyu is deranged and cough is produced. The patient is afflicted only with a sort of dry cough at the outset but begins to spit blood with the progress of the disease. The patient feels an excessive pain in the throat and his Uras (chest) seems to be broken and pricked into with sharp needles, and cannot bear the least touch on account of the pressure of an intolerable aching pain (Śula) in the locality. Breaking pain in the joints, fever, asthma, thirst, and loss of voice are the symptoms which mark the **Kshataja** type of the disease and the patient lies moaning like a pigeon. 10.

Kshayaya-Kása.—The fire of digestion in a person who is addicted to the habit of taking unwholesome and incongenial food or of taking it at improper time and quantity or who is given to sexual excesses or who indulges in grief or disgust or abhorrence (of food) in his mind, or who voluntarily represses any natural urging of his body, becomes affected and diminished. It (thereby) aggravates all the three Doshas of the body, which, in their turn, give rise to a type of cough attended with a gradual emaciation of the body. The disease is called **Kshayaja Kása.** Cramps in the limbs, fever, burning sensation in the body, fainting fits (Moha), loss of strength (Prána) and of flesh, emaciation of the body, spitting blood streaked with pus, and weakness are the symptoms of this type of Kása known as Kshayaja Káśa. It is said by medical experts to be due to the concerted action of all the **three Doshas** and to be included within the category of diseases which are very hard to be cured. A case of cough (in an old man) due to his declining years is only susceptible of palliation. 11—12.

General Treatment :—A compound consisting of *Śringi*, *Vachá*, *Kat-phala*, *Ka-trina*, *Musta*, *Dhanyáka*, *Abhayá*, *Bhárgi*, *Deva-dáru*, *Viśwa* and

Hingu taken in hot water would rapidly cure a case of long-standing cough. A lambative composed of the equal quantity of *Tri-phalá*, *Vyosha*, *Vidanga*, *S'ringi*, *Ra'sna'*, *Vacha'*, *Padmaka* and *Deva'-dáru* pounded together and mixed with a copious quantity of honey, sugar and clarified butter, would speedily conquer a serious attack of cough. 13 - 14.

A patient afflicted with cough should use a lambative composed of *Pathyá*, *sugar*, *Ámalaka*, fried paddy, *Mágadhi*, and *S'unthi* pounded together and mixed with honey and clarified butter, or take *Krishná* and *Saindhava* salt with warm water. He should use *Nágara* and *Pippali* in combination with treacle, or use a lambative of the paste of *Drákshá* mixed with honey and clarified butter. A compound composed of the equal parts of *Drákshá*, sugar and *Mágadhiká*, or of *S'ringa-vera*, *Yashti-madhu*, and *Tugá* (Vams'a-lochana) should be licked with honey and clarified butter ; or a compound consisting of *S'itopala* (sugar) and an equal quantity of *Maricha* should be licked with honey and clarified butter. A compound consisting of *Dhátri*, *Kaná*, *Vis'va* and *S'itopala* (sugar) should be taken with curd-cream (Dadhi-manda). A person suffering from an attack of cough should use *Harenuká* and *Mágadhiká* taken in equal parts and pounded together through the medium of curd. The two kinds of *Haridrá*, *Deva-dáru*, *S'unthi* and the pith of a *Gáyatri*-tree pounded and mixed in equal parts, should be taken with the urine of a goat, or a pulverised compound consisting of *Danti*, *Dravanti* and *Tilvaka* should be taken. Leaves of *Vadara* pasted with *Saindhava* salt and fried in clarified butter should be taken ; or a Kola (two tolás) weight of *Hingu* should be taken with fermented rice-boilings (Souviraka) or with the juice of acid fruit.

Powdered *Maricha* should be likewise licked with honey. 15.

Inhalation of Dhuma :—The patient should be made to **inhale** the smoke of a burning Varti (medicinal stick) composed of *Bhárgi*, *Vachá* and *Hingu*, pounded together and mixed with clarified butter, or of the scrapings of (green) bamboo,* *Elá* and *Lavana* mixed with clarified butter. Similarly, a patient suffering from an attack of cough due to **Váta** and **Kapha** should inhale the smoke of a Varti prepared with *Musta*, bark of *Ingudi*, *Yashti-madhu*, *Mánsi*, *Manah-s'ilá* and *Haritála* pasted together with goat's urine and then take a draught of milk. 16.

In the alternative, Sidhu (a kind of wine) should be taken in combination with *Maricha*, whereby a fit of cough would be instantaneously subdued. Milk duly boiled and cooked with the admixture of *Drákshá*, *Ambu* (Válaka), *Manjishthá* and *Pura*† should be taken with honey. Well-boiled *Mudga* pulse should be taken with powdered *Kanta-Káriká*, Nágara and pippali mixed with honey‡. Utkáráká (a kind of confection) prepared with clarified butter, *Mula* §, *Truti* (Elá), leaves of *Vadara* and a copious quantity of powdered *Nágara* should be used. A thin Peyá prepared with the preceding drugs may be taken cold in combination with honey. 17—19.

Treatment of Vátaja Kása :—The medicated clarified butter mentioned in connection with the

* Dallana explains वेणुत्वक् as वंशदलं (leaves of bamboo).

† Pura means S'allaki (gum) or Guggulu. —Dallana.

‡ Dallana reads कटुकोपगाढान् as a variant and explains that the powders of Tri-katu should be added in a large quantity in place of honey.

§ By the term "मूल" some mean मूलक (raddish), while others take it to mean the drugs of the Pancha-mula group.

medical treatment of Plihodara (enlargement of spleen) and known as Shadanga-Ghrita * proves equally curative in cases of **Vátaja-Kása**. Clarified butter duly cooked with the drugs of the *Vidári-gandhádi* group, or with the expressed juice of *Vásaka,* would also prove beneficial. Applications of purgatives with any Sneha, as well as those of **Ásthápana** or **Anuvásana-Vasti** are recommended. Inhalation of Snaihika (oleaginous) **Dhuma** as well as potions of lukewarm clarified butter, gruels duly cooked with meat-essence, milk and lambatives saturated with clarified butter, may be taken with advantage in such a case. 20.

Treatment of Kaphaja Kása :—Cases of **Kaphaja-Kása** readily yield to the use of emetics, purgatives, medicinal head-purgatives, medicinal gargles, hot and pungent lambatives as well as the inhalation of smoke (Dhuma). Any articles of food which are emaciating (*i.e.*, light, percifying and small in quantity and even fasting) should more particularly be beneficial. A case of cough due to the action of the deranged bodily Kapha is relieved by the use of *Tri-katu,* † or of clarified butter duly cooked with the expressed juice of *Krimighna* ‡ (Vidanga) or with the expressed juice of the leaves of *Nirgundi.* 21.

A clarified butter duly cooked in combination with twice as much juice of *Nidigdhiká* (Kantikári) and with the Kalka of *Páthá*, *Vit-salt*, *Vyosha*, *Vidanga*, *Sain-*

* For Shadánga-ghrita, see chapter XIV, Para 18. It is better known as Shatpalaka-Ghrita.

† According to Vágbhata the clarified butter should be duly cooked with the Kalka of Tri-katu and with the decoction (Rasa) of Vidanga.

‡ Some take 'Krimighna' to mean Vidanga, others take it to mean any antiparasitic drug, *viz.*, the drugs of the Surasádi-gana.—Dallana. The infusion or decoction of Vidanga should be used if its expressed juice be not available.—*Ibid.*

dhava, *Tri-kantaka* (Gokshura), *Rásná*, *Chitraka*, *Valá*, *S'ringi*, *Vachá*, *Mustá*, *Deva-dáru*, *Durálabhá*, *Bhárgi*, *Abhayá* and *S'athi*, proves curative in asthma, dulness of digestion, hoarseness, as well as the violent attacks of the five different types of cough. 22.

Pittaja and Kshayaja Kása :—A case of cough of the **Pittaja**-type, as well as the one due to the wasting (**Kshaya**) brought about by sexual excess, yields to the use every morning of the clarified butter, duly cooked with the decoction of the drugs of the *Vidári-gandhádi*, *Utpaládi*, *Sárivádi* and the *Madhura* (*i.e.* Kákolyádi) groups and with the expressed juice of sugar-cane, water, milk and with the drugs of the *Kákolyádi* group as Kalka and with the addition of sugar as an after-throw. The three cases *viz.*, Pittaja, Kshataja (ulcer-orignied) and Kshayaja (due to any wasting process in the system) of Kása are relieved by the use of the compound prepared with *Kharjura*, *Bhárgi*, *Pippali*, *Piyála*, *Madhuliká*. *Elá* and *Ámalaka* mixed in equal parts, and taken with a copious quantity of clarified butter, honey and sugar. 23—24.

Cases of the **Kshataja** (ulcerated) or **Kshayaja** (consumptive) Kása, would become amenable to the use of a compound consisting of the equal parts of *Raktá* (Manjishthá), *Haridrá*, *Anjana* (antimony), *Chitraka*, *Páthá*, *Murvá* and *Pippali* pounded together and taken with honey, or of clarified butter duly cooked with the expressed juice of sugar-cane. *Ámalaka* powder duly cooked with milk and taken in combination with clarified butter would prove efficacious. Persons afflicted with the three types of cough may take with benefit the fine powders of wheat, barley as well as of the drugs of the *Kákolyádi* group, with milk and clarified butter. Treacle boiled with water should be taken, when cold, with honey and with *Maricha* taken at intervals by biting it. 25—28

Kaláyana-Guda :—Three Prastha measures of the expressed juice of *Ámalaka* and half a Tulá measure (six seers and a half) of treacle should be duly cooked with eight-Pala-weight of powdered *Trivrit* (lightly fried) with eight-Pala measures of oil. Powdered *Granthika* (Pippali-roots), *Chavya, Jiraka, Vyosha, Gaja-pippali, Havashá, Ajamodá, Vidanga, Saindhava, Tri-phalá, Yamáni, Páthá, Chitraka* and *Dhánya*, each weighing a Pichu weight (two Tolás) should then be added to it as an after-throw and the whole compound should be scented with the three scented drugs (Tvak, Elá and Patra). The patient should take an Aksha (two Tolá) weight of this preparation. The medicine thus prepared is called **Kalyanáka Guda** and it proves curative in cases of Grahani, cough, asthma, hoarseness of voice and phthisis. It serves to improve appetite, increase the semen of males and remove sterility in females. There is no special restriction about the regimen of diet and conduct when it is used. 29.

Agastya-Leha :—Two Palas each of the drugs known as *Das'a-mula, Gaja-pippali, Átma-guptá, Bhárgi, S'athi, Pushkara*-roots, *S'unthi, Páthá, Gulancha, Granthika* (Pippali-roots), *S'amkha-pushpi, Rásná, Chitraka, Apámárga, Valá* and *Durálabhá*, and one Ádhaka (half a seer) of *Yava* together with one hundred large-sized *Haritaki* should be boiled with one Drona measure of water and taken down from the oven with its three-quarter part evaporated in the process. It should then be filtered through a piece of linen. A Tulá weight of treacle should be dissolved in the above decoction and duly cooked with the addition of a Kudava measure each of oil and clarified butter. When the cooking is finished, powdered *Pippali* should be added as an after-throw and honey should be mixed with it, when cooled. One Karsha weight of this elixir **Leha** should be licked every day in combination with two Abhayás. It conquers cases of phthisis, Grahani edema, dulness of appetite, hoarseness of voice, cough, Pándu, asthma, head-ache (Śiroroga), Hrid-roga (diseases of the heart)., hiccough and Vishama Jwara. A regular use of this elixir improves strength and memory, imparts vigour of mind and energy of action and removes disinclination to work. It was first concocted by the holy sage, Agastya. 30.

Clarified butter duly cooked with the decoction made by boiling the drugs of the Madhura or any other suitable group with the essence of Kulira (crab), Śukti, Chataka, Ena-deer and Láva proves curative in the case of cough due to the presence of any ulcer (in the lungs) or to any wasting process in the system. The use of clarified butter duly cooked with *S'atávari, Nága-valá* and *Valá* proves beneficial to a person afflicted with cough. 31—32.

Thus ends the fifty-second chapter of the Uttara Tantra in the Sus'ruta Samhitá which deals with the (symptoms and) treatment of cough

CHAPTER LIII.

Now we shall discourse on the chapter which deals with the (symptoms and) medical treatment of hoarseness of voice **(Svara-bheda-Pratishedha).** 1.

Etiology :—The Váyu and the other Doshas are deranged and aggravated by such causes as extremely loud speaking, taking poison, reading at the top of the voice, external hurt or injury and exposure to cold, etc., * and finding lodgment in the sound carrying channels, they affect the voice. The disease is called **Svara-bheda** (hoarseness of voice) and is classified into **six** different types. 2.

Specific Symptoms :—The **Vátaja** type imparts a black colour to the face, eyes, urine and stool and the voice acquires the sound of the rough and hoarse braying of an ass †. The face, eyes and the stool and urine of the patient are tinged yellow in a case of the **Pittaja** type and the voice sounds sunken as if proceeding from the throat with an internal burning sensation. In the **Kaphaja** type the patient constantly feels a sense of constriction in his throat with mucus and is only enabled to speak slowly and softly and that specially in the day. Symptoms specifically belonging to the three preceding Dosha-originated types, are simultaneously present in the type due to the concerted action of the three Doshas (**Tri-Dhoshaja**) together with indistinctness of speech and incapability

* Here Pitta-aggravating and Vayu-aggravating causes also are intended by the word 'आदि' *i.e.*, etc. in 'शीतादिभिः' ।

† Dallana's reading evidently is गद्गदवत् (indistinct).

of articulation. This type should be deemed as incurable. 3—6.

Symptoms of Kshayaja and Medoja types :—In the **Kshayaja** type the voice emits vapour and, becoming lower and lower, it ultimately disappears. This stage of Svara-bheda (loss of voice) should be given up as incurable. In an attack of the **Medoja type** the patient speaks very indistinctly, the voice remaining, as it were, inside his throat. And his throat, lips and palate become sticky. 7-8.

Prognosis :—Svara-bheda in cases of weak, old, emaciated, or fatty patient, as well as a long-standing, congenital or Tri-Doshaja one should be regarded as incurable. 9.

General Treatment :—The body of the patient should be first rubbed wiih a Sneha (clarified butter, lit.—treated with emulsive measures) and the deranged bodily Dosha underlying the root of the attack should be curbed with the help of emetics, purgatives, Vasti, errhines, Avapida-Nasya, lambatives, smoke-inhalations or gargles. Measures and remedies previously mentioned in connection with the treatment of cough and asthma should be as well employed in their entirety in the present disease. Now hear me describe the medicinal remedies which are specifically beneficial to a patient afflicted with an attack of Svara-bheda. 10.

Treatment of Vátaja Type :—In the **Vátaja** type of the disease, the patient should take, after a full meal, clarified butter mixed with the expressed juice of *Kása-marda*, *Vártáku* and *Márkava* with *Ártagala* (Arjua). In the alternative, Ghrita prepared from goat's milk and duly cooked with *Yava-Kshára* and *Ajamodá* or with *Chitraka* and *Ámalaka*, or with

Deva-dáru and *Agni* (Chitraka) should be taken with honey. The **diet** of the patient in such a case should consist of boiled rice taken with treacle and clarified butter, followed by draughts of tepid water. 11.

Pittaja and Kaphaja types :—Clarified butter should be constantly used with milk in the **Pittaja** type of the disease. Páyasa * duly prepared with the admixture of *Yashti-madhu* and clarified butter, should also be taken. Lambatives composed of the powdered drugs of the *Madhura* (Kákolyádi) group saturated with honey and clarified butter, or of powders of *S'atávari* or of *Valá* should be similarly taken. Powders of pungent drugs should be taken with a copious quantity of cow's urine or licked with oil and honey in a case of the **Kaphaja** type of Svara-bheda. 12—13.

Medoja, Kshayaja, etc., Types :—The medical treatment in the case of the **Medoja** type of Svarabheda should be the same as in the Kaphaja type. The medical treatment of the **Tri-Doshaja** and **Kshayaja** types of the disease should be taken in hand without holding out any hope of recovery. Milk † duly cooked with the drugs of the *Madhura* group should be taken in combination with sugar and honey in a case due to the effects of loud speaking. 14—15.

Thus ends the fifty-third chapter of the Uttara-Tantra in the Sus'ruta Samhitá which deals with the (symptoms and) treatment of hoarseness.

* **Páyasa** is a special preparation of rice boiled with milk and sugar.

† Milk of a cow or of a she-buffalo, etc., may be used here.—Dallana.

CHAPTER LIV.

Now we shall discourse on the chapter which deals with the (symtoms and) medical treatment of worms (**Krimi-Roga-Pratishedha**). 1.

Causes :—The Pitta and Kapha of the body are aggravated by such causes as eating before the digestion of a previous meal, excessive use of any indigestible, uncongenial, incompatible or filthy articles of fare, sedentary habits, partaking of cold, heavy or fatty meals, sleeping in the day-time, excessive use of *Másha*, cakes, *Vidala* (cereals), *Visa* (lotus stems), *S'áluka* (bulbous root of the lotus), *Kas'eruka*, pot-herbs, *Surá* (wine) *S'ukta* (a kind of fermented rice-gruel), curd, milk, treacle, sugar-cane, *Palala* (dried plants of corn), flesh of Ánupa animals, Pinyáka (oil cakes), *Prithuka* (Chipitaka), and such other articles of fare as well as by the use of sweet, acid and liquid articles. They help the germination of parasites of various shapes in the different parts of the body, Ámás'aya (stomach) and Pakvás'aya (intestines) being their principal seats or location. 2.

Classification :—The worms or parasites (which are found to germinate and grow in a living human organism) are divided into **twenty** different species, and have their origin either in **feces**, **Kapha** or **blood** *. Now I shall enumerate their names and characteristic features. 2—3.

Names and Symptoms of Purishaja Worms :—The **seven** kinds of worms which are

* Charaka speaks of another kind viz. **Malaja** (produced from the external filth of the body), over and above that kind of worms which are present in every organism from the very birth (**Sahaja**).

known as Ajava, Vijava, Kipya, Tripya, Gandu-pada, Churu and Dvi-mukha, originate from feces (**Purishaja**). They are white and extremely attenuated in their size. They frequent the passage of the rectum and produce a pricking pain (therein). Several of them are thicker and have tails. Cramps (Śula), dulness of appetite, yellowness of complexion, distension of the abdomen, loss of strength, water-brash, aversion to food, heart-disease (Hrid-roga) and looseness of stool, are the symptoms which mark the presence of worms (in the intestines), which originate in the feces. Of these Gandu-pada worms are red and long in their shape producing such symptoms as cutting pain (Śula), rumbling sound in the intestines, looseness of stool, and indigestion and they come out of the anus with an itching sensation. 4—5.

Names and Symptoms of Kaphaja Krimi :—Those known as Darbha-pushpa, Mahá-pushpa, Praluna, Chipita, Pipiliká and Dáruna, have their origin in the deranged **Kapha**. They are either hairy or have hairs only on their heads, or are marked with brown spots on their sides or are provided with tails. They are white and small-sized like fresh paddy-sprouts. They eat away the marrow and bore into the eye-balls, the palate and the ears and produce head-ache, cardiac troubles (Hrid-roga), vomiting and catarrh. 6—7.

Names and Symptoms of Raktaja Krimi :—The names of the worms originating from the vitiated **blood** are Keśáda, Romáda, Nakháda, Dantáda, Kikkiśa, Kushthaja and Parisarpa *. They are either black or blood-coloured, glossy and thick and

* The names of these worms have been derived from the nature of their actions on the different parts of the organism.

generally produce diseases which are peculiar to the vitiated state of the blood * in the body. 8.

Specific Causes:—Worms which have their origin in the **feces** (accumulated in the bowels) are the results of the (excessive) use of such articles of fare as *Másha*-pulse, cakes, salt, treacle and pot-herbs. The **Kaphaja** worms germinate in the system in consequence of eating flesh, *Másha*-pulse (D. R. fish), treacle, milk, curd and Śukta (a kind of fermented rice-gruel). Worms which originate from the contaminated **blood** of the body, are intimately connected with the use of pot-herbs and other indigestible and incompatible articles of fare. 9

General Symptoms:—Fever, paleness of complexion, Śula, cardiac troubles (Hrid-roga), lassitude, vertigo, aversion to food and diarrhoea (Atisára) are the complaints which mark the presence of worms in the system. 10.

Prognosis:—Of these the first thirteen kinds of worms may be seen with the naked eyes, while those beginning with Keśáda (*viz.*, the Raktaja worms) are not so visible and (of these latter) the first two (*viz.*, Keśáda and Romáda) kinds should be given up (as incurable). 11.

A physician should first ascertain the nature of the worms and, with a view to destroy their colony in the body, should treat the patient with a Sneha (clarified butter or oil) and then administer an emetic with clarified butter duly cooked with the drugs of the *Surasádi* group. He should then purge the patient with any strong purgative and treat him with an Ásthápana-vasti prepared with the decoction of *Yava*, *Kola*, *Kulattha*-pulse, and the drugs of the *Surasádi*

* See Chapter xxiv.,—Sutra Sthána.

group, charged with salt and with a Sneha (clarified butter or oil) duly cooked with *Vidanga.* Just after the flowing out of the injected solution (through his anus) the patient should be bathed with lukewarm water and a meal prepared with vermifugal articles should be given to him. Anuvásana-vasti should then be applied with the preceding Sneha (prepared with Vidanga). He should take a potion composed of the expressed juice of *S'irisha* and *Kinihi* (Apámárga) mixed together aud sweetened with honey. The expressed juice of *Kevuka* may be similarly (mixed with and) administered with a meal prepared with the articles of strong (Tikshna) property. 12.

A paste (or powder) of *Palás'a*-seeds or the expressed juice thereof should be taken with the washings of rice. The expressed juice of *Páribhadra*-leaves should be taken with honey. The juice extracted from *Pattura* * or the drugs of the *Surasádi* group should (similarly) be taken, or the powders of dried horse-dung or of *Vidanga* should be licked with honey. Pupuliká-cakes prepared with (pasted Yava and) the pasted leaves of *Mushika-parni* (a kind of Danti) should be taken by the patient followed by draughts of Dhányámla (fermented paddy-gruels). 13—14.

Oil duly cooked with (the paste and decoction of) the drugs of the *Surasádi* group should be given to be drunk. Different kinds of cakes should be prepared for him with (Yava mixed with) powdered *Vidanga.* Sesamum-seeds should be duly soaked in the decoction of *Vidanga* (after the manner of Bhávaná saturation) and oil should be then pressed out thereform (for his use). 15 A.

* Dallana explains "Pattura" as S'epháliká, but S'ivadás'a takes it to be S'álincha.

Powdered excreta of a Śvávidh (porcupine) similarly soaked seven times in (each of) the decoctions of *Tri-phalá* and of *Vidanga* should be licked with honey, followed by draughts of the expressed juice of *Ámalaka, Haritaki*, and *Aksha* (Vibhitaka). Powders of any (dead) metal (Ayas) * may also be prepared and taken in the preceding manner. In the alternative, the expressed juice of *Putika* should be taken with honey, or *Pippali*-roots should be administered through the vehicle of the urine of a she-goat. Trapu (killed lead) should be rubbed in the upper liquid part of curd (Mastu) and should be taken for a week. Worms which have their origin in the accumulated **feces** or aggravated **Kapha** in the body should be destroyed with the help of the aforesaid medicinal remedies. 15.

Medicinal Anjanas, Nasyas and Avapidas should be particularly employed in destroying the different classes of vermins which infest the regions of head, heart and mouth and the nostrils. The liquid expressed out of horse-dung should be dried and then successively soaked several times in the decoction of *Vidanga*. The preperation should be blown into the nostrils (Pradhamana). Powders of killed metal (Ayas, etc.†) may also be applied in the same manner. Oil duly cooked with the drugs of the *Surasádi* Gana should be used in snuffing with the blue part ‡ of Indian bell-metal. 17 A.

Measures and remedies mentioned in connection

* **Ayas**—lit. iron, is also used for all the metals generally.

† Ayas—as in para 15 may mean any metal.

‡ Oil duly cooked with the drugs of the Surasádi Gana should be placed in a pot of Indian bell-metal. When the inner surface of the pot would become blue by being oxidised, the oil should be well stirred and mixed with that blue part and used as an errhine.

with the treatment of alopecia (Indra-lupta) should be employed in cases of **Romáda** worms (*viz.* where the worms would be found to have invaded the hairs of the body). Medicines enumerated in connection with the treatment of the diseases of the mouth should be prescribed in cases of **Dantáda** worms (*viz.* where the vermins would be found to have taken lodgment in the teeth). Cases where the worms would be found to have their origin in the vitiated condition of the blood should be treated as cases of Kushtha to all intents and purposes. The drugs of the *Surasádi* Gana, however, may be used in any shape * in any case (of Krimi). 17.

Diet :—Meals composed of the articles of bitter and pungent tastes as well as draughts of milk mixed with the soup of *Kulattha*-pulse are recommended. A person suffering from any complaint due to the presence of worms (Krimi of whatever kind) and seeking their destruction, should refrain from using milk, cooked meat, clarified butter, curd, pot-herb (edible leaves), things of acid or sweet tastes as well as cold things in general. 18.

Thus ends the fifty-fourth chapter in the Uttara-Tantra of the Sus'ruta Samhitá which deals with the (symptoms and) treatment of Krimi-Roga.

* Both internally and externally e. g. as a drink or bath.

CHAPTER LV.

Now we shall discourse on the chapter which deals with the (symptoms and) medical treatment of the disease due to the retention of any natural physical urging (**Udávarta-Pratishedha).** 1.

Causes :—A wise man valuing his life shall never repress any natural urging of his body, whether upward or downward, *e. g.* that of Váyu, etc. Udávarta is so called from its origin from the repression of any natural urging such as Váta (flatus), evacuation of bowels, micturition, yawning, lacrimation, sneezing, eructation, vomiting and discharge of semen when it makes its appearance (Udita) and urges a person to answer its call. Udávarta is also brought on by the repression of hunger, thirst, respiration and sleep. I shall now fully describe its symptoms and the mode of medical treatment to be pursued therein. It is of **thirteen** different types and are brought about through the aforesaid causes, over and above the one incidental to the habitual use of unwholesome food and drink (Apathyaja). 2-4.

Symptoms of Vátaja Udávarta :—The vital Apána-Váyu (at the anus) anyhow obstructed in its passage gives rise to distension and cramps in the abdomen, oppression and a constricted feeling at the heart, headache, laboured breathing, hiccough, cough, catarrh, catching pain at the throat which makes speaking and Deglutition difficult (Gala-graha), violent movement of deranged Pitta and Kapha all through the body and suppression of stools or emission of fecal matter through the mouth. 5.

Purishaja Udávarta :—A repressed urging for stool is followed by the exhibition of such symptoms, as rumbling in the intestines, severe pain (in the abdomen), cutting pain in the anus, upward coursing of the flatus, suppression of stool or even emission of feces through the mouth. 6.

Mutraja Udávarta :—A repression of the desire of making water is followed by scanty emission of urine which is often given out by painful drops producing distension of the bladder and an excruciating pain in the urethra, anus, scrotum and the inguinal regions and about the umbilicus, and sometimes even in the head, accompanied with distortion of features in consequence. 7.

A repression of **yawning** leads to wry-neck (numbness of the Manyá and of the neck) as well as troubles of the head due to the incarcerated local Váyu and violent diseases affecting the eyes, nose, ears and the mouth. **Tears** born of any mental condition of grief or joy and voluntarily repressed without being given free vent to, give rise to severe distempers of the eyes, heaviness of the head and catarrh (Pinasa). 8–9.

A repression of **sneezing** is followed by acute diseases of the head, eyes, nose and ears. A sense of fulness in the throat as well as the suppression and croaking of the incarcerated Váyu (wind) are also exhibited in this case.* The voluntary repression of any natural urging towards **eructation** gives rise to diseases peculiar to the derangement of the bodily Váyu. 10–11.

A repression of **vomiting** is followed by cutaneous

* The symptoms mentioned in this sentence (which comprises a line in the verse) is taken by Mádhava with the following line which enumerates the symptoms of Udávarta due to the voluntary repression of eructation.

affections (Kushtha) due to the bodily Doshas which, being vitiated, had interfered with the gastric digestion with reactionary acidity and produced the vomiting. Painful swelling of the bladder and of the scrotum, and about the anus as well as suppression of urine, formation of gravels in the bladder and involuntary emission of semen are the symptoms which manifest themselves in a case of repressed **seminal** discharge. 12-13.

Ungratified **hunger** brings on drowsiness, aching pain in the limbs, disrelish for food, sense of exhaustion, and weakness of eye-sight. An ungratified **thirst** brings on dryness of the throat and mouth, dulness of hearing and pain at the heart. A suppression of **breath** in an exhausted person brings on cardiac troubles, fainting fits and an attack of Gulma. An unindulged **sleep** produces yawning, aching pain in the limbs, and a sense of heaviness in the limbs as well as in the head and the eyes. It may also bring on drowsiness. 14-17.

Prognosis :—An Udávarta-patient afflicted with thirst and cramps (S'ula), vomiting fecal matter and suffering from weakness and a distressing exhaustion should be given up by a wise physician. 18.

General Treatment :—In all forms of Udávarta the preliminary treatment generally consists in restoring the deranged and incarcerated bodily **Váyu** to its normal course and direction. Now hear me again describe the specific medicinal remedies to be separately employed in each case. 19.

Specific Treatment :—In a case of **Vátaja** Udávarta the patient should be first treated with a Sneha and Sveda (fomentation) after which medicinal injections should be made into the rectum after the manner of an Ásthápana-vasti. In a case due to the incarceration of feces in the intestines (**Purishaja**), the remedial measures and medicines laid down in connection with the treatment of Ánáha should be employed. 20-21.

Wine charged with a large quantity of *Souvarchala*-salt should be administered in a case due to the retention of **urine**. Milk or *Elá* should also be taken in combination with wine. The expressed juice of *Dhátri* diluted with water should be taken for three successive days; or the expressed liquid of the dung of a horse or of an ass should be taken; or wine made from treacle (Goudika) should be taken with honey and cooked meat should be taken by biting at intervals. One Tolá weight of the compound consisting of *Bhadra-dáru*, *Musta*, *Murvá*, *Haridrá* and *Yashti-madhu* shonld be dissolved in an adequate quantity of rain-water and then be taken. The expressed juice of *Duspars'á* (Durá-labhá) or an infusion of *Kum-kuma* (D. R.—decoction of Kakubha *i. e.* Arjuna) should be taken, or *Ervárukà*-seeds mixed with a little salt should also be taken with water. Milk duly cooked with *Pancha-mula*,* or the expressed juice of *Drákshá* should be prescribed. The medicinal remedies previously described as possessed of the efficacy of disintegrating gravels, (As'mari)† should be administered. Similarly, all the measures to be mentioned hereafter in connection wlth the medical treatment of Mutra-krichchhra ‡ (strangury) and of Mutrágháta § (obstruction of urine) which I shall have occasion to deal with later on should also be adopted in this case. 22.

A case of Udávarta due to the suppression of

* Both Dallana and S'ivadása recommend the use of minor Pancha-mula, but S'rikantha recommeds the Trina-Pancha-mula.

† For As'mari—See Chiktisita-sthána, Chapter VII.

‡ For Mutra-Krichchhra—See ch. LIX., Uttara-Tantra.

§ For Mutraghatá—See ch. LVIII., Uttara-Tantra

yàwning should be conquered with the applications of Sneha and of Sveda (fomentation). The patient should be treated with Sneha and then fomented and lachrymation should then be induced (with appropriate remedies)* in a case where the flow of **tears** has been suddenly checked. Sneezing should be induced with the help of strong Anjanas and Avapidas, or by the application of Vartis, or by holding any strong smell at his nose or by blowing any strong medicinal powder into the nose (Pradhamna) or by making the patient look towards the sun (or such like luminous body) in a case of Udávarta due to the suppression of **sneezing**. 23—24.

In a case of Udávarta due to suppressed **eructation**, the patient should be made to inhale the fumes of oily or lardaceous articles in due order† or to take draught of wine surcharged with *Souvarchala*-salt and the expressed juice of *Vija-pura.* A case of Udávarta due to suppressed **vomiting** should be duly conquered with emulsive measures (treating with a Sneha), etc., according to the nature of the deranged bodily Dosha involved in each case. In the alternative unguents with (Saindhava) salt and (Yava-) Ks'hara should be applied. 25—26.

Milk should be duly cooked with the admixture of four times as much water and with the drugs of bladder-cleansing virtues ‡ and boiled until all the water is evaporated. Draughts of this medicated milk should be prescribed in copious quantities in a case of Udávarta due to the retention of **seminal** fluid and the patient

* These are the applications of strong Anjanas and Avapida-Nasyas.

† The order is (1) Dhuma-inhalation, (2) Nasya (errhine) and (3) Kavala (gargle)

‡ These are the drugs of the Trina-pancha mula as well as of the Viratarvádi groups (Chapter XXXVIII, Sutra Sthána).

should be advised to have sexual intercourse with lovely women. 27.

Fatty (Snigdha) things should be taken lukewarm and in small quantities in a case of Udávarta due to ungratified **hunger**. Cold Manthas or Yavágus should be given to the patient in a case of Udávarta due to the suppression of **thirst**. Food with meat-soup should be given to the patient after sufficient rest in a case of Udávarta originated from the suppression of **breath** in a tired state of the body. Milk* should be given in a case of Udávarta due to the suppression of **sleep** and the patient should be made to sleep with the help of sweet discourses. 28.

Cases of **Ádhmána** (distension of the abodomen), etc., which are the supervening symptoms of Udávarta) should be remedied with appropriate medicines and other measures with an eye to the nature and intensity of the deranged Dosha or Doshas involved in each case underlying at the root. 29.

Udávarta due to errors in diet :—The abdominal (Koshthaja) Váyu deranged and aggravated by such factors as eating dry, astringent, pungent or bitter articles of fare (in inordinate quantities) causes an immediate attack of Udávarta in which the Vàyu (follows an upward course and) obstructs its own channels as well as those of feces, urine, Kapha, fat and blood. It dries up the fecal matter (in the body) causing pain in the heart and bladder, a sense of heaviness in the limbs (D. R —nausea), aversion to food (D. R. unwillingness to do anything) and difficult and scanty emission of stool, urine and flatus. Laboured breathing, cough,

* S'ivadása advises the use of buffalo's milk in this case as being more efficacious in bringing on sleep. But Dallana refutes this and recommends the use of cow's milk.

catarrh, burning sensation in the body, fits of unconsciousness, vomiting, fever, thirst, hiccough troubles in the head, defective functional activity of the Manas (mind) and of the ear and such like symptoms, in consequence, pre-eminently mark the deranged action of the bodily Váyu. 30.

Treatment :—The patient's body should be made emulsive (Snigdha) by the application of unguents composed of salt and oil. Fomentation should then be applied under the circumstances, and intestinal injections should be applied after the manner of a Nirudha Vasti. Intestinal enemas (Vasti) of the Anuvásana kind should also be applied after meal, if the case be attended with loose motions in virtue of the specific nature of the deranged bodily Doshas involved therein. Fatty purgtives should be exhibited after having fully fomented the body of the patient, when the foregoing remedies would fail to give any relief from attacks of Udávarta and he should be made to drink a potion of any acid cordial together with the compound of *Pilu*, *Trivrit* and *Yavâni* or with the compound consisting of *Hingu*, *Kushtha*, *Vacha*, *Svarjika*-kshára and *Vidanga*,* each succeeding drug weighing double the one immediately preceding it in the order of enumeration. These two medicinal compounds may be employed with advantage in relieving attacks of Śula aud Udávarta. 31—32.

The drugs known as *Deva-dáru*, *Chitraka*, *Kushtha*, *Vacha* (D. R—Śunthi), *Haritaki*, *Palamkashá* (Guggulu) and *Pushkara*-roots should be duly boiled with half an Ádhaka measure (thirty-two Palas) of water and taken down from the oven with a quarter part of the original

* Chakradatta reads 'विड़ञ्च' (and Vit salt) in place of 'विड़ङ्ग'.

solution remaining. Draughts of the this decoction would relieve an attack of Udavárta. 33.

A potion of clarified butter duly cooked with the decoction of dried* *Mulaka*, *Árdraka*, *Varshábhu*, *Pancha-mula* † and *Árevata* (Áragvadha) fruits would cure any form of Udávarta whatsoever. 34.

A compound consisting of *Vachá*, *Ativishá*, *Kushtha*, *Yava-Kshára*, *Haritaki*, *Pippali* and *Chitraka* should also be taken with tepid water, or a compound consisting of *Ikshácu*-roots, *Madana*, *Vis'alyá*, *Ativishá*, *Vacha*, *Kushtha*, *Kinva* (sediment of wine) and *Agnika* taken in equal parts should also be taken in the aforesaid manner. A compound of *Deva-dáru*, *Agni*, *Tri-phalá* and *Vrihati*, should be taken with the urine of a cow. The decoction of *Kantakári*-fruits and barley weighing a Prastha cooked in an Ádhaka measure of water and boiled down to half a Prastha only, should be taken in combination with *Hingu*. 35—38.

A compound consisting of the pulverised seeds of *Madana* and of *Alávu*, *Pippali* and *Nidigdhiká* should be blown into the rectum with a pipe. A **Varti** made of *Nikumbha* (Danti), *Kampilla*, *S'yámá* (Trivrit), *Ikshâku*, *Agnika*, (Ajamodá), *Krita-Vedhana* (Kosátaki), *Mágadhi* and salt pounded together, made into a paste with the addition of cow's urine, dried and cut into a proportionate size, should be inserted into the rectum. The last two ambrosial remedies give instantaneous relief in a case of **Udávarta**. 39.

Thus ends the fifty-fifth chapter of the Uttara-Tantra in the Sus'ruta Samhitá which deals with the (symptoms and) treatment of Udávarta.

* Dallana takes dried (S'ushka) with both 'Mulaka and Árdraka.

† Dallana recommends the major Pancha-mula ; but according to Chakrapáni's commentary, "Bhánumati," it should be the minor Pancha-mula.

CHAPTER LVI.

Now we shall discourse on the chapter which deals with the (symptoms and) medical treatment of Vishu-chiká type of cholera, etc. (**Visuchiká-Pratishedha**). 1.

Causes :—Visuchi, Alasaka and Vilambiká are produced from the effects of the three kinds of indigestion spoken of before (in Sutra. chapter XLVI), *viz.*, Ámájirna (indigestion properly so-called), Vidagdhá-jirna (indigestion with acidity) and Vishtabdhájirna (indigestion with undigested food stuffed into the intestines in the form of undigested fecal matter). 2.

Definition :—The disease in which the deranged and incarcerated bodily Váyu produces, owing to the presence of indigestion, a pricking pain in the limbs resembling that produced by the pricking of needles is called **Visuchiká** by the physicians. Men well-versed in the (dietetic) principles and temperate in their diet, enjoy an almost absolute immunity from its attack, whereas fools who are greedy and intemperate and eat like gluttons, fall an easy victim to it. 3.

Symptoms :—Fainting, diarrhœa (loose motions), vomiting, thirst, pain, cramps, vertigo, yawning, burning sensation in the body, discolouring or paleness of complexion, pain (cramps) at the heart and a breaking pain in the head are the symptoms of **Visuchiká**. 4.

Alasaka :—Excessive pain in and stuffedness of the abdomen, rumbling noise (in the intestines),* and the upward coursing of the Váyu incarcerated in the abdomen making a croaking rumbling sound in its way

* According to S'rikantha the commentator on Mádhava's Nidána—the patient himself makes an indistinct sound.

upwards, absolute suppression of stool and flatus, hic-cough * and eructations—a patient suffering from these symptoms is said have an attack of **Alasaka.** 5.

Vilambiká :—The person in whom the deranged and undigested food matter does not find any outlet either through the upper or lower channels of the body owing to the fact of its being obstructed in its course by the action of the deranged Váyu and Kapha, is said to be suffering from an attack of **Vilambiká** by old medical experts and should be given up as in-curable. In whatever part of the body the Áma (undigested food matter) is present, it produces its own characteristic symptoms in that very part and the vitiation of a particular Dosha in such cases should be diagnosed by the presence of the characteristic symptoms (e. g. distension, etc.,) of Áma (indigestion). 6—7.

Prognosis :—A patient exhibiting such symptoms as blackish blue (Śyáma) colour of teeth, nails and lips, diminished consciousness, vomiting, eyes sunk in their sockets, feeble voice and looseness of all the joints, should be regarded as not returning from his journey (to the eternal home). 8.

General Treatment :—In the curable types, cauterization of the regions of Párshni (heels), dry fomentation, exhibition of strong emetics and such like measures are recommended. Fasting should be observed at (the time of) the digestion of the food. Digestive (Páchana) remedies as well as purgatives should also be prescribed. The patient gets instantaneous relief in cases of fainting, diarrhœa, etc., on the cleansing of his body with the medicinal (emetic or purgative) remedies. Intestinal injections after the manner of an Ás'thápana Vasti may be likewise applied in all cases

* Mádhava reads "thirst" in place of "hic-cough."

of the present disease. Now hear me describe the recipes of other medicinal compounds which may be employed in the aforesaid diseases in addition to those already mentioned. 9—10.

A pulverised compound of *Pathyá*, *Vachá*, *Hingu*, *Kalinga* (Indra-yava), *Grinja* (a variety of garlic), *Souvarchala* and *Ativishá* taken with tepid water instantaneously relieves an attack of indigestion, colic, Visuchiká and an aversion to food. The medicine known as **Kshára-gada** (Kalpa—chapter VII) or *Vit*-salt, or mustard-seeds and a profuse quantity of treacle, should be taken (with tepid water). *Saindhava*, *Hingu*, *Vija-pura*, (D. R. seeds of S'áka), clarified butter and the two *Tri-vargas* (Tri-phalá and Tri-katu) in combination with any fermented gruel (Kánjika), or *Tri-katu* and *Saindhava*-salt mixed together with the milky exudation of *Snuhi*, should be taken (with Kánjika). In the alternative, the medicated salt known as **Kalyána-Lavana** described before under the treatment of Váta-vyádhi should be taken (with Kánjika). *Pippali*, *Yamáni* and *Apámárga*, or *Pippali* and *Danti* in equal parts should be similarly taken. *Pippali* mixed with *Danti* should also be used with the expressed juice of *Koshávati* (Ghoshá). *Pippali* and *S'unthi* should also be taken with hot water. 11.

The drugs known as *Vyosha* (*Tri-katu*), *Karanja*-fruits (seeds), the two kinds of *Haridrá** and the root of *Mátulunga* taken in equal parts should be pounded together, made into Gutikás (or pills) and dried in the shade. The application of these pills as an eye-salve (Anjana) along the eye-lids proves curative in cases of Visuchiká.† 12.

* Chakrapáni reads Haridrá in the singular number.

† Some here read the following two compounds as an additional text :— Kushtha, Aguru, Patra, Rásná, S'igru, Vachá and Tvak should be

Diet :—Digestive and appetising Peyá, etc., should be given to the patient when he experiences a good hunger after he had been fully treated with a course of emetic or purgative or kept fasting for a proper period. 13.

Causes and Symptoms of Ánáha :— The disease in which Áma (undigested food) or fecal matter, gradually incarcerated (in the stomach) through the action of the deranged and aggravated local Váyu fails to find its natural outlet, or is not spontaneously evacuated is called **Ánáha** (Enteritis ?).

A case of Ánáha due to the accumulation of undigested food (in the stomach) exhibits such symptoms as thirst, cattarrh, burning in the head, a sense of heaviness and cramps in the stomach, nausea (D. R.—heaviness of the heart) and suppression of eructations. While a case of Ánáha in the Pakvás'aya (intestines) is marked by a sense of stuffedness in the back and waist, suppression of stool and urine, colic, epileptic or fainting fits, vomiting of feces, laboured and difficult respiration (D. R.—swelling), as well as the symptoms mentioned under the head of Alasaka. 14.

Treatment :—In a case of Ánáha due to the presense of Áma, the patient should be treated with emetics and then with digestive medicines and diet according to the prescribed order. The Áma (undigested food) in a case not marked by any vomiting of feces should be treated with fomentation and therapeutic

mixed together and pasted with Kánjika. This would be the best remedy, for rubbing over the body of the patient, in a case of **Visuchiká**.

Oil should be duly cooked with Chitraka, Yuthi-flower, oil-cakes (of sesamum), Bhallátaka, the two Ksháras, Saindhava and two parts of Kushtha. This should be prescribed by an expert to be rubbed, or used as a plaster over the body of the patient.

agents of digestive efficacy. **Vartis** (suppositories) made by pasting the purgative drugs mentioned in connection with the medical treatment of Visuchiká together with the urine of a she-buffalo, or of a she-goat or of a ewe or of a she-elephant, or of a cow, should be used. The body of the patient should be first fomented and then the powders of the drugs used in preparing the afore-said Vartis should be blown (into his intestines) through a pipe inserted into his rectum. Decoction should be duly prepared by boiling the drugs of emetic and purgative virtue in cow's urine. Nirudha Vasti* should soon be applied with the above decoction mixed with half as much of cow's urine† and with honey and adding also the powders of *Trivrit* and salt weighing a Prakuncha (Pala). The procedure laid down in respect of the exhibition of purgatives should be adopted here. Oil duly cooked and boiled with the foregoing drugs should also be injected into the rectum, if necessary, after the manner of an Aunvásana Vasti. 15—16.

Thus ends the fifty-sixth chapter in the Uttara-Tantra of the Sus'ruta Samhitá which deals with the (symptoms and) treatment of Visuchiká.

* The application of this Nirudha Vasti should be prescribed only in the "पक्व" stage of Ánáha and never in its "आम" stage.

† Kártika Kundu does not include "urine" in this list. He reads "मात्रार्द्धयुक्तेन" (added in half dose) in place of "मूत्रार्द्धयुक्तेन".

CHAPTER LVII.

Now we shall discourse on the chapter which deals with the (symptoms and) medical treatment of aversion to food **(Arochaka-Pratishedha).** 1:

Ætiology :—The derangement of the Doshas either several or combined or an apathetic state of the mind (through grief, etc.) tends to block the food-carrying channels *viz.*, the esophagus, etc., as well as the region of the heart causing aversion to all sorts of food, which is designated **Bhaktopaghάta** (lit. aversion to food—popularly known as Arochaka) by the physicians and it is divided into **five** distinct types (according to the different nature of its exciting factor). 2.

Specific Symptoms :—Pain and cramps at the heart and a vapid taste in the mouth are the symptoms which mark the **Vάtaja** type of Arochaka. Excessive burning sensation (in the region) of the heart, sucking pain (in the locality), a bitter taste in the mouth, thirst and fainting fits are the features which mark the **Pittaja** type of the disease. Itching sensation, heaviness of the body, water-brash, lassitude, drowsiness and a sweet taste in the mouth are the indications which characterise the **Kaphaja** type. The **Tri-doshaja** type is characterised by a good many symptoms which severally mark the three Doshas. Indulgence in sensual pleasure, as well as in fear and grief, or the sight of any repugnant article, or of anything that tends to disturb the **mental** (Mánasa) equilibrium, may also usher in an attack of Arochaka. 3-7.

Treatment :—In a case of the **Vάtaja** type, the patient should be first made to vomit with the help of decoction of *Vacha* and then be given a pulverised compound of *Krishná*, *Vidanga*, *Yava-Kshára*, *Harenu*, *Bhárgi*, *Rásná*, *Elá**, *Hingu*, *Saindhava* and *Nágara* through the medium of any Sneha or wine or hot water. Vomiting should be induced with emetics sweetened† with the solution of treacle in the **Pittaja** type of the disease. The use of a lambative prepared with *Saindhava*, *Sitá* (sugar), honey and clarified butter would also be efficacious. In the **Kaphaja** type, vomiting should be induced with the decoction of *Nimba* and the powders of *Yamáni* should then (after the taking of the meal) be administered with the decoction of *Áragvadha* mixed with honey. The pulverised compound mentioned in connection with the treatment of the Vátaja type may also be administered (in this case). All the preceding measures should be employed in the **Tri-doshaja** type of Arochaka. 8-11.

Four Specific Lambatives :—(1) *Drákshá*, *Patola*, *Vit*-salt, *Vetra*, *Karira* (bamboo-sprouts), *Nimba*, *Murvá*, *Abhayá*, *Aksha*, *Vadara*, *Ámalaka*, (barks of) *Kutaja* and seeds of *Karanja* and of *Áragvadha* should be (powdered and) duly cooked with the urine of a cow in the form of a lambative. (2) A similar preparation should be made of *Mustá*, *Vachá*, *Tri-katu*, the two kinds of *Rajani*, *Bhárgi*, *Kushtha* and *Nirdahani*‡ and cooked with the urine of a ewe. (3) Similarly

* Elá—Dallana says that some take Elá in the sense of Ela-váluká (a part used for the whole). S'ivadása, however, refutes this and asserts, on the authority of Vágbhata, that "Ela" should mean Elá.

† According to some, the emetic used should be Madana fruit ; while, according to others, it should be the drugs of the Madhura (Kákolyádi) group—the word 'Madhura' indicating the same. Some, however, read 'Madhuka' (Yashti-madhu) for 'Madhura'.

‡ Nirdahani, according to some, means Chitraka, but, according to others, it means Yamáni. The former sense is the most general one.

Páthá, *Vamsá-lochana*, *Ativishá* and *Rajani* should be boiled together with the urine of a she-elephant. (4) *Manduki*, *Arka*, *Amritá* and *Lángalá* should be similarly boiled by an experienced and practical physician with the urine of a she-buffalo. Whoever licks up any * of the **four** preceding **lambatives** gets rid of Gulma, aversion to food, asthma and diseases affecting the heart and the larynx. 12.

Regimen of Diet :—The patient should partake of fruits, edible roots, etc. which grow in his country and take cordials, Shádavas † Rágas ‡ and other palatable dishes which are congenial to his physical temperament and which he is accustomed to. He should also be made to take (articles of) different Rasas § in different ways and his food should be at the same time light, Ruksha and agreeable to his taste. 13.

The due applications of Ásthápana-Vasti, purgatives and of light head-purgatives (errhines) are efficacious in the disease under discussion. The drugs known as *Tryushana*, *Rajani* (D. R.—the two kinds of Rajani) and *Tri-phalá* pounded together and mixed with powdered *Yava-kshára* and honey, should be used as a **tooth-powder** in washing the mouth. Any other drugs of bitter and pungent taste may be likewise prescribed for the purpose. 14-15.

* According to Dallana the four **lambatives** should be used in cases of **Vátaja, Pittaja, Kaphaja** and **Tri-doshaja** types of Arochaka respectively.

† "Shádava"—It is a preparation with a variety of articles of sweet, acid and saline tastes.

‡ "Râga"—It is a preparation of a cordial with sugar, Souvarchala-salt, Saindhava, turmeric, Parushaka, black-berry and mustard, etc.

§ Dallana interprets "Rasa" by meat-soup but we are inclined to take it in the sense of articles of different tastes (Rasa).

Use of Decoction; Arishta and Ásava: —Decoctions of the drugs of the *Mustádi* and *Áragvadhádi* or *Das'a-mula* groups as well as the different lambatives with honey, the different Ásavas prepared with any officinal urine and with treacle as well as the different Arishtas and the different Ásavas prepared from any *Kshára* and resembling in scent, the wine prepared from honey, should be used in conquering an attack of Arochaka. The aforesaid measures should also be employed for the purpose of re-kindling the digestive fire (appetite) impaired through the action of deranged Váyu and Kapha. 16.

Treatment of Mánasa Arochaka:— In a case of impaired digestion due to the effects of any ungratified desire, fear, grief, etc., the lost longing for food should be restored in the patient by holding out to him the near prospect of its realisation and by consoling him with the prospects of fresh joy and safety. In a case due to the loss of a splendid fortune, the bitter apathy and loathsomeness of the patient towards taking any food should be removed by infusing fresh hopes into his heart and by narrating to him the balmy stories of the Puránas. A case due to dejection or despondency should be conquered by sincere sympathy and cheering up. In short any impairment of appetite due to any disturbed or agitated state of the mind should be remedied with discourses gratifying to the patient under the circumstances. 17.

Thus ends the fifty-seventh chapter in the Uttara-Tantra of the Sus'ruta Samhitá which deals with the (symptoms and) treatment of Arochaka.

CHAPTER LVIII.

Now we shall discourse on the chapter which deals with the (symptoms and) medical treatment of the suppression of urine (**Mutrá-gháta Prati-shedha**). 1.

The disease is of **twelve*** **kinds**, *viz.*, Váta-kundaliká, Ashthilá, Váta-vasti Mutrátita, (Mutra-) Jathara, Mutrotsanga, (Mutra-)Kshaya, Mutra-granthi, Mutra-śukra, Ushna-váta and the two forms of (*viz.* Kaphaja and Pittaja) Mutraukasáda. 2.

Symptoms of Váta-kundaliká:—The bodily Váyu deranged and aggravated through an extremely parched condition or through the voluntary repression of an urging towards micturition affects and retains the urine in the bladder, causing it to revolve in eddies within the cavity of that organ. It allows the urine to pass in small quantity or (even) to dribble out in drops with pain. This disease is known as **Váta-kundaliká** and is of a violent type. 3.

Vátáshthilá:—The deranged and aggravated bodily Váyu incarcerated or lodged in the region lying between the bladder and the anus gives rise to a thick lumpy tumour like a pebble (Ashthilá), which is hard and non-shifting in its character, producing suppression of stool, urine and flatus, distension of the abdomen and pain in the bladder. It is known as **Vátáshthilá**. 4.

Váta-vasti:—The bodily Váyu in the locality, aggravated by a voluntary repression of a propulsion to urination enters into the bladder of the ignorant

* Mádhava reads thirteen different kinds of this disease. He reads only one kind of Mutra-sáda and adds Vid-vigháta and Vasti-kundala.

person doing the same and also obstructs the orifice of that organ causing retention of urine with an oppressive pain in the bladder and loins. The disease is known as **Váta-vasti** and is extremely hard to cure. 5.

Mutrátita:—The urine of a person voluntarily suppressing it does not flow out at all or only dribbles out in drops or in scanty jets with slight pain, when he strains. The disease is called **Mutrátita.** 6.

Mutra-jathara:—The vital Apána Váyu is deranged and aggravated by the Udávarta produced by a checked desire for urination and completely fills up and distends, with an excruciating pain in the abdomen below the umbilicus. The disease is called **Mutra-jathara** and the lower orifices* (*viz.* the anus and the urethra) are obstructed in this disease. 7.

Mutrotsanga:—The disease in which the stream of urine gliding along the bladder and urethra is gradually emitted in scanty jets or runs down the exterior surface of the glan penis with blood, whether with or without pain, is called **Mutrotsanga** (lit. gliding urination) and is an outcome of the deranged and aggravated action of the bodily Váyu. 8.

Mutra-kshaya and Mutra-granthi:—The deranged and aggravated Pitta and Váyu in the bladder of an extremely fatigued person already suffering from an extreme parchedness of organism, finds lodgement in the bladder producing, in concert, a sensation of local burning and pain attended with a scanty accumulation of urine in the cavity of the organ (lit. absence of micturition). The disease which can be made to yeild only to the virtue of therapeutic agents

* Some read "अधोवस्तिनिरोधकम्" the lower part *viz.*, the neck of the bladder is obstructed.

with the greatest difficulty is called **Mutra-kshaya**. A small round painful fixed Granthi suddenly occurring on the interior side (of the orifice) of the bladder and exhibiting by its characteristic pain, etc., all the symptoms of the presence of gravels (urinary calculii) in that organ, and which stands completely obstructing its orifice without letting out a single drop of urine, or admits only of its being dribbled out in scanty jets, is called **Mutra-granthi**. 9-10.

Mutra-Śukra and Ushna-váta:—A person visiting a woman in the presence of a strong urging towards urination and by voluntarily repressing the same is found to pass urine highly charged with semen which is sometimes seen to precede or follow the discharge of urine. The urine in this case resembles the washing or solution of ashes in colour. The disease is called **Mutra-śukra** (lit. semen-charged urine). The disease in which the Pitta of a person deranged by such factors as over-fatiguing physical exercise, exposure to the sun, or arduous pedestrian journey, gets into his bladder completely wrapped in the deranged Váyu of his body, and produces an intense burning sensation in his bladder, penis and the anus, setting up a painful flow of a dark yellow or blood-streaked urine or of blood alone through the urethra in its stead, is designated as **Ushna-váta**. 11-12.

Two kinds of Mutraukasáda:—A non-slimy and thick flow of yellow-coloured urine attended with a burning sensation, and leaving a sediment like powdered Rochaná when dried, is called (Pittaja) **Mutraukasáda**. The wise ascribe the origin of this disease to the action of the deranged **Pitta**. The type in which a pale sediment resembling the powders of conch-shell is deposited when the urine is dried and in which the flow is painful and the urine is slimy, thick and white, should be attributed to the action of the deranged **Kapha**. It is but another variety of the disease described immediately before. 13.

General Treatment :—Medicinal decoctions, Kalkas, (medicated) Ghritas, (various kinds of) foods, lambatives, preparations of milk, alkalis, honey, Ásavas, fomentation and Uttara-vasti should be employed according to their indications in coping with an attack of any of the aforesaid ailments. An intelligent physician shall resort, in these cases, to measures which are efficacious in cases of As'mari, or shall employ in their entirely the medicinal compounds which have been described as curative under the treatment of urinary Udávarta. 14.

A case of Mutra-krichchhra would be relieved by the use of pasted *Erváru*-seeds and *Saindhava* weighing an Aksha and taken with the fermented paddy-boilings. A person afflicted with Mutra-krichchhra should take wine (prepared from Pishta or pasted rice) in combination with *Souvarchala*-salt, or he should take wine prepared from honey by biting meat at intervals, or take any wine made from treacle. In the alternative, a Karsha measure of *Kumkuma* should be kept saturated with honey and water during the night and this should be taken in the morning, whereby the patient would be relieved of the trouble (of Mutra-krichchhra). By taking the principal wine (*viz.*, that prepared from Pishta or pasted rice) with salt, powdered *Elá*, *Jiraka and Nágara* and saturated with the acid juice of pomegranade one would get rid of Mutra-krichchhra. 15—16.

Half a Prastha measure of water with four times as much of milk together with the drugs of the *Prithak-Parnyádi* (Vidári-gandhádi) group and *Gokshura*-roots should be kept boiling till all the water is evaporated. A person suffering from an attack of Mutrá-gháta due to the concerted action of deranged Váyu and Pitta should use this medicated **milk**, when cooled, with sugar and honey. The dung of an ass or of a horse should he squeezed through a piece of linen and a Kudava measure of this expressed liquid should be taken for the cure of an attack of painful urination. 17—18.

An Aksha measure of the compound made by pasting *Musta, Abhayá, Deva-dáru, Murvá and Yashti-madhu*, should be taken with the decoction of *Drákshá. Abhayá, Ámalaka* and *Aksha* (Vibhitaka) together weighing a Vadara measure should be taken with salt and water for getting relief in cases of painful urination. An Udumbara measure of *Drákshá* should be kept saturated in water for the whole night and this cold infusion should be taken (in the morning) for getting relief in cases of painful urination. A Kudava measure of the expressed juice of *Nidigdhiká* or the Kalka of the same should be taken with honey as a relief from the urinary complaints. 19.

By taking a Kudava measure of the expressed juice of *Ámalaka*, a person suffering from uninary complaints would get rid of his troubles. In the alternative, the patient should drink a potion consisting of powdered small *Elá*, dissolved in the expressed juice of *Ámalaka* (and mixed with honey), or he should take a paste of the tender roots of *Tála* (palm) with cold rice-washing. The expressed juice of *Trapusha* and white *Kaikataka* should also be prescribed to be taken with milk in the morning. In the alternative a person should take a potion consisting of milk duly boiled with the drugs of the *Madhura* group saturated with clarified butter as the compound is possessed of excellent diuretic properties and tends to remove the seminal troubles (*e. g.*, Mutra-s'ukra) as well. 20.

A compound consisting of *Valá*, *S'vadamshtrá*, seeds of lotus (Krouncha)*, Tandula (*i.e.*, seeds) of *Kokiláksha* †, roots of *S'ata-parvan* ‡, Devadáru, *Chitraka* and stone of *Aksha*, pasted together and dissolved in wine should be taken by a person under the circumstances inasmuch as it removes the defects of urine and eliminates the gravels from the bladder. 21.

The ashes of burnt *Pátalá* wood, which are efficacious in relieving all sorts of urinary troubles, should be strained seven times in succession (after the manner of Kshára preparation) and taken with a small quantity of oil. In a similar way a paste of *Nala*, *Ikshu*, *Darbha*, *As'ma-bheda* and the seeds of *Trapusha* and *Ervúruka*, should be duly washed in milk and filtered and taken in combination with clarified butter. Powders of *Tvak*, *Elá* and *Tri-katu* should be taken by the intelligent one in combination with the alkaline solution of the ashes of *Pátalá*, *Yava-kshára*, *Páribhadra* and *Tila*. Lambatives made of the powders of the above-mentioned drugs should be separately licked with treacle. 22—24.

Now I shall describe the measures which are beneficial in **Mutra-dosha** (urinary defects). Purgatives should be administered to a patient after the due application of Sneha and Sveda. Uttara-vastis should be injected after he has been duly purged. 25.

Sexual intercourse should be refrained from by a person afflicted with a discharge of blood from the

* Dallana explains Krounchásthi as bones of a Krouncha bird, but we are not inclined to accept this explanation.

† Some explain "Kokilákshaka-tandula" as meaning Kokiláksha and Tandula (rice) which meaning may also be accepted.

‡ "S'ata-parvan" may mean Durbá-grass or bamboo.

urethra owing to sexual excesses, and he should be treated with remedies which are constructive tonics (e. g., meat-soup, milk, clarified butter, * etc.). Uttara-vastis should be applied into the urethra, under the circumstances, with cock's lard and with oil, the process of applying which has already been elaborately described. (See Chikitsá, XXVII). 26-27.

Half a Pátra measure of honey, one Pátra measure of clarified butter churned from milk (Kshira-sarpis) † and equal parts of sugar, and powdered *Drákshá*, *Átmaguptá*-seed, *Ikshuraka* and *Pippali*, together weighing one half part (i.e., half of half a Pátra) should be thoroughly mixed by stirring the compound with a laddle. A Páni-tala (two Tolás) measure of this compound should be licked, followed by draughts of milk. By using this Ghrita, a man is relieved of all injurious principles of his body, and gets rid of distressing and dreadful urinary troubles which cannot otherwise be easily cured by any other remedy. It acts as an excellent blood-purifier, and, by using it, even a barren woman may get rid of her sterility and of all other vaginal and uterine complaints which usually obstruct or retard conception in females. 28.

* Dallana says that Kârtika does not read this, in as much as this would increase the number originally mentioned, as also because this case has already been mentioned in Prameha. But according to Jejjata, this is mentioned here to make the case more clear.

† Dallana's reading here evidently is 'Kshira-sarpishah', but according to a variant the reading would be "Kshira-sarpish u" i.e., milk and clarified butter (taken together). The latter reading has the support of Chakrapáni and Vrinda who, however, read these lines in a different way and prescribe the drugs in somewhat different proportions. The former reading 'Kshira-sarpishah' with the sixth case-ending is, however, more grammatical.

Equal parts of *Valá*, stones of *Kola*-fruits, *Yashti-madhu*, *S'vadamshtrá* (Gokshura), *S'atávari*, *Mrinála* (lotus-stem), Kas'eru, seeds of Ikshuraka, Sahasra-viryá (Durbá), Ams'umati (S'ála-parni), *Payasyá* (Vidári), *Kálá*, *S'rigálavinná* (Pris'niparni), *Ati-valá* and the drugs of the *Vrimhaniya* (Kákolyádi) group should be duly boiled with four times of water of their combined weight and a Tulá masure of treacle. When only a Drona measure of water would remain, it should be taken down and strained through a piece of linen. It should then be duly cooked with an Ádhaka measure of clarified butter. The medicated Ghrita (thus prepared) with a Prastha measure of honey added to it (when cooled) should be kept in an earthen pitcher. By using this medicated Ghrita, one would be cured of all urinary troubles.* 29.

Thus ends the fifty-eighth chapter in the Uttara-Tantra of the Sus'ruta Samhitá which deals with the (symptoms and) treatment of the suppression of urine (Mutràghàta).

* **Additional Text** :—Powders of Tugá-kshiri and sugar should be mixed together with honey and licked in an auspicious day according to the digesting capacity of the patient and a draught of milk should then be taken. By its use the patient would be able to conquer all seminal troubles if he observes a perfect continence. One whose semen has been wasted by sexual excesses would get instantaneous relief; and a man who is possessed of vigour (Ojas) and strength would be refreshed and cheerful.

CHAPTER LIX.

Now we shall discourse on the chapter which deals with the (symptoms and) medical treatment of the defects of urine **(Mutra-dosha-Pratishedha).*** 1.

Classification :—The disease known as **Mutropagháta** is divided into **eight** different types according as an attack is induced by the deranged action of the bodily Váyu, Pitta and Kapha separately, or is due to the concerted action of all of them, or to the effects of an external blow or hurt (on the locality), or to the pressure of the feces incarcerated (in the intestine),—*i.e.* to the constipation of the bowels—or to the presence of any stone (As'mari in the bladder). The eighth is the one due to the presence of gravels (S'arkará in the bladder). This disease is one of the most painful and distressing ailments which assail the human body. 2.

Specific Symptoms:—A scanty flow of urine coming out in drops and producing an oppressive and bursting pain in the scrotum, penis and bladder, is the specific feature of the **Vátaja** type of the disease. The **Pittaja** type is characterised by the emission of bloody or high-coloured (lit. dark yellow) and (very) warm urine which produces a burning sensation in the scrotum, bladder and penis being burnt by fire, as it were. A

* Dallana's reading evidently is **Mutra-krichchhra** (Strangury), for he says that the variant here in some *Mss.* is Mutra-dosha. He says further that some do not read this chapter at all on the ground that the matter in this chapter is included in the chapters on As'mari, Mutrágháta and Udàvarta, etc. But, according to him, it must be read here for treatment's sake as well as on the ground of its being separately treated in other authoritative works. Màdhava, Chakra-páni, Vrinda and other compilers have read this as Mutra-krichchhra in a separate chapter as here.

sense of weight or heaviness in the scrotum, penis and bladder, an appearance of goose-flesh (on the skin) and the emission of cold, white and glossy (oily) urine, are the features which mark the **Kaphaja** type. Burning sensation (in the urethra, etc.), shivering (of the body), frequent emission of urine of varied colours, painful micturition and loss of consciousness are the indications which point to the **Sánnipátika** origin of the disease which is very hard to cure. 3-6.

The presence of any **ulcer** in or an **injury** to the urethra, by any external object gives rise to an extremely distressing stricture in the case of which the characteristic symptoms of Váta-vasti manifest themselves. The suppression of the **feces** leads to the aggravation of the local Váyu which, in its turn, produces a distension of the abdomen and a suppression of urine accompanied with cramps (in the bladder). 7-8.

Aśmarija and Śarkarája :—Mutrá-gháta (obstructed urination) due to the presence of Aśmari (stone) has been already mentioned (in the Nidána Sthána). Stones and gravels are of similar origin and exhibit similar symptoms. Now hear me describe the symptoms which are the distinguishing traits of a case of Sarkará (gravel or urinary calculus in the bladder). Flakes or particles of deranged and condensed Kapha when baked (dried ?) by the action of the deranged and aggravated Pitta and severed in pieces by the deranged bodily Váyu, are called **Sarkará** (gravels) giving rise to such symptoms as cardiac troubles (pain in the heart, etc.), shivering, cramps in the loins, great diminution of the digestive fire, fainting fits and painful and obstructed urination. The pain, however, subsides with the subsidence of the desire for micturition (full evacuation of the bladder), the relief from the pain continuing until the orifice of the organ (urethra) is not again obstructed by the presence of other calculii. These are the symptoms which characterise a case of Mutrághála (obstructed urination) due to the presence of gravels in the bladder. 9.

General Treatment :—Now I shall describe the mode of medical treatment and active therapeutic agents to be employed in the eight cases of Mutrághála. Medical measures and remedies mentioned in connection with the treatment of As'mari (stone) should also* be employed in the present instance in due succession—commencing with the application of Sneha, etc. —with proper regard to the Dosha or Dhosas involved in each case. 10.

Treatment of Vátaja Type :—Oil, clarified butter and lard mixed together should be duly cooked with *S'va-damshtrá*, *As'mabheda*, *Kumbhi* (a kind of moss), *Hapushá*, *Kantakári*, *Balá*, *S'atávari*, *Rásná*, *Varuna*, *Giri-karniká* and the drugs of the *Vidári-gandhádi* group. Oil or clarified butter alone may also be similarly cooked and prepared with the above drugs. The above preparations should be internally administered, or injected into the intestines after the manner of an Anuvásana-vasti, or into the urethra as an Uttara-vasti for giving relief in cases of **Vátaja** Mutra-krichchhra. 11-12.

Pittaja and Kaphaja Types :—The internal use of the clarified butter duly cooked with the drugs of the *Trina-pancha-mula*, *Utpaládi*, *Kákolyádi* and *Nyagrodhádi* groups would give an instantaneous relief in a case of **Pittaja** Mutra-Krichchhra. The use of this Ghrita as an Uttara-vasti would also similarly give

* Dallana says that the presence of the particle "च" (meaning also) indicates that the mode of medical treatment prescribed in cases of Mutrághála should also be applied in this case.

relief in a case of the present type. Any Sneha duly cooked with the preceding drugs should be similarly used after the manner of any of the three Vasti-applications. Purging with milk and the expressed juice of *Ikshu* and of *Drákshá* is also beneficial. Oils and Yavágus duly cooked with the drugs of the *Surasádi*, *Ushakádi*, *Mustádi* and the *Varunádi* groups would prove curative in a case of **Kaphaja** Mutra-krichchhra. 13—14.

Tri-doshaja Type :—The foregoing measures and remedies should be employed in the **Tri-doshaja** type of Mutra-krichchhra according to the nature and intensity of the predominance of the Doshas involved. Pulverised compound of *Phalgu* (Kákodumbara), *Vris'chika* (white Punarnavá), *Darbha and As'ma-sára* (dead iron) taken with water, potions of Surá (wine), the expressed juice of *Ikshu*, and the decoction of *Darbha* would relieve pain in a case of Mutra-krichchhra. 15.

Medicines and medicinal measures mentioned in the chapter on the treatment of Sadyo-vrana should be employed in a case of stricture due to any hurt (**Abhigháta**) to the urethra. Váyu-subduing remedies should be constantly used, and baths, fomentations, unguents, applications of Vasti and powders should be employed in a case of **Purishaja** Mutra-krichchhra. The treatment of the last two kinds (*viz.* As'mari-ja and S'arkará-ja) has already been described. 16-17.

Thus ends the fifty-ninth chapter of the Uttara-Tantra in the Sus'ruta Samhitá which deals with the (symptoms and) medical treatment of Mutra-dosha.

Here ends the Káya-Chikitsá.

CHAPTER LX.

Now we shall discourse on the chapter which deals with the (symptoms and) medical treatment of the disease brought on through super-human* influences **(Amánusha-Pratishedha).** 1.

Now we dilate upon the dictum which has been put forward in the first portion of the present work, and which is to the effect that a patient suffering from ulcers should always be protected from the evil influences cast by night-rangers (*i. e.* ghost, monsters, and malignant spirits, etc.). Whoever produces super-human character in a man by making him exhibit uncommon fortitude and marked irrelevancy in his dealings and the power to know the private and future events.is called a **Graha.** 2–3.

Causes of influence by a Graha :— Innumerable are the Grahas and their tutelary divinities who roam about in the world in quest of offerings or out of their innate tendency for mischief and cruelty and choose their victims from among persons who are impure in body, mind and acts—be they ulcerated or otherwise. These Grabas though possessed of various shapes and figures are mainly classified under **eight** groups or families. The Devas (deities) and their enemies (*viz.* the Asuras), Gandharvas, Yakshas, Pitris (manes), Bhujangas, (Serpent-dieties), Rákshasas (monsters) and Piśáchas (filthy goblins) are the eight classes of Grabas. 4–5.

Indications of attack by Grahas :— A person possessed by a **Deva** (divine) Graha is cleanly,

* Amánusha—lit. non-mánusha, *i. e.* other than human. It includes the deities, demons, ghosts, monsters and the manes and even the serpent-deities.

contented, vigorous and with little sleep. He speaks in good and pure Sanskrit, betrays a strong and decided liking for flowers and perfumes, grants boons (after the fashion of a divine being) to all and is devoted to Bráhmanas, and stares with a fixed gaze (in his eyes). A person labouring under the malignant influence of an **Asura** Graha (devil) perspires copiously, speaks ill of the gods, Bráhmanas and preceptors, knits his brow with arched eyes, has no fear, becomes satisfied with all kinds of food or drink and exhibits vicious propensities. A person under the influence of a **Gandharva** Graha moves about happily along lovely river-banks, or in lovely forest. Always cleanly in body and acts, he shows fondness for songs, flowers and sweet scents, laughs merrily and croons sweet songs and dances. Copper-coloured eyes, partiality for wearing thin red garments, vigour and fortitude, repeated offers for granting boons or gifts to persons, taciternity, restiveness (D. R.—fastness in walking) and gravity of the mind are the symptoms which are manifested in a person coming under the influence of a **Yaksha** Graha. 6–9.

A person similarly affected by a **Pitri** Graha becomes calm and quiet as well as reverent towards the manes. He offers oblations on *Kus'a*-grass and libations of water for their satisfaction, with the upper garment worn in a fashion so as to fall under his left arm and exhibits a liking for cooked meat as well as sesamum, treacle and Páyasa. A person struck by the malignant influence of a **Bhujanga** Graha, sometimes moves on his breast along the ground like a serpent, always licks the corners of his lips with the tip of his tongue, becomes drowsy (D. R. irritable) and shows a marked predilection for treacle, honey, milk and Páyasa. 10–11.

A fondness for flesh, blood and various kinds of ardent spirit, blank shamelessness, extreme cruelty, courageousness, irritability, extraordinary strength, stirring out in the night and an entire disregard of cleanliness are the traits which mark a person attacked by a **Rákshasa** Graha. Haughtiness, emaciation of the frame, roughness of behaviour, garrulousness, fetid smell from the body, extreme uncleanliness and restiveness, voracious eating, fondness for cold water and lonely places, stirring abroad in the night (D. R. fondness for walking about the out-skirts of forest) and roaming about weeping and engaged in vicious pursuits (D. R. anxious looks) are the features which show that a person has been possessed by a **Pisácha** Graha. 12–13.

Prognosis :—If a person possessed by a Graha, has swollen eyes, quick pace, foam at the mouth which he licks himself, drowsiness, staggering gait which sometimes compels him to fall down on the ground or if he is possessed by a Graha after his fall from a hill, an elephant, a tree or such other high place, or if he be old,* he should be regarded as incurable. 14.

Times of possession :—A Deva Graha strikes *i. e.* possesses a man at full moon ; an Asura Graha at the meeting of day and night *i. e.* in the morning and evening twilights ; a Gandharva generally on the eighth and a Yaksha on the first day of the fortnights. A Pitri Graha possesses a man on the new moon day ; and a Sarpa Graha (serpent-devil) enters on the fifth day of the new or full moon. A Rákshasa Graha possesses a man at night and a

* In place of "वार्द्धकेन जुष्टः" Mádhava reads 'त्रयोदशाब्दे' *i. e.* (it is also incurable) when it has continued for thirteen years.

Pis'ácha Graha on the fourteenth day of the fortnights. A Graha imperceptibly enters into the body of the patient in the same way as an image imperceptibly enters into (the surface of) a mirror, as heat or cold penetrates into the body of an organic being and as the rays of the sun are collected in the crystal lens known as the Surja-kánta gem and as soul enters the body unseen. 15-16.

Austere penances and vows, self-control, truthfulness, charities and religious practices as well as the eight qualities* are either wholly or partially present in the Grahas according to the degree of their respective power. These spiritual bodies never come in contact with, nor do they themselves strike human beings. Those who hold contrary opinion, must be ignorant of the mysteries of demonology. It is the thousands and hundreds of thousands and hundreds of millions of the followers of the Grahas, who are fierce-looking and fond of flesh and blood, and who stir abroad in the night and possess the men on earth. 17.

Of these malignant spirits (Grahas) those who are associated with the gods should be regarded as of celestial essence in virtue of their partaking of a tinge of divine virtues. Those who are known as Deva Grahas and are cleanly should be worshipped and homaged and prayed like the other gods of our Pantheon. The Grahas should be credited with those powers, virtues and characteristics which are the attributes of

* The eight qualities referred to are :—(1) Animan or the superhuman power of becoming as small as an atom at will. (2) Laghiman—power of becoming excessively light at will. (3) Vyápti—expansiveness. (4) Prákàmya—irrisestible will. (5) Mahiman—power of increasing the size at will. (6) Is'itva—greatness. (7) Vas'itva—self-control and (8) Kámávasàyità—suppression of passion.

their respective masters. They are the issues of Nairiti's daughters and their living has been fixed as such by the various Ganas (or groups of gods and demi-gods) as they are always adverse to truthfulness, *i. e.* the true performance of the dictates of the Śáśtra. Those that roam about in quest of evil and mischief in spite of the celestial nature of their own divine essence and temperament have been termed **Bhutas** (spirits). Hence that branch of medical science which treats of the therapeutics of diseases which originate from the influences of Bhutas (or Grahas) is called the **Bhuta-Vidyá**. 18-20.

General Religious Treatment :—Japas (mental repetition of a Mantra sacred to any deity), Homas (offering of oblations to the gods) and other religious rites in accordance with the proper rules should be undertaken by a careful physician for their propitiation. Offerings of garlands of red flowers with red scents (such as red Sandal paste, Kumkuma, etc.), seeds (such as mustard, barley, etc.), honey, clarified butter and all sorts of victuals are the articles required generally for (propitiation of) all classes (of Grahas). 21.

Specific Religious Treatment :—Clothes, wine, blood, flesh or milk should be offered to them according to their respective likings*. Offerings to the respective Grahas should be made on the day corresponding to that in which they generally strike their victims. Homas in the fire with the offerings of *Kus'a*, Svastika, cakes (Pupa), clarified butter, umbrella and Páyasa (porridge) should be made to the **Deva** (celestial) Grabas in divine temples. To the **Asura** Grahas the offering should the made in the yard

* This S'loka corresponding to "cloth......likings" is only a variant according to Dallana. He does not seem to read this S'loka.

48

(Chatwara), etc. of a house at the proper time (*viz.* at evening); offerings to the **Gandharva** Grahas should be made with wine and the soup of Jángala animals in the midst of a gathering; while those to the **Yaksha** Grahas should be made inside a house with the cakes of boiled *Másha* pulse (Kulmásha), blood, wine, etc. The **Pitri** Grahas should be propitiated with the offerings made on *Kus'a* grass together with *Mádhavi* and and *Kunda* flowers on the banks of a river; offerings to the **Rákshasas** should be dedicated in dreadful lonely forests or at the crossing of two roads, while to the **Pis'áchas** cooked or uncooked flesh should be offered in a lonely chamber. 22.

Medical Treatment :—In case the prevalent Mantras enjoined to be recited on such occasions (in works on Demonology) are found to be ineffective the following medical measures, should be employed. Skin and hairs of a goat, a bear, a Śalyaka (porcupine), or of an owl pasted togother with *Hingu* and goat's urine and made into incense sticks, should be burnt before the patient, who would be fumigated with the fumes emitted therefrom. The attack even of a violent Graha would readily yield to it. The drugs known as *Gaja-pippali*, *Pippali*-roots, *Tri-katu*, *Ámalaka* and *Sarshapa*, duly soaked in the biles of a lizard, mungoose, cat and bear should be employed as unguents, snuffs and wash by an experienced physician. Dungs of an ass, horse, mule, owl, camel*, dog, jackal, vulture, crow and boar pasted together with the urine of a she-goat should be duly cooked with an adequate quantity of oil. The oil thus prepared would be beneficial if used (as snuff, etc.) in the preceding manner. 23–25.

* The word in the text is 'Karabha' which many mean a camel or an elephant. Dallana explicitly explains the word as a camel.

S'irisha-seed, *Las'una*, *S'unthi*, *Siddhárthaka*, *Vacha*, *Manjishthá*, *Rajani* and *Krishná* should be pasted together with goat's urine and dried in the shade. Vartis (sticks) prepared with this should be applied with the bile (of a cow) along the eye-lids as an Anjana. Vartis prepared with *Naktamála*-fruit, *Tri-katu*, roots of *S'yonáka* and of *Vilva* as well as the two kinds of *Haridrá* should be used as an Anjana in a similar way. *Saindhava*, *Katuka*, *Hingu*, *Vayasthá* (Guduchi) and *Vachá*, pasted together with goat's urine and with the bile of a fish, should be similarly used as an Anjana in cases of attacks by the Grahas which would not otherwise yield. 26-28.

Matured clarified butter, *Las'una*, *Hingu*, *Siddhárthaka*, *Vacha*, *Golomi*, *Ajalomi*, *Bhutakes'i* (Jatámámsi), *Jatá* (Gandha-mámsi), *Kukkuti* (a kind of bulb), *Sarpagandhá*, *Kána*, (Kshira-kákoli), *Vishánikd* (Madhuriká), *Rishya-prokta*, *Vayasthá*, *S'ringi*, *Mohana-Valli*, (Vatapatriká), *Arka*-roots, *Tri-katu*, *Latá* (Priyangu), *Anjana* (Rasánjana), *Srotonjana*, *Naipáli*, *Haritála* and other articles which have the efficacy of exorcising evil spirits, as well as the dungs, hairs, skin, Vasá, urine, blood, bile nails, etc. of lions, tigers, bears, cats, elephants, horses cows, dogs, Śalyakas, lizards, camels, mongooses, etc., should be used in the preparation of oil and clarified butter which should be used internally as well as in snuffing and as unguents. Pills made of the above drugs should be used in sprinkling (wash) and their powdered compound in dusting (the body of the patient). A paste prepared with the above drugs should be used as plasters. The due and proper application of the oil, Ghrita, etc. thus prepared would, in a very short time, surely cures all sorts of mental disorders. 29.

Unholy and improper articles should not be employed in a case due to the influence of any Deva Graha (divine spirit). No hostile measure should be adopted in a case of possession by a Graha other than that due to the influence of a Pis'ácha Graha in as much as the mighty Grahas, if offended, might kill both the patient and the physician for the act. A physician, treating such a case with discretion according to the rules laid dawn in the chapter known as the Hitáhita (Ch. XX, Sutra-Sthána) may acquire both fame and wealth. 30–31.

Thus ends the sixtieth chapter of the Uttara-Tantra in the Sus'ruta-Samhitá which deals with the (symptoms and) treatment of the disease brought on through super-human influences.

CHAPTER LXI.

Now we shall discourse on the chapter which deals with the (symptoms and) medical treatment of Apasmára **(Apasmára-Pratishedha)**. 1.

Derivative Significance :—The word "Smriti" signifies the faculty of past sense-perceptions and (the prefix) "Apa" denotes the privation (of any object or attribute). Hence, this disease (in which an individual loses the faculty of past cognitions) is termed **Apasmára** (Epilepsy) and it turns fatal. 2.

Causes :—Excessive, inadequate and improper attention to the objects of the sense as well as to their actions, partaking of filthy, impure, incompatible and uncongenial articles of fare and regimen of conduct, repression of any natural urging of the body or aggravation of the Rajas and Tamas (nescience), or going in unto a woman in her menses, or indulgence in amorous fancies, fright, anxiety, anger, or grief, etc., leads to an aggravation of the bodily Doshas which in their turn affect the mind (Chetas) very greatly and give rise to **Apasmára**. 3.

The sense-carrying Srotas (channels) of the body overwhelmed by the concerted action of the deranged Doshas bring in a predominance of Rajas and Tamas (Nescience) causing the patient unconscious and forgetful of all past memories. He writhes in agony and throws his hands and legs in convulsive jerks with contracted eyes (D. R. tongue) and eye-brows. He gnashes his teeth, with foams at the mouth, etc., and falls to the ground with open eyes, the consciousness returning a short while after. The disease is called **Apasmára** which is classified into **four** distinct types—*viz*., Vátaja, Pittaja, Kaphaja and Sannipátaja. 4.

Premonitory Symptoms :—The throbbing of the heart, emptiness or lightness (of the chest *i.e.* a sense as if the external world is vanishing away fastly), perspiration, pensiveness, fainting, stupid appearance and sleeplessness are the symptoms, which are usually found to usher in an attack (of Apasmára). 5.

Symptoms of Vátaja and Pittaja types :—In the **Vátaja** type of Apasmára the patient fancies that a dark supernatural being is coming after him to seize his person and is frightened and faints in consequence with shivering grinding of the teeth *i. e.* lock-jaw, laboured breathing and foaming at the mouth. Fainting is excited by a terror of being seized by a yellow and fierce-looking being in the **Pittaja** type which is further marked by thirst, increased heat of the body, perspiration, fainting, mild tremor of the limbs and restlessness. 6—7.

Kaphaja and Sannipátaja Types :—Where the patient is excited by a fancied dread as if a supernatural being of white colour is coming to apprehend him, it is a case of the **Kaphaja** type which is moreover characterised by the exhibition of such symptoms as shivering, nausea, sleepiness, falling prostrate on the ground and vomiting of mucus. Pain in the heart, thirst and nausea are the specific characteristics of the three types respectively. But delirious talk and the making of indistinct and moaning sounds are present in all the types The specific features of all the three foregoing types manifest themselves in concert in a case of **Sánnipátika** type. 8—10.

Discussion on its cause :—The sudden appearance of the disease without any apparent cause and also its sudden and spontaneous disappearance after a short while without any apparent treatment, have induced several medical authorities to hold that Apasmára is not due to any (aggravation of the) Dosha. Several authorities, on the contrary, have described, on the authority of other works on the subject, the gradual aggravation of the (suddenly) deranged Doshas as well as the concomitant symptoms of the disease in its various phases with the spontaneous and speedy nature of its abatement (though only temporary). Hence it may be presumed that as seeds sprout in autumn only, when the rains make the ground ready to receive them, the shortness of time being counted as no factor potent enough to obstruct the process (of sprouting), so the deranged Doshas of the body though gradually aggravated bring on, as a matter of fact, an attack of Apasmára with all its concomitant symptoms, only under conditions favourable to its appearance which may, however, be short and transitory in its duration. Hence this dreadful Apasmára is certainly a disease of **idiopathic** origin. 11.

General Treatment :—Medicinal agents and remedies to be mentioned in connection with insanity (Unmàda) may be as well employed in the present disease. The use of matured clarified butter both internally and as unguents is recommended. Medicinal measures and compounds mentioned under the head of possession by the Grahas are also specially beneficial in the present disease. Oil duly cooked with *S'igru*, *Katvanga*, (Śyonáka), *Kinna* (sediment of wine) and with the expressed juice of *Nimba*-barks and with cow's urine weiging four times as much, should be employed as unguents. Draughts and embrocations of oil duly cooked (separately) with the biles of a lizard, a mongoose, an elephant (or snake), a deer of the Prishaṭa class, a bear and a cow, are recommended. Strong medicinal errhines (S'iro-virechana) as well as strong emetics and purgatives should be administered. The divine Rudra god and the host of his followers should be regularly worshipped and propitiated every day. 12—15.

Specific Treatment :—Clarified butter duly cooked with goat's urine and with the decoction of *Kulattha, Yava, Kola, S'ana-seeds, Palankashá* (Guggulu), *Jatámámsi, Das'a-mula* and *Pathyá* may be given with advantage in a case of the **Vátaja** type (of Apasmára). Clarified butter duly cooked with the decoction of the drugs of the first (*i.e.* Vidári-gandhádi) group and with the drugs of *Kákolyádi* group (as Kalka) if administered with milk, honey and sugar would be beneficial in a case of the **Pittaja** type. The use of (the medicated) Ghrita duly cooked with *Krishná, Vachá* and the drugs of the *Mustakádi* group (as Kalka) and with the decoction of the drugs of the *Áragvadhádi* group* and with the five officinal kinds of animal urine is recommended in cases of the **Kaphaja** type of Apasmára. 16—18.

Siddhárthaka Ghrita :—Clarified butter duly cooked with (the Kalka of) *Sura-druma, Vacha, Kushtha, Siddhártha, Vyosha, Hingu, Manjishthá,* the two kinds of *Rajani, Samangá, Tri-phalá, Ambuda* (Musta), *Karanja*-seeds, *S'irisha*-seeds, *Giri-karná* (white Aparájitá) and *Hutás'ana* (Chitraka) and with four times as much of cow's urine is called **Siddhárthaka** Ghrita, which proves curative in cases of poisoning, worms (in the intestines), Kushtha, asthma, derangements of Kapha, Vishama-Jvara, Bhuta-graha, insanity and Apasmára. 19.

* According to Dallana, the Ghrita should be cooked with the decoction of Krishná and Vacha, while the drugs of the Áragvadhádi group should be used as Kalka.

Pancha-gavya Ghrita :—Clarified butter duly cooked with the Kalka of *Das'a-mula*, barks of *Indra-vriksha*,* *Murvá*, *Bhárgi* †, *Tri-phalá*, *Sampáka*, (Áragvadha), *S'reyasi* (Gaja-pippali), *Sapta-parni*, *Apámárga* and *Pilu*, and with the decoction of *Bhu-nimba*, *Putika* (Karanja), *Vyosha*, *Chitraka*, *Trivrit*, *Páthá*, the two kinds of *Haridrá*, the two kinds of *Sárivá*, *Pushkara*-roots *Katuka*, *Madayanti* (Mallika), *Ugrá* (Vachá), *Nilini* and *Vidanga*, and with the milk, curd (Dadhi), urine and the expressed liquid of dung of a cow is called **Pancha-gavya** Ghrita. It proves curative in all forms of Apasmára, Bhuta-graha, Cháturthaka (quartian) fever, Phthisis, Asthma and Insanity. 20.

General Treatment :—Vastis should be applied in the Vátaja, purgatives, in the Pittaja and emetics, in the Kaphaja types of Apasmára. 21.

Milk should be duly cooked with *Bhárgi* and Páyasa (porridge) should be prepared by cooking grains of Śáli rice with this milk. This preparation should be given to a boar kept fasting for three days. When it is assured that the food taken has acquired a sweet taste (*i.e.* that the process of digestion has begun in the stomach of the boar) and when the symptoms of poisoning come to be exhibited in the boar, the contents should be taken out (of the boar's stomach) and (should be dried and) powdered. Three parts of this powder and one part of Kinva (the sediment of wine) should be mixed together and made to ferment in a cleansed earthen pitcher with the addition of the cooled decoction of *Bhárgi* The wine (Surá) thus prepared should be given in proper doses to

* By the term 'Indra-vriksha-twak' some mean (barks of) Kutaja and Twak (cinnamon).

† Bhárgi—Dallana explains it as Goshthodumbara—the wild fig.

the patient as soon as it would acquire its (particular) taste and aroma. **Venesection** (in the forehead) as recommended before (Śárira-sthána, Chap. VIII, 25-26) should be resorted to and prophylactic and auspicious articles should be used (by the patient). 22-23.

Thus ends the sixty-first chapter in the Uttara Tantra of the Sus'ruta Samhitá which deals with the (symptoms and) treatment of Apasmára.

CHAPTER LXII.

Now we shall discourse on the chapter which deals with the (symptoms and) medical treatment of Insanity **(Unmáda-Pratishedha).** 1.

Derivation :—In as much as (in this disease) the deranged bodily Doshas traversing the upper part of the body affect the up-coursing nerves and produce thereby a distracting state of the mind, it is called **Unmáda** (Insanity), and it is a disease of the Manas (mind). 2.

Classification :—This disease is divided into five different types according to the nature of their origin—*viz.*, the three types due to the several actions of the three deranged and aggravated Doshas, the one due to their concerted actions and the one due to grief, etc. (real or imaginary). There is a sixth kind also, *viz.*, that due to the effects of poison, which should be treated according to the nature and intensity of the deranged Dosha or Doshas lying at the root and which in its early stage, if not abnormally aggravated, goes by the name of **Mada.** 3.

Premonitory Symptoms :—Fits of unconsciousness, agitated state of the mind, ringing of the ears, emaciation of the body, excessive energy of action aversion to food, eating filthy things in dreams, perturbation *i.e.* palpitation (of the heart) due to Váyu and vertigo or giddiness are the symptoms in a patient which forebode a speedy and impending attack of insanity. 4.

Specific Symptoms of Vátaja, Pittaja and Kaphaja types :—Shaggy appearance, use of harsh language, appearance of a number of Dhamanis (nerves) over the body, laboured breathing (D. R. experience of excessive coldness), emaciation of the body and throbbing of the joints of the limbs are the specific features of a case of the **Vátaja** type (of Unmâda) and the patient in such a case reads clapping his hands, or sings while dancing, or shouts or wanders about Excessive thirst, perspiration, burning sensation, voracious eating, insomnia, desire for shade, cold, wind and walks on the banks (of rivers or tanks), fits of anger, fancying fire in cold water and fancied sight of stars in the heavens in the day are the symptoms which characterise a case of the **Pittaja** type. Vomiting, dulness of appetite, lassitude or gone-feeling in the limbs, aversion to food, fondness for sexual propulsion and loveliness, stupidity, somnolence, reservedness in speech, eating little, fondness for warm things and aggravation of the disease in the night mark a case of the **Kaphaja** type of insanity. 5-7.

Tri-doshaja Type :—A case of **Sánnipátika** insanity exhibits all the symptoms belonging to the three aforesaid types origined from the three Doshas, *viz.*, Váta, Pitta and Kapha. A case in which the specific symptoms of the disease are manifested in full should be deemed as incurable. Several authorities, however, hold the Sannipátika type to be sometimes curable. 8.

Śokaja and Vishaja types :—A person frightened by a thief, a king's officers or his own enemy or any such person, or suffering from any distracted state of the mind owing to a loss of wealth, or from any **grief** (**Śoka**) or bereavement or from any disappointed love would likely have an attack of mental distraction (insanity). In such cases he would unconsciously talk incoherently about subjects uppermost in his mind or would sing in a stupid fashion or laugh or weep. (These are the symptoms of **Sokaja** insanity). Redness of the eyes, dulness of complexion and of the perceptive faculties, diminution of bodily strength, extreme dejection, blush on face and loss of consciousness are the symptoms which mark a case of insanity due to the effects of **poisoning**. 9–10.

General Treatment :—A patient suffering from insanity should be first treated with Sneha and Sveda and then subjected to a course of emetics, purgatives and head-purgatives (Śiro-Virechana). Powders of various sorts of (drugs used in) Avapida snuffing should be mixed with mustard oil and employed for the purpose of snuffing). Fumigation with burnt putrid beef or dog's flesh should be constantly employed. Snuffing and unguents of mustard oil are also efficacious in all cases. The patient should be surprised with wonderful sights and the news of the death of any of his dear ones should be related to him. He should be constantly frightened with sights of fierce-looking men, well-trained elephants or non-venomous snakes. The patient should be threatened with being fastened with ropes or being flogged, or frightened with bundles of blazing hay, after being fastened, while asleep. He should also be pierced in his body with pointed instruments, avoiding, however, the vulnerable parts*, or he should be made to reside constantly in a dry well with a cover over it. Barley gruel, powders of parched barley mixed with water alone should be given to him on every third day by an intelligent physician. The diet of the patient should consist also of palatable and appetising articles. 11.

* **Additional Text :**—The patient should likewise be threatened with being forced into a burning hut. He should be also kept immersed in water or threatened with the fall of a thunder bolt.

Mahá-Kalyána Ghrita :—Clarified butter duly cooked with twice as much of milk and with *Vidanga, Tri-phalá, Musta, Manjishthá, Dádima, Utpala, S'yámá, Ela-váluká, Elá,* (red) *Chandana, Deva-dáru, Barhishtha* (Bálaka), *Haridrá, Kushtha, Parnini* (Sála-parni), *Sárivá, Harenuká, Trivrit, Danti, Vacha, Tálisa-patra, Nága-kes'ara* and *Málati* flowers as Kalka (is called **Kalya'na Ghrita*** and) proves curative in cases of Gulma, cough, fever, asthma, phthisis and insanity. Clarified butter duly cooked with four times as much of milk and with the aforesaid drugs as Kalka and with the drugs of the *Kákolyádi* group added to it by way of an after-throw is called **Mahá-kalyána Ghrita**. The range of its therapeutic application includes (such ailments as) Apasmára, (attack by) Graha, consumption, impotency, emaciation and sterility as well as the diseases mentioned above. 12.

Phala Ghrita :—Clarified butter duly cooked with *Bálaka, Kushtha, Manjishthá, Katuka, Elá, Haridrá, Tri-phalá, Hingu, As'vagandhá, Deva-dáru, Vacha, Yamáni, Kákoli, Medá, Yashti-madhu* and *Padmaka* (as Kalka), and with four times as much of milk and with sugar as an after-throw would be beneficial. It should also be prescribed for infants struck by malignant stars as well as for male adults of evil propensities and short intellect. This is known as **Phala-Ghrita*** and removes barrenness of women 13.

Bráhmi (Manduka-parni), *Aindri, Vidanga, Tri-katu, Hingu, Surá* (Deva-dáru), *Jatá* (Jatá-mámsi), *Vishaghni* (Haridrá), *Las'una* (garlic), *Rásná, Vis'alyá* (Guduchi), *Surasá, Vacha, Jyotishmati, Nága-vinná* (a kind of

* According to Dallana the mentions of these two recipes (Kalyána Ghrita and Phala Grita) are interpolations.

Indra-váruni), *Anantá*, *Abhayá* and *Souráshtri* taken in equal parts should be pounded together and made into a paste with the addition of elephant's urine. It should then be dried in the shade, and **Vartis** should be prepared thereof. These should be used by an intelligent person as an Anjana, unguent, snuff, fumigation and Avapida. 14.

Blood-letting from the Uras (chest), Apánga (outer corner of the eye) and Laláta (forehead) should be resorted to. Measures and drugs mentioned in connection with the treatment of Apasmára and Graha-roga may be likewise employed in the present instance. Oily purgatives (Sneha-vasti) should be administered after the subsidence of the deranged Dosha. 15.

In a case of the fifth kind (*viz.* **Śokaja**) of insanity the cause of grief should be first removed. In all forms of insanity the restoration of the serenity of mind should be first attempted. Mild and gentle forms of these remedies should be resorted to in a case of Mada (preliminary stage of insanity). Mild anti-venomous (anti-toxin) measures should be resorted to in a case (of insanity, due to the effects of **poison**. 17–18.

Thus ends the sixty-second chapter in the Uttara-Tantra of the Sus'ruta Samhitá which deals with the (symptoms and) treatment of Insanity.

Here ends the Bhuta-vidyá-Tantra.

CHAPTER LXIII.

Now we shall discourse on the chapter which deals with the different combinations of the (six) different Rasas **(Rasa-bheda-vikalpa-Adhyáya).** 1.

The fifteen different combinations of the Doshas already spoken of (in Chapter XXI, Sutra-Sthána) are meant only for the **sixty-three** different combinations of the (six) Rasas (taken one, two, three, four, five or all at a time). They (*viz.* the different Doshas) may be manifest separately (Avidagdha) or combinedly (Vidagdha) with one another and the number of their combinations should be taken to be sixty-three *pari passu* with the sixty-three different combinations of the (six) different Rasas. In other words, the combinations of the Doshas with one another already spoken of should be considered by an intelligent person to be sixty-three in all (and not fifteen only, as spoken of in Chapter XXI, Sutra-Sthána). 2—3.

Enumeration—Taken two at a time:— The Madhura Rasa (sweet taste) coming first in the order of enumeration has got **five** combinations (with the other five Rasas) taken two at a time. Similarly Amla Rasa (acid taste) has got four combinations and Lavana Rasa (saline taste) has got three. Katuka Rasa (pungent taste) has got two and Tikta Rasa (bitter taste) has got only one with Kasáya Rasa (astringent taste). The different combinations taken two at a time are thus fifteen in all. They are as follows :—

(1) Sweet and acid, (2) sweet and saline, (3) sweet and pungent (4) sweet and bitter and (5) sweet and astringent—these are the five combinations of Madhura

(sweet) Rasa. (1) Acid and saline, (2) Acid and pungent (3) Acid and bitter, and (4) Acid and astringent—these are the four combinations of Amla (acid) Rasa. (1) Saline and pungent, (2) Saline and bitter, and (3) Saline and astringent—these are the three combinations of Lavana (saline) Rasa. (1) Pungent and bitter, and (2) Pungent and astringent—these are the two combinations of Katuka (pungent) Rasa. Bitter and pungent is the only combination of Tikta (bitter) Rasa. Thus the **fifteen** different combinations (of the six Rases) taken two at a time have been enumerated. Now we shall speak of their combinations taken three at a time. 4.

Taken three at a time :—The Madhura Rasa (sweet taste) coming first in the list has got ten combinations (with the other Rasas taken three at a time). Similarly Amla Rasa (acid taste) has got six; Lavana Rasa (saline taste) has got half that number *i. e.* three; and Katuka Rasa (pungent taste) has got only one combination. They are as follows:—(1) Sweet, acid and saline, (2) Sweet, acid and pungent, (3) Sweet, acid and bitter, (4) Sweet, acid and astringent, (5) Sweet, saline and pungent, (6) Sweet, saline and bitter, (7) Sweet, saline and astringent, (8) Sweet, pungent and bitter, (9) Sweet, pungent and astringent, and (10) Sweet, bitter and astringent—these are the **ten** combinations of the Rasas taken three at a time and beginning with Madhura (sweet) Rasa. (1) Acid, saline and pungent, (2) Acid, saline and bitter, (3) Acid, saline and astringent, (4) Acid, pungent and bitter, (5) Acid, pungent and astringent, and (6) Acid, bitter and astringent—these are the **six** combinations (taken three at a time and) beginning with Amla (acid) taste. (1) Saline, pungent and bitter, (2) Saline, pungent and astringent, and (3) Saline, bitter, and astringent—these are the **three** combinations (taken three at a time) beginning with Lavana (saline) taste. (1) Pungent, bitter and astringent is the only **one** combination (taken three at a time and) beginning with Katuka (puugent) taste. Thus the **twenty** different combinations (of the six Rasas) taken three at a time have been explained. Now we shall speak of their combinations taken four at a time. 5.

Taken four at a time :—The Madhura (sweet) Rasa has got ten different combinations of four at a time. Similarly Amla (acid) Rasa has got four, and Lavana (saline) Rasa only one. They are as follows :—(1) Sweet, acid, saline and pungent, (2) Sweet, acid, saline and bitter, (3) Sweet, acid, saline and astringent, (4) Sweet, acid, pungent and bitter (5) Sweet, acid, pungent and astringent, (6) Sweet, saline, pungent and bitter, (7) Sweet, acid, bitter and astiingent, (8) Sweet, saline, pungent and astringent, (9) Sweet, saline, pungent and astringent, and (10) Sweet, pungent, bitter and astringent—these are the **ten** combinations (taken four at a time and) beginning with Madhura (sweet) Rasa. (1) Acid, saline, pungent and bitter, (2) Acid, saline, bitter and astringent, (3) Acid, pungent, bitter and astringent, and (4) Acid, saline, pungent and astringent—these are the **four** combinations beginning with Amla (acid) taste. (1) Saline, pungent, bitter and astringent—this is the only **one** combination beginning with Lavana (saline) taste. Thus the **fifteen** different combinations (of the six Rasas) taken four at a time have been enumerated. Now we shall speak of their combinations taken five at a time. 6.

Taken five at a time :—There would be five combinations (of the six Rasas) taken **five** at a time and beginning with the Madhura (sweet) Rasa, and only one with Amla (acid) Rasa. They are as follows :—(1) Sweet, acid, saline, pungent and bitter, (2) Sweet, acid, saline, pungent and astringent, (3) Sweet, acid, saline, bitter and astringent, (4) Sweet, acid, pungent, bitter and astringent, and 5) Sweet, saline, pungent, bitter and astringent—these are the **five** combinations (of the six Rasas) taken five at a time beginning with Madhura (sweet) Rasa. (1) Acid, saline, pungent, bitter and astringent is the only **one** combination of the kind beginning with Amla (acid Rasa. Thus the six combinations taken five at a time have been enumerated. Now we shall speak of their combination with (all the) six at a time. 7.

The combination (of the six Rasas) taken (all the) **six** at a time is only **one**. The only combination of this kind is (1) Sweet, acid, saline, pungent, bitter and astringent. 8.

Separately taken one at a time, the six Rasas will be—(1) Madhura (sweet), (2) Amla acid), (3) Lavana (saline), (4) Katuka (pungent), (5) Tikta (bitter, and (6) Kashàya (astringent). 9.

Memorable Verse :—Sixty-three combinations of the (six) different Rasas have been enumerated by the experts on Rasa and these sixty-three combinations should be prescribed by experienced physicians with due regard to (the aggravation or diminution of one or more of) the (three) different Doshas. 10.

Thus ends the sixty-third chapter of the Uttara-Tantra in the Sus'ruta Samhitá which deals with the different combinations of the (six) different Rasas.

CHAPTER LXIV.

Now we shall discourse on the chapter which deals with the Rules of Health **(Svastha-Vritta-adhyáya).** 1.

Health indicates a normal condition of the (three) Doshas (fundamental principles), Agni (the digestive fire), Mala (excrements *viz*, feces, urine, etc)*, and the (seven) Dhátus or root-principles of the body as well as a serene state of the body, mind and the sense-organs. It has already been stated in the Sutra-sthána, that the primary object of medical treatment is to maintain this healthy state (of the body and of the mind) in its normal equilibrium. A brief outline of the means to be applied and of the rules to be observed for the realisation of that end, has also been given before. Now we shall enter into a lengthy and elaborate dissertation on the subject. 2–3.

Regimen of diet and conduct in the Varshá (rainy) season :—Articles of particular tastes which are remedial to the specific deranged bodily Dosha should be used or employed by experienced persons in the particular season of the year in which the Doshas are respectively aggravated. The bodily Váyu, etc, of a person is generally aggravated during the Varshá (rainy) season owing to a slimy condition of the organism, producing an impairment of the digestive fire as well as goose-flesh on the skin. Articles of astringent, bitter and pungent tastes should therefore be prescribed for a king and king-like personages during those months of the year for

* Some explain 'Kriyá' separately as the organic functions *e. g.* sleep and awakening, etc.—Dallana.

correcting or remedying the altered slimy condition of (things which obtain inside) the body, as well as for mitigating the aggravation of the bodily Doshas. The food should be non-liquid and made neither too emollient (fatty or lardacious) nor too Ruksha (dry), and should be composed of articles which are appetising and heat-making in their potency. Water for drinking should be prescribed according to the rules laid down before (in chapter XLV, Sutra-sthána), or water, heated and subsequently cooled, should be taken in combination with honey, if the sky is overcast with clouds and the air is charged with humid vapours, making the water consequently very cold. 4-5.

The herbs and vegetables being newly grown in this (rainy) season, are (over-juicy and) consequently not very easy to digest ; a wise man should, therefore, avoid the excessive use of physical exercise, water, dew, sexual intercourse and the sun's rays (which might lead to indigestion). One should, in this season, lie upon some higher place to avoid the cold damp due to the emission of earthly vapours at this time. When feeling cold one should protect oneself from it with warm clothes and should lie inside a room free from blasts of wind and with fire burning within. Fine *Aguru* should be used as pastes, and elephants should be used as conveyance in this season. Sleep at day-time and eating before the previous meal is digested should be strictly avoided. 6.

Rules for Autumn :—Articles of astringent, sweet and bitter tastes, different preparations of milk and of sugar-cane-juice as well as honey, *S'áli*-rice, *Mudga*-pulse, oil and the meat of Jángala animals should be used in the Autumn (S'arat) season. All kinds of water are recommended in this season as they are all clear and pure at this time of the year. Swimming and (immersion) in ponds full of *Kamala* (lotus) and *Utpala* (water lily), enjoying the moon's rays at dusk and the use of sandal-pastes are recommended. The aggravation of Pitta in the (previous) rainy season should, in this season, be duly remedied by the use of Tikta-Ghrita (Chapter IX, Chikitsita sthána), by means of venesection or by the use of purgatives. Tikshna (sharp-potencied or pungent), acid, hot and alkaline articles (of food) as well as the sun's rays, sexual excess and sleep at day-time and keeping late hours should be avoided. Sweet and cold water and purified wine as transparent as crystals are also recommended. All kinds of water are in this season washed, as it were, by the clear white rays of the autumnal moon and being purified by the rising of the Agastya star,* become very clear and transparent and consequently beneficial. Clean and thin clothes scented with sandal-pastes or with camphor as well as garlands of autumnal flowers should be worn, and the Sidhu class of wine should be judiciously taken In short, all Pitta-subduing measures should be taken in this season. 7.

Rules for Hemanta and winter seasons :—The season of Hemanta is cold but dry (Ruksha). The sun is weak and the atmosphere is very airy. Hence, owing to the outside cold, the bodily Váyu is also aggravated in this season. The abdominal fire becomes dull owing to the internal cold and dries up the bodily Rasa (liquid portion of the system). The use of oleaginous things is, therefore, beneficial in this

* The waters in the rainy season are generally muddy and impure. When, after the rains, the waters become purer, it is said in Hindu mythology that owing to the rise of Agastya (a star making its appearance in the horizon after the rains—generally in the beginning of September) the waters become clear and transparent.

season. The use of saline, alkaline, bitter, acid and pungent articles of diet (prepared) with the addition of clarified butter or oil are beneficial. Food should not be taken cold, and drinks prepared with tikshna (hot-potencied) articles (such as strong wine should be taken, after pasting the body all over with Aguru-pastes. Baths should be taken in tepid water after rubbing in oil all over the body. Large inner apartments completely surrounded by rooms on all sides and containing fire-pots (serving the purpose of chimneys) should be used as bed-rooms, and the bed-sheets should be silken. Sufficiently warm coverings for the body should be used. Kings (and king-like personages) should lie within the sweet embraces of maidens with big breasts and thighs and scented with the fumes of *Aguru*, and they can, in this season, enjoy the sexual pleasures to their heart's content and should take proper soothing food. Sweet, bitter, pungent, acid and saline articles of food and drink, as well as *Tila* (sesamum-seeds), *Másha*-pulse, pot-herbs, curd, different modifications of sugar-cane-juice, scented and newly husked *S'áli*-rice, flesh of Prasaha, Ánupa, Kravyáda, Biles'aya, Audaka (aquatic), Plava and Pádin classes* of animals, as well as clear transparent wines and all other invigorating articles of diet should be used to his content at the advent of cold by a person wishing vigour (of the body and of the mind). The rules for Hemanta enumerated above would hold equally good for the S'is'ira (winter) season. 8-9.

Rules for Spring :—The bodily Kapha already stored in the organism owing to the coldness of the body during the Hemanta season is aggravated during the spring by the (increasing) heat (of the sun

* For a list of the animals of the different classes mentioned here, see Chapter XLVI, Sutra-sthána, pages 480 &c., Vol. I

and consequently of the organism) and gives rise to many diseases. Acid, sweet, demulcent and saline articles of food and drink as well as those that are heavy (of digestion) should, therefore, be avoided, and recourse should be had to vomiting, etc. *Shashtika*-rice, barley, articles of cold potency, *Mudga*-pulse, *Nivára* rice, and *Kodrava*-rice, should be duly prescribed after the cold *i. e.* in the spring with the soup of the meat of the animals of the Vishkira class, such as Láva, etc., as well as with the soup of *Patola*, *Nimba*-leaves, bringals and other bitter vegetables. All sorts of **Ásava** and especially the Ásava and Sidhu prepared from honey should be freely used in the spring. Physical exercise should be had recourse to, **Anjana** (collyrium) should be applied (to the eyes), strong smokes should be inhaled and strong gargles used in the spring. Everything should be used with tepid water and a diet consisting of Tikshna (strong-potencied), Ruksha (non-demulcent), pungent, alkaline, astringent, tepid and non-liquid articles and especially the preparations of barley, *Mudga* pulse and honey would be beneficial in the spring. Physical exercise in the shape of mock-fight, walk, or the throwing of stones would be beneficial. Utsádana (massage) and bath should be had, and groves should be resorted to. Sexual pleasure may be enjoyed in this season. The bodily Kapha stored in the body during the Hemanta season should be eliminated by means of Śiro-Vireka (errhines), vomiting, Niruha-vasti and gargles, etc. Day-sleep and sweet, demulcent aud liquid articles of fare as well as those hard to digest should be strictly avoided. 10.

Rules for Summer :—Physical exercise, toil, hot and excessively drying articles of fare (*e.g.* those prepared with pulses), as well as those abounding in heat-producing (*e. g.* pungent, acid and saline) tastes should be avoided in summer. Large tanks, lakes and rivers as well as charming gardens and cold rooms should be resorted to, and the finest (refreshing) sandal-pastes and garlands of flowers of lotuses and lilies, soft breeze from palm-leaf-fans and necklaces (of precious stones and pearls) as well as light clothes should be used in summer. Sweet-scented and cooling Pánakas and Manthas with abundance of sugar should be used. Sweet, liquid and cold food mixed with clarified butter, and boiled milk sweetened with sugar, etc, taken at night-time would be found (tasteful and) beneficial at that time. One should at that time lie on a bed strewn over with full-blown and fresh flowers in some palatial building with his body besmeared with sandal-pastes and refreshed by cooling breeze. 11.

Rules for Právrit (rainy) season*:— Articles of the three (*viz.* sweet, acid and saline) heavy Rasas as well as milk, tepid meat-soup, oil, clarified butter, and everything which is Vrimhana (fat-making) and Abhishyandi (secreting) in its nature are beneficial after the end of the summer season *i. e.* in the rainy season. The bodily Váyu which is liable to be aggravated and which actually begins to aggravate in the summer should be pacified by wise men with Váyu-subduing remedies. 12 A.

River-water, Ruksha (non-demulcent) and heat-producing articles, Manthas prepared with abundance of water, the sun's rays, physical exercise, day-sleep and sexual intercourse should be avoided in this season. Old barley, old *Shastika*-rice, old *S'áli*-rice, and old wheat

* A period of four months has been ascribed to the rains. Of these the first two months are ealled Pràvrit, and the last two Varshá—both meaning the rainy season. See chapter VI, Sutra-sthána.

should be used as food, and the bed to lie upon should be stretched inside a room where there is no blast of wind and should be covered over with a soft bed-sheet. The rain-water (in and after its descent on the earth) becomes poisoned with the excretions, urine, salivation, sputum, etc., of poisonous animals as well as with the poisonous atmosphere peculiar to the rainy season; its use should, therefore, be strictly avoided in this season. The naturally aggravated bodily Váyu (in this season) should be duly pacified, or the rules for Varshá (*i.e.* the rainy season) should be duly observed in this season*. 12.

Whoever observes these rules for the different seasons of the year does not suffer from the evil consequences due to the change of seasons. 13.

Different kinds of food :—Now we shall deal with the twelve different kinds of food (and drink). They are—Cold, hot, Snigdha (demulcent), Ruksha (non-demulcent), liquid, dry, taken once a day, twice a day, taken with medicine, taken in smaller quantity, taken for the pacification of (any aggravated Dosha) and taken for subsistence. 14.

Persons afflicted with thirst, heat, alcoholism, burning sensation, Rakta-pitta, poisoning and epileptic fits as well as those suffering from the effects of sexual excess should be treated with **cold** food (and drink); while persons afflicted with the aggravation of bodily Kapha and Váyu as well as those already treated with purgatives or Sneha and those whose bodies are full of Kleda (physical moisture) should be treated with **warm** food (and drink). 15-16.

Persons suffering from the aggravation of bodily Váyu and from a parched (Ruksha) condition of the

* The whole of this Para is an interpolation in as much as Jejjata does not read this.—Dallana.

body as well as those suffering from the effects of sexual excess and those accustomed to physical exercise should be treated with **Snigdha** food (and drink); while persons with an excess of bodily Medas and Kapha as well as those suffering from Meha and those previously treated with a Sneha should be treated with **Ruksha** (or non-demulcent) food and drink. 17-18.

Weak, parched and thirsty persons should be given **Drava** (liquid) food; while those suffering from Meha and ulcers as well as those whose bodies are full of Kleda (bodily moisture) should be given **dry** (non-juicy) food. Persons with impaired digestion should be given only **one meal** every day, so that the digestive fire may have opportunities to) be rekindled; while persons with the proper amount of digestion should be given **two meals** a day. 19-20.

Medicine should be given with food and drink to a person averse to it, while food and drink in **smaller** quantity would be beneficial to persons suffering from impaired digestion or any other disease. Food and drink administered with due regard to the bodily Doshas is called **Dosha-prasámana**; while any kind of food and drink taken for the preservation of life by a healthy person would be called **Vrittayrtha** food and drink. These are the twelve different kinds of food and drink. 21-22.

Proper times for the administration of Medicines:—We shall now speak of the ten specific times (*i. e.* proper occasions) for the administration of medicines. They are—Nir-bhakta, Prág-bhakta, Adho-bhakta, Madhye-bhakta, Antará-bhakta, Sa-bhakta, Sámudga, Muhur-muhuh, Grása and Grásántara. 23.

Of the above medicines what is applied alone (with or without some vehicle but not with any food or drink) is called **Nirbhakta** medicine. A medicine not applied with any food (but applied by itself with or without any vehicle) would have greater effect and would soon and certainly destroy the disease it is applied in; but a medicine should not be applied in this way to a child, an old man, a young woman and persons of mild temperament, for it is likely to produce lassitude and weaken the patient (in such cases). 24.

A medicine taken (in an empty stomach) just before a meal, is called **Prágbhakta**. A medicine taken in such a manner, is easily digested, does not lead to any diminution of strength and is not ejected out of the mouth owing to its being covered over with the meal. On the other hand, taken before the meal, it adds to the bodily strength and proves the most convenient form in which a medicine can be administered to old men, infants, females and persons of timid disposition. A medicine taken just after a meal is called **Adhobhakta**. It conquers diseases which affect the upper part of the body and gives strength in many ways. 25-26.

A medicine taken in the course of a meal is called **Madhyebhakta**. A medicine taken in this manner fails to be diffused all through the organism and hence proves beneficial only in those ailments which are confined to the middle part of the body. A medicine taken between the two meals (*i. e.* after the morning-meal but before the evening-meal) is called **Antarábhakta**. It is invigorating to the mind, greatly appetising and Hridya (agreeable) and is beneficial in every respect. A medicine applied with* any food is called **Sabhakta**. It is most convenient to administer

* "A medicine applied with food" may mean a medicine prepared before and taken with the meal; or, it may mean that the meal is cooked (while being prepared) with the medicines to be applied.

a medicine with food in cases of female, old and infant patients as well as in cases of those averse to taking any medicine. 27–29.

A medicine taken at the beginning and again at the close of a meal is called **Sámudga.** This form of administration is most beneficial in cases where the deranged bodily Doshas take both the (upward and downward) courses. A medicine taken at intervals, either with or without food, is called **Muhurmuhuh.** This mode is to be adopted in severe cases of asthma, cough, hiccough and vomiting. A medicine taken with every morsel (Grása) of food is called **Grása.** In this form the medicine in the shape of a powder is administered for increasing the appetite in cases of weak patients. Vájikara (aphrodisiac) medicines are also better administered in this form. A medicine taken with each alternate morsel of food is called **Grásántara.** Emetics and Dhumas as well as the well-known and well-experimented lambatives for cases of asthma should be administered in this form. These are the ten proper occasions for administering medicines. 30–33.

Proper time for taking food :—The proper time for giving diet to a patient is when he gets free stool, urine and eructations, and feels his body and sense-organs light and free, when he gets free actions of the heart as well as natural courses of his bodily (Apána) Váyu, when he feels hungry (D. R. feels easy) and has got relish for food and when his Kukshi (belly) becomes light (*i. e.* when his belly appears to be empty on account of hunger). 34.

Thus ends the sixty-fourth chapter in the Uttara-tantra of the Sus'ruta-Samhitá which deals with the Rules of Hygiene.

CHAPTER LXV.

Now we shall discourse on the chapter which deals with the technical terms used in this treatise **(Tantra-Yukti-Náma-Adhyáya).** 1.

Names of the technical terms :—There are thirty-two technical terms in this Treatise. They are—(1) Adhikarana, (2) Yoga, (3) Padártha, (4) Hetvartha, (5) Uddes'a, (6) Nirdes'a, (7) Upades'a, (8) Apades'a, (9) Prades'a, (10) Atides'a, (11) Apavarga, (12) Vákya-s'esha, (13) Arthápatti, (14) Viparyaya, (15) Prasanga, (16) Ekánta, (17) Anekánta, (18) Purva-paksha, (19) Nirnaya, (20) Anumata, (21) Vidhána, (22) Anágatá-vekshana, (23) Atikrántá-vekshana, (24) Sams'aya, (25) Vyàkhyána, (26) Sva-samjná, (27) Nirvachana, (28) Nidars'ana, (29) Niyoga, (30) Samuchchaya, (31) Vikalpa, and (32) Uhya. 2.

Necessity :—What is the necessity of the use of these **technical terms** (Tantra-Yukti)? The answer is—For connecting words together, *i. e.*, making up sentences and giving a sense or meaning to them. 3.

Memorable verses :—By the use of technical terms in a scientific treatise the points of argument of the opposite party are frustrated and the points of one's own argument are established. The meanings of the words, whether clearly used or not, whether direct or indirect, or partially used, if there is any such, in the treatise are also made distinct (by the use of the technical terms). Just as the sun shows a cluster of lotus and a lighted lamp (the inside of) a room at their best, so the technical terms used in a treatise clearly show *i. e.*, explain the intended meaning. 4.

Of these terms **Adhikarana** is the subject about which something is spoken of. For example—on (the subject of) Rasa or on (the subject of) Dosha. 5.

The term "**Yoga**" is the union of words or sentences together. For example—an oil duly cooked with *Amrita-valli*, *Nimba*, *Himsrá*, *Abhayá*, *Vrikshaka*, *Pippali*, the two kinds of *Balá* and with *Devá-dáru* should be prescribed for drinking as being efficacious in all cases of Gala-ganda. Here the main idea is 'Siddham pivet' *i. e.* should be cooked and taken internally; but the word 'Siddham' is used in the first half of the second hemistich, far away from the word 'Pivet' in the sentence. This combining together of the different words, however distant in a sentence, is called a Yoga. 6.

The term "**Padártha**" is the meaning implied by a word or an aphorism (*i. e.* a sentence). Padárthas are innumerable. For example—Sneha, Sveda, or Anjana, when used in a sentence, would each imply two or three meanings; but only one meaning which tallies with the use of the previous or subsequent word (in the text) should be understood in each case. Thus, in the sentence "Vedotpattim Vyákhyá syámah" *i. e.* we shall discourse on the origin of the 'Veda', the use of the word "Veda" would put the hearer at a loss to understand which of the Vedas is going to be discoursed on, for there are several Vedas, *viz*, Rigveda, etc. But when we try to understand the expression in connection with the previous or subsequent use of the expression—for the root 'vid' may mean either 'Vichárana' (discussion) or 'Vindati' (to get)—we can afterwards come to the conclusion that the subject to be discoursed upon is the origin of Áyurveda. This is what is meant by the term Padártha. 7.

Hetwartha is the meaning indirectly implied by a

word. For example—as earth is moistened by water, so an ulcer is moistened (and consequently secretes) by (the taking of) *Másha*-pulse, milk, etc. 8.

Uddeśa is the statement in brief. For example—Śalya (ordinarily any foreign matter but secondarily implying any obstructing matter in the body). 9.

Nirdeśa is the statement in detail. For example—"Śalya" is of two kinds "Śárira" (idiopathic) and "Ágantu" (traumatic). 10.

Upadeśa is an instruction for the doing of a thing in a particular way. For example—one should not sit up at night and one should give up sleep at the day time. 11.

Apadeśa is the statement of reason. For example—it has been specified that Śleshmá is increased by the use of the articles of sweet taste. 12.

Pradeśa is the determination of a present action from past events. For example—Devadatta's Śalya has been extracted by this person, hence Yajnadatta's Śalya will also be extracted by him. 13.

Atideśa is the determination of some future event from some present event. For example—one's bodily Váyu courses upwards by such and such an action, hence one may get (an attack of Vátaja) Udávarta by such an action. 14.

Apavarga is the extraction—*i. e.* exception of (something) from something more comprehensive or extended, that is to say, it is an exception to the general rule. For example—fomentation should not be applied to persons suffering from the effects of poisoning excepting those suffering from insect-poison. 15.

Vákya-śesha is the word the absence of the use of which does not make the sentence incomplete. For example—when we say of the head, the hands, the legs, the sides, the back, the abdomen (Udara) and the chest" it becomes evident that these (parts) *of a 'person'* are intended. 16.

Arthápatti (presumption) is the term used when the sense (of a sentence), though not specifically mentioned, can yet be indirectly presumed or deduced. For example*—when one says to another 'this rice (solid food) can be taken,' it *becomes evident* that he is not willing to drink a (liquid) Yavágu or gruel. 17.

Viparyaya (reverse) is the term used when the words used (in a sentence) convey quite a different or opposite sense. For example,—when it is said that 'emaciated, weak and frightened persons are very difficult to be medically treated', the opposite sense becomes evident, *viz.*, that strong, and such-like persons are very easy to be medically treated. 18.

Prasanga (connected reasoning) is the term used when a different subject is introduced at the end. It is also the term used when the same sense is repeated in different words in different places (in the same topic). For example—it is said in the chapter on Vedotpatti (Chapter I, Sutra-Sthána) that "Purusha" (living organism) is the sum-total of the "Mahá-bhutas" (or the five primary elements—*viz.*, earth, water, fire, air and ether) and the Śariri (or the soul), that medical treatment should be made of him (Purusha) and that he is the subject matter of every action); and it has been repeated in the chapter on Bhuta-vidyá (demonology) that the Purusha has therefore been said to be the combination of the five Mahá-bhutas and the soul and

* The common example of an Arthápatti (presumption) in Sanskrit philosophy is 'Pino Devadatto divá na bhumkte,' (*i. e.*, **Fat** Devadatta does not eat at day-time), from which it is evident that he certainly eats at night, otherwise he could not have become fat.

that he is the subject-matter of all sorts of medical treatment. 19.

Ekánta is the term used to denote a thing which is certain in every case. For example—*Trivrit* causes purgation, and *Madana*-fruit produces vomiting. 20.

Anekánta is the term used to denote certainty in some cases and uncertainty in some other cases. For example—many authorities hold that 'Dravya' or the thing itself is the principal factor, some hold the Rasa' or taste (in a thing) to be the principal factor, some again hold the "Viryya" or potency to be the principal factor and others hold "Vipáka" or digestive reaction to be the principal factor. 21.

Purva-paksha is (the putting of) a question with an apparent objection. For example—(the question' why are the four kinds of Vátaja-Prameha incurable. 22.

Nirnaya is the reply to a Purva-paksha or question. For example—the (bodily) Váyu affects *i. e.* spreads over the (whole) body and then forces the urine through (the passage with the (vitiated bodily Vasá (grease), Medas (fat) and Majjan (marrow). The Vátaja cases (of Prameha) are, therefore, incurable. As has been said—the (bodily) Váyu affects *i e.* spreads over the whole body and coming in contact with the (bodily) Medas (fat), Majjan (marrow) and Vasá (grease) becomes vitiated and courses downward. The Vátaja cases (of Prameha) are, therefore, incurable. 23.

Anumata is the term used when an opinion of another is (quoted but) not refuted. For example—some authorities hold that there are seven Rasas or tastes. (Now, as this is not refuted it is said to be **Anumata** or sanctioned by the author). 24.

Vidhána is the act of mentioning, at the beginning, the fact to be established. For example—the vulnerable or vital parts (Marmans) in the thigh are eleven in number, and this has already been stated to be established. 25.

Anágatávekshana is the term used when something in the future is referred to in such terms as 'this will be dealt with hereafter'. For example—it can be said in the Sutra-sthána 'it will be dealt with in the Chikitsita-sthána'. 26.

Atikrántávekshana is the term used when something in the past is referred to. For example—it can be said in the Chikitsita-sthána 'it has already been said in the Sutra-sthána'. 27.

Samsaya is the term used when examples of two opposite and dissimilar subjects are cited. For example—hurt to the Tala-Hridaya (Marmans in the hands and legs) is fatal ; amputation of the hand and of the leg is not fatal. 28.

Vyákhyána is the description or explanation of the details. For example—Purusha as the twenty-fifth factor has been dealt with in this book. While only the twenty-four factors constituting this body have been dealt with in other works 29.

Sva-samjná denotes the specific terms specially used in any work and not in common with any other work. For example – the term 'Mithuna' (in medical works) means the two things, *viz.*, honey and clarified butter. 30.

Udáharana* is the example of what is well-established or well-known in the world. For example—

* Udáharana has been recognised here as a technical term. But it should not have been recognised as such, since it has not been included in the list (see para 2). Had it been so, the number would have been 31 and not 32. Dallana prefers to regard the portion सर्वोषभयात् etc. as an interpolation and adding a वा after the sentence लोके प्रथितमुदाहरणम् takes it in continuation of the example of स्वसंज्ञा

cooling measures should be had recourse to to guard against warmth. 31.

Nirvachana is the derivation of a term. For example—Áyus (life) is the subject-matter of this work, and a man gets (the means of) Áyus (longevity) from this work and hence it is called Áyurveda. 32.

Nidarśana is the term used when the meaning (of a word or sentence) is supported by examples. For example—just as the (digestive) fire in the Koshtha (abdomen) increases in contact with (the local bodily) Váyu, so also an ulcer increases when assisted by the (bodily) Váyu, Pitta and Kapha. 33.

Niyoga is the enjoining of something to be done as a duty. For example—only what is beneficial (Pathya) should be taken. 34.

Samuchchaya is the joining (of two or more connected but independent ideas) as such and such. For example—in the group of flesh, (those of) Ena and Harina (two kinds of deer), Láva and Tittira (two kinds of birds) and Sáranga (spotted deer) are the principal ones. 35.

Vikalpa is the term used when something is said to be this or that, *i. e.*, when alternatives are used. For example—either meat-soup or Yavágu (gruel) cooked with clarified butter (should be used in such and such a case). 36.

Uhya is the term used when something more can be understood by an intelligent man, though not definitely used. For example—it has been said in the chapter on Anna-pána-vidhi (Chapter XLVI, Sutra-Sthána) that Anna (food) is of four kinds, *viz.*, (1)

in the previous para. His meaning is that the word मिद्दृष being not found in the sense referred to in para. 30, the reader is asked to find out a popular example.

Bhakshya (masticable) or the solid food that has to be bitten with the teeth before eating, (2) **Bhojya** (edible) or the solid food proper *i. e.*, which has not to be bitten with the teeth, (3) **Lehya** (lambative) or the semi-liquid food that has to be licked like an electuary, and (4) **Peya** (drink) or the liquid food proper that has to be drunk ; but of these four kinds, two kinds only (*viz.*, Anna and Pániya) have been mentioned (in naming the chapter). Here it is (said that the other two kinds) are) understood. For, when only two are mentioned in respect of food and drink, the inclusion of all the four therein is easily comprehended. And why? Because the term 'Bhakshya' is included in the term 'Anna'—both being of the same kind, *viz.*, solid food ; and the term 'Lehya' is included in the term 'Peya'—both being of the same kind, *viz*, liquid. And the articles of food, though they are really of four kinds, are usually spoken of in the common language as being of two kinds only (*viz*, solid and liquid). 37.

Here have been fully described by me the **thirty-two** technical terms for the investigation into the essence of this Tantra (work). The intelligent man who is fully conversant with these technical terms—which work like lights, as it were,—is to be regarded as the greatest physician and to be held in great esteem.—This is what the Sage Dhanvantari says. 38.

Thus ends the sixty-fifth chapter of the Uttara-Tantra in the Sus'ruta-Samhitá which deals with the technical terms used in this work

CHAPTER LXVI.

Now we shall discourse on the chapter which (deals with and) is called the different modifications (combinations) of the different Doshas—**Dosha-Bheda-vikalpa-námádhyáya.**

Revered Sus'ruta, the son of Vis'vámitra, asks (the following to) the high-minded Divodása, well-versed in all the eight divisions of Áyurveda, with intellect sharp and as deep as an ocean, as it were, and with all the difficulties in the meanings of the S'ástras fully solved. The question is—It has been already said that there are sixty-two* varieties of the Doshas, but how are they divided when taken one, two or all the three at a time'? 2—3.

On hearing his word the great sage and king (Divodása) with all his difficulties solved was greatly pleased and thus narrated the true conditions to Sus'ruta. 4.

The three Doshas, the (seven) Dhátus, feces and urine—these, in their normal state, hold together the corporeal frame in conjunction with the (six Rasas necessary (for the constitution). 5.

Puru-ha or human body has sixteen sub-strata†. The Pránas (*viz.* the organs of sense) are eleven in number while the number of diseases is **one thousand one hundred** and **twenty** and that of elementary sub-

* The reference is to chapter LXIII, but there the number is sixty-three and not sixty-two. The three Dhátus Váyu, Pitta and Kapha, in their normal state, cannot properly be called Doshas. The state in which all the three Dhátus are in their normal state, is said to be the 63 rd. combination (see also para. 8 below).

† The sixteen sub-strata are the five elementary principles, (*viz* —Earth, Water, Fire, Air and Ether) and the eleven sense-organs.

stances (Dravya) is five hundred and seventy-three, – these have already been explained in detail. The three qualities (*viz.*, Sattva, Rajas and Tamas) have also been explained in connection with the (three) different Doshas (*viz.*, Váyu, Pitta and Kapha) which are generally said to have **sixty-two** combinations. 6—8.

Different Combinations of Doshas :— The three Doshas separately have **three** combinations, *viz.*, where one of the Doshas is aggravated and the other two are in their normal state. Taken two at a time, both of them aggravated, whether equally or unequally (with the third in its normal state), the number of combinations would be **nine** ; while the number of combinations would be **thirteen** if they are taken three at a time—all of them aggravated, both equally and unequally (thus making twenty-five in all with the aggravated Doshas). With an equal number of combinations in cases of the diminution of the Doshas (taken one, two or three at a time) we have fifty combinations. The number of combinations (taken one, two and three at a time) with the aggravated and diminished Doshas mixed together would be twelve only.— Thus making **sixty-two** in all. 9

The number of combinations, when mixed together, would be innumerable. It, therefore, behoves a physician to treat a patient with the different combinations of the (six different) Rasas after properly diagnosing the disease with a due regard to the aggravation of the different Doshas and without going into any further details. In ameliorating a disease, the physician is the doer of that action the effect whereof is health and the instruments with which the action is performed are the Rasas while the Doshas are the causes. The opposite hereof is want of health. 10.

The Uttara-Tantra, enriched with the sixty-six chapters wherein have been described and explained the order of the words and their meanings, and wherein have been explained very clearly the hidden meanings of the terms for making them clear to persons of weak intellect, has thus been duly explained to you in accordance with your question. 11.

Persons reading, according to the rules laid down, this treatise together with the Uttara-Tantra coming from (the mouth of) Brahmá himself, are not abondoned by their wished for objects, that is to say, they are sure to obtain them. This word of Brahmá is perfectly true. 12.

Thus ends the sixty-sixth chapter of the Uttara-Tantra in the Sus'ruta-Samhitá which (deals with and) is called the different combinations of the different Doshas.

Here ends the Uttara-Tantra.

THE END

AN ENGLISH TRANSLATION

OF

THE SUSHRUTA SAMHITA

INDEX & APPENDICES, Etc.

BY

KAVIRAJ KUNJA LAL BHISHAGRATNA, M. R. A. S. (LONDON).

PUBLISHED BY

S. L. BHADURI, B. L.

10, KASHI GHOSE LANE, CALCUTTA.

1918.

INDEX

A

C

E

H

O

APPENDIX No. 1.

GLOSSARY OF IMPORTANT WORDS.

A

	Abhishyandi ...	... Anything that produces a sliminess in the channels and a consequent heaviness of the limbs. Causing defluxions or watery effusion; secreting.
	Abhyanga ...	... Smearing the body with oily substance.
II—532	Áchamana ...	... Rinsing the mouth; sipping water before religious ceremony, or before or after meal. Washing.
I—287	Adhvaryu ...	... One of the priests at a Vedic sacrifice. See note Vol. I P. 305.
II—549	Adequate quantity	... See Vol. II. 549.
	Ágneya	... Pertaining to fire. See Vol. I P. 108. Digesting.
I—196, 319	Agni... ...	... The Fire-god. See Vol. I intro. XLVII; Vol. II P. 3.
II—531	Agni-shtoma ...	... A religious sacrifice.
	Aksha	... A weight equal to two Tolás.
II—311	Akshi-Tarpana ...	... A fluid medicine to be dropped into the eye. Eye-lotions. See Vol. III. P. 85.
	Akrita-yusha ...	... Unseasoned soup
II—735	Alarka	... A mad dog.
	Alakta	... Lac.
	Álepa Álepana } ...	... Plaster—see Vol. I Ch. XVIII.
III—155	Andha-putaná ...	... A demoness supposed to cause diseases to children.
	Anila	... See Váyu
	Anjali	... A measure weighing half a seer. 32 Tolás.
	Anna	... Boiled rice; solid food; food.
II—391	Antar-dhuma ...	... (Burning) in two covered pitchers—i.e. in the abscence of air.
I—487	Ánupa	... Belonging to a marshy place. See Vol. I. P. 325, 487.
	Anuloma ...	... In regular or natural order or course.

II—394	Anulomana ...	... Medicines which help the digestion of the Doshas, esp. the Váyu and set them free. Purgative.
	Anu-rasa... ...	... A secondary flavour. An after-taste.
	Anuvásana ...	... Oily enema. See Vol. II P. 594.
	Anuvellita ...	... Bandage. See Vol. I P. 167.
	Ápa	... Water or liquid. See Vol. I P. 374 ; Vol. II P. 121.
	Apána-Váyu ...	... See Vol. II P. 3. Flatus.
	Apa-Tarpana ...	... Depletory measures ; fasting ; food that does not gratify.
II—209	Ápta-vák ...	... Persons or words of authority.
	Apupa	... Cakes.
	Áranála	... The acid fermentation of the wheat-boiling. A variety of kánjika.
	Árdrá	... One of the 27 constellations.
	Arishta	... A variety of liquor. See Vol. I. 266.
I—287	Arundhati ...	... Pole-star ; one of the Pliades.
II—75	Arvuda	... A tumour.
	Ásava	... Fermented liquor.
	Ás'chyotana ...	... The process of dropping a liquid into the eye. Eye-drop. See Vol. III P. 84.
	As'leshá	... One of the 27 constellations.
	Ásthápana ...	... Non-oily enema. See Vol. II Ch. XXXVII.
	As'vini	... The first of the 27 constellatons.
	Atharvan ...	... The fourth Veda.
	Átreya	... The founder of the school of Áyurvedic medicine.
	Audaka	... Pertaining to water.
	Aupadrava ...	... Pertaining to an Upadrava or the side-issue of a disease.
I—317	Aupasargika ...	... Pertaining to an Upasarga ; sympathetic.
I—425	Avanti	... Name of a city—modern Ujjaini.
	Avapida-nasya ...	... A kind of errhine. II. P. 659.
	Avasechana ...	... Sprinkling.
	Ayana	... Half year : the solstice.
	Ayaskánta ...	... Magnet. Vol. I. 256.
	Áyuh	... Vital condition ; natural span of life. See Vol. II.—Intro. VIII.

Ayurveda ... ... The Science of life ; See Vol. I. P. 2 ; Vol. II. Intro. ii.

B

III—162 Bhaga ... ... A god of that name.

Bharadvája ... ... The founder of the School of Áyurvedic medicine.

Bharani ... ... The second of the 27 constellations.

Bhávaná ... ... A process of saturating. See Vol. II. note P. 312.

Brahmá ... ... The supreme Being. The creator ; the first Deity of the sacred Hindu Trinity to whom is entrusted the work of creating the world. The founder of the Áyurveda.

Bráhmana ... ... A person belonging to the highest (original) caste of the Hindus ; A Bráhmana was born from the mouth of the Purusha—cf. Manu. ch. I P. 30.

Brahmadeva ... ... A commentator of Sushruta Samhitá.

II—128 Brahma-chárini ... A woman ovserving the vow of continence...Manu-samhitá—ch I.

Brahmarshi ... ... A Bráhmana ascetic.

C

Chakra-taila ... ... Oil pressed out from a wooden oil-mill.

Chakradatta ... ... A shortened form of Chakrapáni Dutta, commentator of Charaka and Sushruta Samhitá and the clebrated compiler of a medical treatise named "Chakradatta."

Chaitya ... ... A Buddhist temple. See note Vol. II. P. 216.

Chatuh-Sneha ... ... Oil, clarified butter, fat and marrow.

II—405 Chitra-bhánu ... ... The name of Surya, the Sun-god.

D

Dárvi-homa ... ... A kind of Vedic religious sacrifice.

Das'a-mula ... ... See Vol. I. P. 355.

J—230 Dauhrida ... ... The longing of an enciente (for some thing or other).

Dhátus ... ... Root or fundamental principles. See Vol. I. Ch. XV. See Intro. XLI.

Dhányámla ... ... A fermented acid gruel prepared from paddy.

I—546 Dháná ... ... Parched barley.

Dhamani ... ... See Vol. II. P. 209. A vessel, artery or duct.

II.—653 Dhuma-pána ... ... Smoking ; fumagative inhalation.

Dhruva ... ... Immutable Being ; the pole-star.

Dipana ... ... Appetising.

II—120 Dosha ... ... The fundamental principles ; morbid diothesis. See Dhátu I. P. 120 Intro. XLVII.

Drona ... ... A measure of sixteen seers ; when used in respect of a liquid substance, it would mean double that quantity i.e. thirty-two seers.

Dundubhi ... ... A sort of large kettle-drum ; a drum.

Dvandaja ... ... Dvi-doshaja ; Produced from the morbid affection of any two Doshas.

Dvi-dosha ... ... A combination of any two of the three Doshas.

G

Gangá ... ... One of the sacred rivers of the Hindus ; the modern Ganges. The river Ganges personified.

II—127 Garbhádhána ... ... The ceremony of impregnation ; one of the principal Samskáras (rites) of the Hindus.

Garuda ... ... The name of the king of birds. It is the carrier of Vishnu.

Garuda-Purána ... ... One of the principal Puránas.

Gáyatri ... ... The sacred vedic hymn.

Ghata ... ... A measure of thirty-two seers ; when used in respect of liquid substances, it would mean double the quantity—i e. 64 seer.

I—437 Ghola ... ... Curd-whey. See Takra.

I—442 Ghrita-manda ... ... Upper layer of clarified butter ; cream-feather.

II—26 Gomeda ... ... A kind of gem

Gotra ... ... Lineage, family or race.

Gophaná ... ... A kind of bandage. See Vol. I. P. 168.

III—141 Graha... ... ... Stars, planets or spirits. An evi. spirit.

Gráhi ... ... Astringent, lit. any medicines which is both stomachic and digestive and dries the fluid of the body through its heat-producing properties.

H

II—127 Havishya ... ... A particular course of food consisting of Ghrita, etc., esp. without meat and fish as prescribed in the Hindu Smriti.

Himálaya ... ... A mountain.

Homa ... ... Offering oblations to gods by throwing Ghee into the consecrated fire.

Hotri ... ... A sacrificial priest, esp. one who recites the prayers of Rig-veda at a sacrifice. See note Vol. I. P. 305.

Hridya ... ... Cordial ; pertaining to the heart ; exhilarant.

I

Indra ... ... The king of the gods of Hindu mythology. The preceptor of the different branches of Hindu medicine.

I—105 Indramada ... ... A kind of disease peculiar to the leeches.

II—180 Indra-vasti ... ... The name of a Marma.

Is'ána ... ... The presiding diety of the north-east quarter. One of the different manifestations of S'iva.

J

Jángala ... ... Pertaining to the forest ; See Vol. I. P. 326, 480.

II—133 Játismara ... ... One who remembers his conditions in a former life.

K

I—46 Kalá ... ... A division of time ; thirty Káshthás make one Kala, i.e. one hundred and forty-four seconds.

I—164	Kalka	... A paste of any drug. In connection with any medicated oil or Ghrita this term is used to mean the pasted drugs with which the oil or Ghrita is cooked. See Vol. II 549.
I—541	Kámvalika ...	... A kind of soup.
	Kánjika	... A fermented acidgruel. The water of boiled rice &c. preserved in a closed pitcher for spontaneous fermentation.
II—530	Kandarpa ...	... The cupid of the Hindu mythology.
I—17	Karana	... An astrological division of the day.
	Karma	... Physiological action. Action of medicine.—Vol. I.P. 377.
I—522	Karisha	... Dry cakes of cow-dung.
I—46	Káshthá	... A measure of time ; $4\frac{4}{6}$ seconds.
	Kapha	... See Vol. I. P. 121 ; Intro. P. XLI.
I—202	Katvara	... Curd mixed with oil.
	Khattá	... Bandage. See Vol. I. Ch. 18.
I—540	Khada } Khala } ...	... A kind of soup.
,,	Khada-Yavágu ...	... A kind of soup.
,,	Khada-yusha ...	... A kind of soup.
I—439	Kiláta	... Condensed milk.
	Kos'a	... Bandage. See Vol 1. Ch. 18.
I—530	Krisará	... A kind of food prepared by cooking rice and pulse together. See Vol. I. P. 178.
	Krita-yusha ...	... A seasoned soup.
	Krishna	... An incarnation of Vishnu.
III—146	Krittikás	... One of the constellations of the Hindu astronomy. The supposed nurse-mother of Kumára.
	Kshatriya ...	... The second of the four original castes of the Hindus. The warrior and ruling caste of the Hindus.
	Kshiti	... Earth or solid See Vol. I. P. 375 ; Vol. II. P. 121.
I—442	Kshira-Ghrita } Kshira-Sarpih }	... Clarified butter churned out of milk itself without turning it into curd.
	Kudava	... A measure of weight equal to half a Seer.

	Kulmásha ...	... A preparation of food from Másha pulse. Half-boiled Chanaka or gram. I—546.
	Kumára ...	... The name of Skanda, originally the chief of Grahas, afterwards the god of war—Vol. iii. Ch. 37.
I—443	Kumbha-Ghrita	... Clarified butter one hundred and ten years old. According to Charaka one hundred years old.
I—439	Kurchiká ...	... Coagulated or inspissated milk.
	Kuvera	... The god of riches and treasure, son Visravá ; Crœsus.
	Kás'i	... The seat of ancient Hindu surgery. It was here that the holy Dhanvantari gave lessons on Áyurveda to Susr'uta and others. The greatest place of Hindu pilgrimage. The modern Benares.
	Kavaliká ...	... Plug. Medicated tow. Vol. I. Ch. 18.

L

	Lekhana ...	... Liquefacation as opposite to Vringhana ; attenuated ; Scarification.
	Loha	... The seven principal metals ; also it means iron.
	Lunchaka ...	... One who plucks or tears off.

M

I—456	Madhu-S'arkará	... Sugar prepared from concentrated honey.
I—544	Madhu-Mastaka	... A kind of confection having for its ingredients powdered rice, barley, Ghrita and honey.
	Maghá	... One of the constellations of Hindu Astronomy ; the liones.
	Magnet ...	... Vol. I. 256.
	Mahá-agada ...	... The name of an antitoxic preparation. See Kalpa-sthána Ch. 5. 21 Sloka.
	Mahá-vyádhi ...	... See Vol. I. P. 287, 297.
	Mahendra ...	... One of the seven principal chains of mountains in India.
I—443	Mahá-ghrita ...	... Older even than Kumbha-ghrita.
	Mala	... See Vol. I. P. 119; also Intro. P. LII.

I—425	Malaya	... One of the seven principal chains of mountains in India. It is said to be teeming with sandal trees.
	Mantra	... Incantations.
I—42	Manu	... The progenitor of the human race. Author of "Manu-Samhitá."
	Mandala ...	... A kind of circular bandage. See Vol. I P. 167.
I—439	Manda	... The residuary sediment of a compound made of Kurchiká and Dadhi.
I—533	Manda	... Rice, Barley etc. boiled in water weighing fourteen times of rice and strained through a piece of linen.
	Mantha	... See Vol. I. 542.
	Máruti	... Air or Ether. The wind-god. See Vol. I. P. 375.
I—425	Maru-des'a ...	... Lit.—a desert-land; the name of a country.
	Mastu	... The upper part of a thickened sour milk; the watery part of curd, whey &c.
	Másha	... A weight equal to twenty grains.
	Masi	... A lamp-black; anything burnt in a covered pitcher or vessel.
	Mastulunga ...	... Brain materials.
	Mastishkya ...	... Any medicine or substance acting on the brain.
	Mátrá	... A dose.
	Mercury	... Vol. II. 508 and 698.
	Morata	... See note Vol. I. P. 439.
I—544	Modakas ...	... Sweets.
	Muhurta ...	... A measure of time i.e. twenty Kalás make one Muhurta, i.e. equal to forty-eight minutes.
I—544	Mudga-vesavára	... Vesavára prepared with the addition of Mudga pulse—see Vesavára.
III—111	Mukhamandiká graha ...	An evil goddess often doing harm to children.
	Mulá	... One of the constellations of Hindu astronomy.
	Mushti	... A measure equal to eight Tolás.

N

II—140	Nádi	... Umbelical chord. Senus.
	Nága	... The celestial serpent.
II—236	Nágodara ...	... False pregnancy. See Vol. II. P. 236.
II—236 III—111	Naigamesha Naigamesha Graha	... An evil god often doing harm to children.
I—42	Nárada	... The name of a divine sage.
	Nasya	... Snuff, errhine ; anything taken through the nostrills. See Vol. II. P. 659.
I—439	Navanita ...	... Butter.
I—42	Nimesha ...	... Time taken in closing the eyelids.
	Niyama	... Certain minor duties to be observed by every man.
	Nirudha-Vasti ...	... Same as Ásthápana. See Vol. II. P. 627.

O

	Ojah	... Strength ; Vitality. See Vol. I. 130. Intro. P. LVI.
	Omkára ...	... The mystic syllable "Om".

P

	Páchana	... Process of setting up suppuration. Anything that digests the undigested food without increasing the appetite.
	Panchangi ...	... A five-tailed bangage I- 168.
	Pala	... A measure equal to 8 Tolás.
I—545	Palala	... A preparation of treacle, pasted sesamum and corn flour.
	Palala	... Powdered sesame.
I—101	Pándya	... The Deccan.
,,	Pautana	... Mathurá.
	Panchángi ...	... A kind of Bandage. See Vol. I. P. 168.
	Pancha-karma ...	... It is a technical term used for the application of the five medical measures viz. Emetics, Purgatives, Errhine, Ásthápana and Anuvásana.
I—542	Pánaka	... Syrup ; drinks ; cordials.

	Pancha-kola ...	... The five officinal drugs Pippali, Pippali-root, Chavya, Chitraka-root and S'unthi.
	Pancha Lavana ...	... The five different officinal salts. See Vol. I. 527.
	Párada	... Mercury. Vol. II. 508, 698.
I—425	Páripàtra ...	... The name of a mountain in the Deccan. The Western Range.
I—41	Parjanya	... The rain-god ; a cloud.
I—42	Parvata	... Mountain ; the presiding god of the mountain.
II—499	Parvan	... See foot-note, P. 499, Vol. II.
I—180	Pas'upati... ...	... The name of S'iva of the Hindu Trinity.
	Pavana	... The wind-god ; Váyu.
	Páyasa	... A preparation of rice, milk and sugar cooked together.
I—533	Peyá	... A preparation of rice, barley &c., boiled in 15 times of water.
I—455	Phánita	... The inspissated or half boiled juice of sugar-cane ; a variety of treacle.
I—439	Piyusha	... The milk of a cow during the first seven days after calving.
I—195	Pitta	... See Vol. I, P. 120. Intro, P. XLIII.
I—41	Pitris	... The *Manes*, the deceased forefathers.
I—41	Pis'ácha	... A kind of demon.
	Prajápati ...	... The first progenitor.
	Pradeha ...	... Thick plaster. See Vol. I, Ch. 18.
	Pralepa	... Plaster. See Vol. I, Ch. 18, P. 163.
	Prána	... Strength or Protoplasm. One of the five vital Váyus.
I—253	Pránáyáma ...	... The regulation of the breath preliminary to the practice of Yoga.
	Pratoli	... A form of broad bandage. See Vol. I, P. 167.
	Pratiloma ...	... Against the natural direction or bending of the hair, i.e. against the hair, hence against the natural course or motion of anything.
	Prána-Váyu ...	... See Vol. II, P. 3.
	Prakuncha ...	... A weight equal to eight Tolás or one Pala.

	Prás'a	... A form of medicine—lit. that which is eaten, e.g. Chyavana-prás'a.
	Prasrita	... A measure equal to sixteen Tolás.
I—547	Prithuka ...	... Thrashed or parched paddy.
I—544	Pupa	... Cakes. See Apupa.
	Purusha	... Vol. I, P. 9, 14; Vol. II. P. 117.
I—42	Purushottama ...	... The foremost of beings.
	Purva-rupa ...	... Premonitory symptoms or indications of a disease. Vol. I. 317.
III—89	Puta-páka ...	... A process of preparing medicine by burning something inside two pots hermetically closed, one placed upside-down over the other.
II—312	Phala-varti ...	... A kind of purgative plug. Suppository.

R

I—538	Rága-shádava ...	... Soup prepared with grapes and the expressed juice of pomegranate.
	Rajas	... The Principle of action and co-hesion. See note Vol. II, P. 114, 120.
I—41	Rájarshi	... A royal sage.
	Rakshá-karma ...	... Incantations for the cure and safety of a patient. See Vol. I. Ch. 5.
II—543	Ráma	... The eldest son of Das'aratha, king of Ajodhyá, better known as Ráma Chandra.
	Rasa	... The water-origined flavour. Expressed juice. Essence; serus fluid. Vol. I. P. 107 and P. 382; Vol. III. 392.
	Rasa-kriyá ...	... A process for preparing medicine by thickening the decoction of any drug or drugs.
I—541	Rasálá	... A kind of sweetened drink.
	Rati	... A measure equal to two grains.
	Revati-graha ...	... The name of an evil goddess often doing harm to children.
	Rik	... The name of one of the Vedas.
	Rishi	... A sage; a hermit.
	Rudra	... The name of a god. The god of destruction.

S

I—425	Sahya	... The Ghâta mountains.
	S'akra	... Indra, the king of the gods.
	S'aktu	... Powdered barley.
	S'alya	... See Vol. P. 56, 245.
II—291	S'álvana-Upanáha	... A kind of fomentation by plastering.
	Sams'odhana ...	... A medication which purifies the system by purgative or vomiting. Vol. I. Intro. LXI. P. 358.
I—358	Sams'amana ...	... A medicine or measure which neutralises the Doshas in the system. Vol. I. Intro. LXI.
	Sáma	... The name of one of the Vedas.
	Samána-Váyu ...	... See Vol. II, P. 3.
	S'anaka	... The name of a sage.
	Sánnipátika ...	... Pertaining to the Sannipáta or the simultaneous aggravation of all the three Doshas.
I—544	Sanyáva	... A preparation of wheat boiled with milk, clarified butter &c.
	Sánkhya	... One of the six schools of Hindu philosophy.
I—314	Sára	... The pith. Physical temperament.
	Saráva	... A weight equal to 8 Palas or one seer.
	S'arkará	... Sugar.
	S'arkará	... Gravels ; concretions ; calculi.
	Sárodaka ...	... The decoction of the drugs of the Sála-sárádi group. See note Vol. II. P. 387.
	Sarpih	... Clarified butter.
	Sattva	... An illuminating or psychic principle. See note Vol. II. P. 114.
	S'átaka	... Linen ; cloth.
	S'ata-dhauta Ghrita	... Clarified butter washed 100 times in water.
	Sattaka	... Vol. I. P. 544.
	Shádava	... I. P. 549.
	Sauvira	... A kind of fermented gruel prepared by boiling huskless barley.
I—545	Shashkuli ...	... A kind of confectionary.
	Siddhas	... A class of demi-gods.
I—461	Sidhu	... Wine prepared from Madhuka flower.

I—541	S'indáki	A special combination of some spices. A kind of firmented gruel prepared from radish, mustard &c.
	S'iro-Virechana	Sternutatoric. see Vol II. P. 659.
II—92	S'iro-Vasti	An applieation over the scalf. An application of medicated oil on the head by tying a piece of leather all round the head, luting its margin to the skin by pasted Másha pulse and then filling the cavity thus formed with oil.
	S'leshmá	See Kapha.
	Sneha	See Vol II. P. See 546.
	Sneha-Karma	The applying, whether internally or externally, of any oily (fotty) substance to the body. II. Ch. 31.
	Sneha-páka	See Vol II. P. 549.
	Soma	See note Vol. II. 530.
	Soumya	Pertaining to Soma or the moon-god; cold.
II—527	S'ree-S'ukta	A number of holy Mantras dedicated to S'ree or the goddess of fortune.
	Stambhana	Constipator. Stuffing.
Ch. II.	Sthandila	The bare ground.
	Sthagiká	A sort of bandage. See Vol I. P. 168.
	S'udra	One of the first four castes according to the Hindu S'ástras.
II—290	Supta-Váta	A kind of nervous disease. See Vol. II. P. 290.
I.—465	S'ukta	Acid fermentation of any article.
	S'ukti	A weight equal to four Tolás; an oyster.
	Supa	Soup.
	Sutára	Mercury. Vol. II. P. 698.
I. P. 18	Sváhá-mantra	The uttering of the holy word 'Sváhá' in connection with the dedication of anything to a god.
	Sveda-Karma	Diaphoretic measures. Vol. II. P. 558.
	Svastika	A circular cross bandage. See Vol. I. 167.
I—275	Svastika	A cross-shaped religious insignia.
	Sva-gotra	One belonging to the same family.

Sveda ... ... See Vol. II P. 558.
S'yámá stri ... ... A young lady of middle age.

T

Takra ... ... Vol. I 438.
Takshaka ... ... The name of the king of serpents.
Tamas ... ... Princple of nescience. Illusion. See note—Vol. II. P. 114, 120
Tarpana ... ... A pleasing tonic. A soothing measure. Vol. III. 84.
Tarpana ... ... Flour of barley or parched grain dissolved in water. Vol. II. P. 303.
II—121 Tejas ... ... Fire or gas. See Vol. I. P. 375.
II—413 Traivrita ... ... Clarified butter, oil and lard.
Tri-páda Gáyatri ... The holy mantra of Gáyatri which is divided into three parts.
Tri-phalá ... ... See Vol. I. P. 353.
Tri-sugandhi ... ... The three aromatic drugs viz. Tvak, (cinnamon), Elá (cardamom) and Tejapatra.
Tri-dosha ... ... Váyu, Pitta and Kapha.
II—529 Tripáda ... ... Three-footed.
III—161 Tripura ... ... The three ærial cities of the demon, generally known as Tripura for possessing those three cities.
II—481 Tri-Varga ... ... Tri-katu, Tri-phalá and Tri-mada.
Tri-Katu... ... ... Pippali, Maricha and S'unthi.
Tryushana ... ... Same as Tri-Katu.
I—408 Tushodaka ... ... See Vol. I. 408.
I—465 Tushámbu ... ... Fermented liquid of unboiled barley with husks.
Tulá ... ... One hundred Palas or twelve seers and a half.
Tvak ... ... Serum ; skin ; cinnamon.

U

II—405 Uchchaihs'ravs ... ... The name of Indra's horse.
Udána-Váyu ... ... See Vol. II. P. 3.
Udgátri ... ... See note Vol. I. P. 305.
Ulumba ... ... Mudga-pulse etc., boiled over a fire.
III—146 Umá ... ... The consort of Mahádeva.
Upa-drava / Upa-sarga } ... ... Supervening symptoms.

	Upanáha ...	... A kind of fomentation ; poulticing.
	Utkáriká ...	... Porridge-like preparations used as food. A massive poultice.
II—536	Uttara-Kuru ...	... The country round the North Pole.
	Uttara-Vasti ...	... Urethral and vaginal injection. See Vol. II. P. 628. 624.

V

I—42	Vais'vánara ...	... The fire-god.
	Vais'ya	... One of the 4 classes of men according to the Hindu S'ástras.
I—42	Varuna	... The god of water (Neptune).
II—225	Varna	... Caste. Colour.
I—42	Vasundhará ...	... The earth.
	Vasti-s'odhaka ...	... Diuretic.
II—405	Vásava	... Indra.
	Vasti-karma ...	... Application of enema. See Vol. II. P. 590.
	Vasá	... The oily substance of the flesh.
	Váta	... See Váyu.
I—541	Vataka	... A kind of food. Pill. 8 Másha.
	Váyu	... The one of the three fundamental morbific principles of human body. Vol. I. P. 120. Intro. P. XLI. Vol. II. P. 3.
I—538	Ves'avára... ...	... A poultice prepared with boneless pasted flesh—Vol. II. P. 30. A cooked preparation of boneless pasted meat mixed with treacle Ghrita, Pippali and Maricha.
	Vidáha } Vidagdha } ...	... A sluggish digestion due to the production of acidity. Imperfect digestion.
	Vidyádhara ...	... A class of demi-gods.
	Videha	... The modern Tirhoot ; The name of an author of S'álákya Tantra (esp. the eye-disease).
	Vilepi	... Rice, barley etc. cooked with water weighing four times.
	Vipáka	... Digestive transformation ; digestive or chemical reaction. Vol. I. 369.
I—42	Vishnu	... The second god of the Hindu Triad.

Vitána ... ... A Canopy-bandage. See Vol. I. P. 168.

Vishyandana ... ... Secretion. See note—Vol. I. P. 544.

III—148 Vis'ákhá ... ... Name of an evil goddess bent upon doing harm to children.

Vilva ... ... A weight equal to eight Tolás.

Vi-yoni ... ... A woman of an inferior caste.

Vrimhana ... ... Constructive or restorative.

Vrishya ... ... An agent stimulating the sexual passion ; aphrodisiac.

Vyosha ... ... Trikatu.

Vyoma ... ... The sky or etherin. See Vol. I. P. 375 ; see Vol. II. P. 121.

Vivandha ... ... A circular chest-bandage—Vol. I. 167.

Vyána-váyu ... ... Vol. I. 120 ; Vol. II. P. 3.

Vyasana... ... ... See note—Vol. II. 539.

Y

Yajna ... ... Religious sacrifice.

Yamaka ... ... A double bandage. See Vol. I. P. 168.

Yamaka ... ... Two things viz., oil and clarified. butter ; rice and pulse.

Yaksha ... ... A class of demi-gods.

I—291 Yama ... ... Pluto, the god of death.

I—101 Yavana ... ... Turkisthána. The Jonians, generally used for the Greeks and the Mahomedans.

I—456 Yavása-S'arkárá ... Sugar prepared from the decoction of Durálabhá.

Yavágu ... ... A gruel prepared with rice, barley, wheat &c.

Yoga ... ... Religious meditation. Medicinal preparations. Compounds.

Yojana ... ... Equal to eight miles.

I—46 Yuga ... ... Twelve complete years count as a Yuga.

Yusha ... ... Soup.

APPENDIX No. 2.

NAMES OF ANIMALS

(With English equivalents or explanations).

A

Ajágara ... ... A python (rock-snake) ; a boa.
A'lahvaya ... ... A bird belonging to the group that kill or strike with beaks.
Ambu-Kukkutiká... ... ... A water-fowl.
Anjali-karna ... ... One of the birds of prey.
Arnaya Gavaya ... ... A wild cow
As'wa... ... ... A horse.
As'watara ... ... A mule.
A'ti (*Turdus Ginginiamus*) ... A kind of bird living in marshes.
Aundra ... ... An otter.
Avabhanjana ... ... One of the birds of prey.
Avakus'a ... ... A sort of ape.

B

Bhalluka ... ... A particular class of shells.
Bhalluka ... ... A bear.
Bhása ... ... A vulture.
Bhedáśi ... ... A bird of the genus that kill or strike with bills.
Bhramara ... ... A bumble-bee.
Bhringarája (*Lanius malabaricus*) A kind of bird, probably a shrike or thrush.
Brika ... ... A wolf.
Byághra (*Tigris regalia*) ... ... A tiger.

C

Chakora ... ... A Greek partridge.
Chakra-báka (*Anas casarca*) ... Ruddy goose generally known in India as Brahminy duck or goose.
Chamara (Bos or yak Grunniens)... A sort of deer.
Chandraka ... ... A silver-fish (a sea-fish) ; (turbot ?).
Charaki ... ... A kind of poisonous (?) fish.
Chárushkara ... ... A kind of deer.
Chásha (*Coracias Indica*) ... ... The blue jay ; a king-fisher (according to some).

Chataka ... ... A sparrow.
Chátaka ... ... A kind of bird ; a sky-lark.
Chilli... ... ... A kite.

D

Darbbikara Sarpa... ... ... A class of venomous snakes with expanded or broad hoods—e. g a cobra—(26 species).
Dátyuha ... ... One of the several wading birds ; a gallinule.
Dhushaka ... ... A bird of the genus that kill or strike with beaks.
Dindimánaka ... ... A kind of bird whose cry is very harsh and loud.
Dvipi (*Felis pardus*) ... ... A panther ; a leopard.

E

Ena ... ... A kind of deer having black colour, beautiful eyes and short legs.
Ervâruka (*Cervus elephas*) ... A deer.

G

Gaja ... ... An elephant.
Gardabha ... ... An ass.
Gargara (*Pimelodus gagora, Ham*) A kind of sea-fish
Gavaya (*Bas gavœus*) wild on ... A kind of ox, the *gayal*.
Girisa... ... ... A kind of mountain-bird.
Go ... ... A cow.
Godhá ... ... An iguana.
Gokarna ... ... An animal frequenting a marshy place ; (the Nilgan ?).
Gokshada ... ... A kind of heron.
Gomatsya ... ... A huge sheat-fish.
Gridhra (*Perogine falcoon*) ... A female vulture.
Griha-godhiká ... ... A lizard.
Griha-Kulinga ... ... A sparrow.

H

Hansa ... ... A goose or duck.
Harina ... ... A red deer ; a spotted deer.
Hárita (*Columba hariala*) ... ... The green or wood pigeon.

J

Jivan-jivaka ... ... A variety of heion (Vaka) with blackish white feathers or wings.

K

Kadali ... ... A kind of antelope.
Kádamba ... ... A kind of goose with dark grey wings.
Káka (*Corvus corone*) ... ... A crow or raven.
Kála-Kapota ... ... A wild dove.
Kála-puchchhaka... ... ... A black-tailed bird.
Kalavinka (*Lonius malabaricus*)... A variety of bird.
Kanka (*Ardea cenerea*) ... ... A heron.
Kapinjala (*the francoline partridge ?*) A sort of bird.
Kapinjala ... ... A brown partridge.
Kapota ... ... A dove.
Karála ... ... A musk-deer.
Kárandava ... ... A variety of white goose.
Karkataka ... ... A crab.
Khadgi ... ... A rhinoceros.
Khanjaritaka (*Motacilla alba*) ... The wag-tail.
Konálaka ... ... A kind of aquatic bird.
Koyashthika ... ... A bird of the genus that kill or strike with bills.
Krakara (*Perdix Sylvatica*) ... A sort of partridge.
Krauncha (*Ardea jaculator*) ... A kind of heron.
Krishna-Karkataka ... ... A variety of crab.
Krishna-matsya ... ... A kind of fish (lit. a black fish).
Kritamála ... ... A kind of deer.
Kukkuta ... ... A cock.
Kulinga ... ... A kind of bird (a fork-tailed shrike ?).
Kulis'a ... ... A kind of sea-fish.
Kumbhira ... ... A crocodile.
Kuranga ... ... An antelope.
Kurara (*Pandion haliaectus*) ... A chakraváka ; an osprey (whose cry resembles a plaintive note).
Kurma ... ... A tortoise ; a turtle.
Kura-Váhuka ... ... A kind of bird.
Ku-Tittira ... ... A sort of partridge.
Kuvara ... ... A kind of water-bird.

L

Láva (*Perdix chinensis*) ... ... A kind of quail.
Lomas'a-karna ... ... A sort of burrower (lit. one having hairy ears).
Lopáka ... ... A fox.
Lutá ... ... A spider.

M

Madgu ... ... A shag ; a cormorant.
Mahábhru ... ... A variety of mungoose.
Mahá-mina ... ... A kind of sea-fish.
Mahisha ... ... A buffalo.
Makara ... ... A Dolphin shark or a shark with a proboscis.
Makshiká ... ... A fly.
Mallikáksha ... ... A sort of goose.
Márjjára (*Filus domestica*) ... A cat.
Mátri-nindaka ... ... A bird belonging to the group that kills or striks with bills.
Mayura (*Celosin crestola*) ... ... A pea-cock.
Medahpuchchha ... ... A fat-tailed sheep.
Meghavara (*Acuculus Milanohuercas*) A kind of aquatic bird.
Mesha ... ... A sheep.
Mrigairbbáruka ... ... A species of animal (probably a jackal-like tiger dwelling in a cave or hole and feeding on a deer) ; glutton (?).
Mriga-mátrika ... ... A doe.
Mriga-priyaka ... ... A boa (lit. one fond of a deer).
Mrigodara ... ... A big-bellied deer.
Murala ... ... A kind of fish (fry-fish ?).
Mushika ... ... A mouse ; a rat.

N

Nakula (*Mungoose viverra ichneumon*) A mongoose.
Nandi-mukha (*Turdus Ginginianus*) A sort of bird.
Nandi-váralaka ... ... A kind of marine fish.
Naptriká ... ... A kind of dove.
Nirálaka ... ... A kind of sea-fish.
Nyanku ... ... An antelope.

P

Páka-matsya ... ... A kind of sea-fish.
Parabhrita ... ... A cuckoo.
Párávata ... ... A pigeon.
Parna-mriga ... ... A kind of arboreal animal; a monkey.
Páthina (*Siburus pelorius boalis*) A kind of trout (with many teeth) ; a Boál fish.
Plava ... ... A diver (?).

Prishata ... ... The porcine deer (?) ; birds that roam together.

Pundarika ... ... A kind of white-eyed bird.

Pushkara-S'áyiká (*Ardea Sibcreca*) A species of crane.

Putighása ... ... A civet-cat.

R

Rájiva ... ... (1) A species of fish (2) a kind of sea-fish.

Raktaráji ... ... A species of poisonous insect.

Riksha (*Ursus Amiricanas*) ... A bear.

Rishya ... ... The painted or white-footed antelope ; a blue deer.

Rohita (*Cyprinus Rohita*) ... ... A Rohita or red fish (2) a doe (3) a kind of red deer.

Ruru ... ... A sort of many-horned deer (it sets up a plaintive cry at the time when the horns fall off).

S

Sahasra-danshtrá ... ... A huge trout (lit. one having 1000 teeth).

S'akuli-matsya (*cyprinus Mrigal*) A kind of fish.

S'alyaka ... ... A porcupine.

S'ambuka ... . A small conch-shell ; a snail.

S'amkha ... ... A conch-shell.

S'mkha-nakha ... ... A small shell.

S'arabha ... ... A species of deer of the size of a camel (fabulously supposed to have 8 legs).

Sáranga (*Ardea Sarunga*) ... ... A large kind of crow.

Sárasa (*Ardea Siberice*) ... ... An Indian crane.

S'arári-mukha ... ... A kind of bird.

S'árddula ... ... A tiger

Sáriká (*Gracula religiosa or turdus Salica*) ... ... A kind of Indian mimic bird ; a Mainá.

S'as'a ... ... A hare ; a rabbit.

S'as'a-gháti ... ... A bird of prey (lit. one killing a hare) ; an eagle (?).

S'atapatra ... ... A wood-pecker.

S'atapatra ... ... A peacock ; " Raja-s'uka".

Sinha ... ... A lion.

S'is'u-mára ... ... A porpoise.

S'rigála (*Conis aureas*) ... ... A jackal.
Srimara ... ... A kind of young deer.
Sugrihi ... ... A tailor-bird.
S'uka ... ... A parrot.
Śukláksha ... ... A white-eyed bird.
S'ukti ... ... A pearl-oyster.
S'wadanshtrá ... ... A four-horned deer.
S'wávit ... ... A hedge-hog.
S'wetacharana ... ... A kind of edible bird (lit. one having white legs).
S'yena (*Vulture cinereas*) ... ... A hawk or falcon.

T

Tarakshu ... ... A hyena.
Timi ... ... A kind of whale.
Timingila ... ... A large whale.
Tittira ... ... A partridge.

U

Uchchitinga ... ... A sort of cricket.
Uluka (*Strex flammea*) ... ... An owl.
Upachakra ... ... A variety of ruddy goose.
Ushtra ... ... A camel.
Utkros'a ... ... An osprey.

V

Vágunjára ... ... A kind of fish.
Vaka (*Ardea Niveda*) ... ... A heron ; a crane.
Valáka ... ... A crane ; a kind of edible crane.
Valgudi ... ... A bird of the genus that kill or strike with bills ; a *Bool-bool* (?).
Vánara ... ... A monkey ; an ape.
Varáha ... ... A boar.
Varati ... ... A wasp.
Varmmi ... ... An eel.
Vartaka, **Vartiká** ... ... A quail.
Vartira ... ... A kind of bird.
Vatika ... ... A kind of tick (?).
Vrika (*Conis lupus*) ... ... A wolf.
Vriksha-S'áyiká ... ... A squirrel.
Vris'chika ... ... A scorpion.
Vris'a-dans'a ... ... A cat.

APPENDIX NO. 3.

NAMES OF DRUGS.

(WITH LATIN SYNONYMS).

A

Abhayá	... Terminalia Chebula.
Abhraka	... Talc.
Ádhaki	... See Tuvara.
Áditya-Vaktrá	... Cleome Viscosa. Gynandropsis pentaphylla.
Árdraka	... Zingiber.
Ágára-dhuma	... Soot.
Agasti	... Sesbana grandiflora.
Agastya	... Agati.
Agni	... See Chitraka.
Agniká	... See Ajamodá.
Agni-mantha	... Premna Serratifolia ; ,, Integrifolia.
Aguru	... Aquilaria agallocha.
Ahifena	... Papaver Somniferum. Opium.
Ahigandhá	... Aristolochia Indica. Indian birthwort.
Airávata (Nárengá) ...	... Citrus Aurantium. Orange.
Ajagandhá...	... Ocymum gratissimum.
Ajamodá	... Pimpinella Involucrata.
Aja-Śringi	... Gymnema Sylvestre.
Ákáśa-Valli	... Cassayta filiformis.
Ákhu-parni	... Salvinia cucullata.
Aksha	... Terminalia belerica.
Akshota	... Juglans regia.
Alarka	... Calotropis gigantia.
Alávu	... Lagenaria Vulgaris.
Ámalaka } **Ámalaki** }	Phyleanthus emblica ; Emblica officinalis.
Amara-pushpi	... Andropogon acicularis.
Ambhoja	... Nelumbium speciosum.
Ambashthá	... Stephania hernandifolia.
Ambu	... Pavonia odorata.
Amla-loniká	... See Chángeri.
Amla-Vetasa	... Ruxem vesicarius.

Amliká	Tamarindus Indica. Tamarind.
Ámra	Mangifera Indica. Mango.
Ámra'taka	Sapondias Mangifera.
Amritá	See Guduchi.
Anantá / **Ananta-mula**	Hemidesmus Indicus.
Ankotaka	Alangium hexapetalum.
Apámárga	Achyranthis Aspera.
Aparájitá	Clitoria Ternatia.
Áragbadha	Cassia Fistula.
Aravinda	See Ambhoja.
Árevata	See A'ragvadha.
Arimeda	Accacia Farnesiana.
Arishta	Sapindus trifoliatus, Soap-nut.
Arishta	See Nimba.
Arjaka	Ocimum Album.
Arjuna	Terminalia Arjuna.
Arka	Calotropis gigantia.
Arka-mula	Aristolochia Indica.
Arka-pushpi	Gynandropsis Pentaphylla.
Arushkara	See Bhallátaka.
Asana	Terminalia Tomentosa.
Aśma-bheda	Kalanchoe Laciniata.
Aśoka	Saraca Indica.
Ásphota'	Salvodora Persica.
Asthi-samháraka	Vitis quadrangularis.
Aśva-Balá	Basella Bubra.
Aśva-gandhá	Withania Somnifera ; Physalis Flexuosa.
Aśva-karna	See S'ála.
Aśva-máraka	Nerium Odorum.
Aśvattha	Ficus Religiosa.
Atasi	Linum Usitatissimum.
Atipatrá	Sida Cordifolia.
Ativalá	Sida rhombifolia.
Ativisá	Aconitum heterophyllum.
Átma-guptá	Macuna pruriens.

B

Badara	See Vadara.
Badarámalaka	Andropogon Schoenantteus.

Bahu-mulá	... See S'atávari.
Bahu-vára	... Cordi Myxa.
Bahu-vija	... Citrus Medica.
Baka	... See Agasti.
Bákuchi	... Psoralea Corylifolia.
Bakula } **Vakula** }	... Mimusops Elengi.
Bala-bhadrá } **Balá** }	... Sida Cordifolia.
Bála	... Pavonia Odorata.
Balgá	... Jasaminum curiculatum.
Bandhu-jiva	... Pentapetes phoenicea.
Bandhuka	... Pentapetas phoenicea.
Bandhyákotika	... See Karkati.
Barbura } **Barbula** }	... Accacia Arabica.
Bhadra-káli	... See Prasárani.
Bhallátaka	... Semecarpus Anacardium.
Bhándi	... Rubica Cordifolia.
Bhandira	... Amaranthus Spinosus.
Bhantáki	... Solanum Indicum.
Bharadváji	... Hibiscus Vitifolius.
Bhárgi	... Clerodendron Siphonanthus.
Bhanjana	... Calartroptis gigantia.
Bhavya	... Dilenia Indica.
Bhringa-rája	... Wedelia Calendulacea ; Eclipta Erecta.
Bhu-champaka	... Kemferia Rotunda.
Bhu-Kadamba	... Blumnia lacera.
Bhumi-Kushmánda ...	... Batatas paniculata ; Ipomœa Digitata.
Bhumyámalaki	... Phyallanthus Niruri.
Bhu-Nimba	... Swertia Cherata.
Bhurja-patra	... Betula Bhojapattra.
Bhuta-kes'i	... Corydalis Govoniana.
Bhu-trina	... Andropogon Schoenanthus.
Bilva	... Aegle Marmellos.
Bimbiká	... Coccinia Indica.
Brahmadandi	... Mimosa pudica.
Brahma-yashtiká	... Clerodendron Siphonanthus.
Bráhmi	... Siphonanthus Indica ; Herpestis Mouniera.
Briddha-dáraka	... Argyreira speciosa.

C

Chakramarda	... Cassia Tora.
Champaka	... Michelia Champaca.
Chanaka	... Cicer Arietinum.
Chandana	... Santalum Album.
Chángeri	... Oxalis Monadelpha ; O. corniculata.
Chavya / **Chaviká** / **Chavyaka**	... Piper Chaba.
Chhatriká	... Agaricus Campestris.
Chira-villa	... Pongamia Glabra.
Chitraka	... Pleumbago Zeylanica.
Chitraka-phala	... See Indra-váruni.
Choraka / **Chora-pushpi**	... Andropogon Acicularis.
Chuta	... See Ámra.

D

Dádima / **Da'dimba**	... Punica Granatum. Pomegranate.
Dandálu	... Dioscorea Alata.
Dandotpala	... Canscora decussata.
Danti...	... Baliospermum Montonum ; ,, Axillare.
Darbha	... Poa cynosuroides.
Dadru-marda / **Dadrughna** ...	... Cassia alata.
Dáru / **Dáru-Haridrá** / **Dárvi** ...	... Berberis Asiatica ; ,, Lycium.
Dási	... Barleria cristata ; B. Caerulea.
Deva-dáru	... Cedrus Deodara.
Dhánya	... Oryza sativa. Paddy.
Dhanyáka	... Coriandrum Sativum.
Dhátaki	... Woodfordia floribunda.
Dhátri	... See Ámalaka.
Dhava	... Anogeissus latifolia.
Dhustura	... Datura fastuosa.
Dirgha-patoliká' ...	... Luffa Cylindrica.
Dirgha-vrinta	... Calosanthes Indica.
Drákshá	... Vitis Vinifera. Grapes.

Dravantiká / **Drávanti**	... ... Anthericum Tuberosum.
Drona-pushpi	... ... Leucas Linifolia.
Dugdhika'	... ... Oxystelma esculentum.
Durálabhá	... ... Alhagi Maurorun.
Durvá	... ... Cynodon dactylon.

E

Elá	... ... Elettaria Cardamomum. Cardamom.
Eranda	... ... Ricinus communis.
Erváruka	... ... Cucumis utillissimus.

G

Gairika	... ... Red ochre.
Gaja-Pippali	... ... Scindapasus officinalis.
Gámbhári	... ... Gmelina arboria.
Gandha-Trina	... ... See Katrina.
Gángeruki	... ... Hedysarum lagopodioides.
Gauri	... ... See Haridra'.
Gáyatri	... ... See Khadira
Godhápadi	... ... Vitis pedata.
Godhuma	... ... Triticum Vulgare. Wheat.
Goji	... ... Elephantopus Scaber.
Gokshura	... ... Tribulus terestris.
Guda-Tvak	... ... Cinnamomum zeylanicum.
Gudnchi	... ... Tinospora Cordifolio. Coculus cordifolius.
Guggulu	... ... Balsamodendrom Mukul.
Gunjá	... ... Abrus precatorius.

H

Hamsa-padi	... ... Vitis pedata.
Haridrá	... ... Curcuma longa.
Hari-Mudga	... ... Phaseolus mungo.
Haritaki	... ... Terminalia chebula. Chebulic Myrobalan.
Hasti-karna-Paláśa	... ... Butea Superba.
Hasti-Pippali	... ... Scindaspus officinalis.
Hasti-sundá	... ... Heliotropium Indicum.
Haya-máraka	... ... Nerium odorum.
Hijjala	... ... Barringtonia acutangula.
Hila-mochiká	... ... Enhydra Heloncha.

Hingu ... ... Ferula asafoetida.
Hingu-patri ... ... Balanites Roxburghii.
Hrivera ... ... Pavonia odorata.

I

Ikshu ... ... Saccharum officinarum. Sugarcane.
Ikshu-gandhá ... ... Tribulus terrestris.
Indra-Váruni ... ... Citrulus Colocynthis. Cunnis melo.
Indra-Yava... ... ... (Seeds of) Hollarrhena anti-dysenterica
Indra-vriksha ... ... Wrightia Tinctorea.
Ingudi ... ... See Putranjiva.

J

Jambira ... ... Citrus medica.
Jambu ... ... Eugenia gambolana.
Jata'-ma'nsi ... ... Valeriana Jatámánsi.
Ja'ti ... ... Jasminum Grandiflorum.
Jatila' ... ... See Jatamansi.
Ja'ti-phala ... ... Myristica Fragrans.
Javá ... ... Hibiscus Rosa sinensis.
Jayapa'la ... ... Croton tiglium.
Jhinti ... ... Barlarea Cristata.
Jiraka ... ... Cuminum Cyminum. Cumin seed.
Jivaka ... ... Pentaptera tomentosa.
Jayanti ... ... Sesbania aculatia ; S. Ægyptiaca.

K

Kachu (Mána) ... ... Arum Indicum ; A. Colocasia.
Kachchhurá ... ... See Átmaguptá.
Kadali ... ... Musa Sapientum. Plantain.
Kadamba ... ... Anthocephalus Kadamba.
Kaivarta-Mustaka ... ... Cyperus Rotundus.
Káka-janghá ... ... Leea hirta.
Ka'ka-ma'chi ... ... Solanum nigrum.
Káka-násá ... ... Cocculus Suberosus; Solanum Indicum
Kakkola ... ... (Fruit of) Cocculus Indicus.
Kákoli ... ... Tizyphus Napeca.
Kalambi ... ... Convobrelus repens.
Kalinga ... ... See Kutaja.
Kamala ... ... Nebembium Speciosum. Nymphaea Lotus.
Kampilla ... ... Mallotus Philippensis.

Ka'nchana	Bauhinia Variegata.
Kankarola	Alangium Hexapetalum.
Kanku **Kangu**	Panicum Itailcum.
Kantakári	Solanum Xanthocarpum ; S. Jaquinii.
Kapi-kachchhu	See Átma-Guptá.
Kapittha	Feronia Elephantum.
Karanja	Pongamia Glabra.
Ka'ravella	Momordica charantia ; M. Muricata.
Karavira	Nerium Odorum.
Kari-Pippali	See Gaja-pippali.
Karkáru **Karka'ruka**	Cucumis utilatissimus ; Convolvulus Panicutatus. Mello.
Karkata-S'ringi	Rhus succedanea ; Pistaca Integerruna.
Karkati	Cucumis utilatissimus.
Karmaranga	Averrhoa Arambola.
Kárpási	Gossypium Harbeceum.
Karpura	Cinamomum Camphora.
Kás'a	Soccharum Spontaneum.
Kása-marda	Cossia Saphora.
Ka's'mari	See Gámbhári.
Kataka	Strychnos Potatorum.
Katphala	Myrica Sapida.
Ka-trina	Andropogon Schoenanthus.
Katuká **Katuki** **Katu-Rohini**	Picrorrhiza Kurroa ; Helleborus Niger.
Kes'a-rája	Eclipta Erecta.
Ketaki	Pandanus Odoratissimus.
Khadira	Accacia Catechu.
Kharjura	Phoenix sylvestris. Dactylifera.
Kims'uka	Butea frondosa.
Kira'ta **Kira'ta-tikta**	Swertia Chirata.
Kodrava	Paspalum Scrobiculatum.
Kokila'ksha	Hygrophila Spinosa.
Kovida'ra	Bauhinia Variegata.
Koranta	Barleria Prionitis.
Kosha'taki	Luffa Amara ; L. Acutangula.
Kramuka	Areca Catechu.
Krishna'	See Pippali.
Krishna-jiraka	Nigella Sativa.

Krita-vedhana ... ... See Koshátaki.
Kshetra-Parpata ... ... Oldenlandia herbacea.
Kshira-kanda ... ... See Vidári.
Kshudra-mallika' ... ... Oxalis Corinculata.
Kulattha ... ... Dolichos Biflorus ; D. uniflorus.
Kuma'ri ... ... Aloe Barbadensis. Indica.
Kumbhiká ... ... Pistia Stratiotes.
Kumkuma ... ... Crocus Sativus. Saffron.
Kumuda ... ... Nymphaea Esculenta.
Kunda ... ... Jasminum Multiflorum.
Kuruvaka ... ... Barleria Cristata.
Kuśa ... ... Poa Cynosuroides.
Kushmánda ... ... Benincasa Cerifera.
Kustumburu ... ... See Dhanya'ka.
Kushtha ... ... Sausurea Auricnlata ; Lappa.
Kutaja ... ... Holarrhena Antidysenterica.

L

Lajjálu ... ... Mimosa Pudica.
La'kshá ... ... Coccus Lacca. Lac.
Lakucha ... ... Artocarpus Lakucha.
Lámajjaka ... ... Andropogon Muricatus.
Lángali, Lángaliká ... ... Gloriosa Superba.
Lasuna ... ... Allium Sativum.
Latá-Kasturi, Lata'-Kasturiká ... ... Abelmoschus Moschatus.
Lavanga ... ... Caryophylius Aromaticus.
Lavali ... ... Phyllanthus distichus.
Lavani ... ... Anona Reticulata.
Likucha ... ... Rnmex Vesicarius.
Limpáka ... ... Citras acida. Lemon.
Lodhra (Rodhra) ... ... Symplocos racemosa.
Loni ... ... Portulaca oleracea.

M

Madana ... ... Randia dumetorum.
Ma'dhavi ... ... Hiptage Mádhablatá.
Madhuka ... ... Glycyrrhiza Glabra. Liquorice.
Madhuka ... ... Basia Latifolia.
Madhu-Karkatika' ... ... Citrus Acida.
Madhurika' ... ... Pimpenella Anisum. Anisi.

Ma'gadhi	... See "Pippali."
Maha'-kosha'taki ...	... Luffa Pentandra.
Mahá-nimba	.. Melia Azedarach.
Mahá-Tikta	... Andrographis Paniculata.
Mahá-valá...	... Sida Rhomboidea.
Mahá-vriksha	... See Snuhi.
Makushtha	... Phaseolus Aconitifolius.
Málati	... Aganosam Crayophyllata ; Jasminun Grandiflorum.
Mallika	... Jasminum Samboc.
Mána / **Mánaka** }	... Arum Indicum.
Mandára	... See "Paribhadra."
Manduka-parni	... Hydrocotyle Asiatica.
Manduki	... See Bráhmi.
Manjishtha'	... Rubia Cordifolia.
Ma'nsi	... Nardostachys Jatámánsi.
Maricha	... Peper Nigrum, Black pepper.
Márisha	.. Amaranthus obraceus.
Markati	... See "S'uka-s'mbi."
Márkava	... Wedelia Calendulacea.
Maruvaka	... Ocymum Caryophyllatum.
Másha	... Phaseolus radiatus, Roxburghii.
Másha-parni	... Teramnus labialis.
Masura	... Vicia lens, Lens Esculenta. Ervum Lens.
Mátulunga...	... Citrus Medica.
Mesha-S'ringi	... Gymnema Sylvestre.
Methi / **Methiká** }	... Trigonella foenum graecum.
Mishi (Madhuriká)... ...	... Foeniculum vulgari Anisi.
Muchukundu	... Peterospermum Suberfolium.
Mudga	... Phaseolus Mungo.
Mudga-parni	... Phaseolus Tribolus.
Mulaka	... Raphanus Sativus. Redish.
Munditiká	... Saphoerontheus Hirtus.
Munja	... Saccharum Munja.
Murá-mánsi	... Murraya Exotica.
Murva'	... Sanseviera Zeylanica.
Mushali / **Mushalika'** }	... Curculigo Orchioides.
Mushika-parni	... Salvina Cucullata.

Mushkaka	... Schrebera Switenioides.
Mustaka / **Musta**	... Cyperus Rotundas.

N

Na'diká	... Corchorus Olitorius.
Nága-dantiká	... Helistropium Indicum.
Nága-Keśara / **Nága-pushpa**	... Mesua Ferrea.
Naganá	... See "Jyotishmati."
Nágara-mustaka ...	... Cyperus pertinuis.
Nága-valá	... Sida spierosa. Graveolens.
Nága-valli	... Betelo, Coevica Betel, Piper Betel.
Naktá	... Gloriosa Superba.
Nakta-mála	... Pangamia Globra.
Nákuli	... Vanda Roxburghii.
Nala	... Phragmites Karka.
Nalada	... See "Us'ira."
Nandi	... Ficus Cingalensis.
Nárikela	... Cocos Nucefera. Cocoa-nut.
Nichula	... Calamus rotang.
Nidigdhiká	... See "Kantakári."
Nikumbha	... See "Danti."
Nila / **Nili** / **Nilini**	... Indigofera Tinctoria. (Indigo plant).
Nilotpala	... Nymphea Stellata.
Nimba	... Melia Azadirachta Indica (Neem).
Nimbuka	... Citrus Medica. (Lemon).
Nirbishá	... Kyllingia Monocephala.
Nirgundi	... Vitex Negundo.
Niśá	... Curcuma Longa.
Nishpáva	... Vigna Catjang.
Nivára	... Wild variety of Oryzo sativa.
Nyagrodha	... Ficus Bengalensis

P

Padma	... Nelumbium Speciosum.
Palándu	... Allium sepa. Onion.
Pálanka	... Beta Maritima.
Palankashá	... See Guggulu.
Paláśa	... Butea Frandosa.

Pálindi	... See "Trivrit."
Panasa	... Artocarpus Integrifolia.
Páribhadra **Párijáta**	... Erythrina Indica.
Parkati	... Ficus Infectoria.
Parna	... Coevika betel.
Parpata **Parpataka**	... Oldenlandia herbocea.
Parusha **Parushaka**	... Zyllocarpus Granatum.
Páshána-bheda **Páshána-bhid** ...	... Colemes Amboinicus.
Pátalá **Pátali**	... Stereopermum Suaveolens.
Páthá	... Stephanea Hernandifolio.
Patola	... Tricosanthus Diocia.
Patra	... See "Tejpatra."
Pattanga **Patranga**	... Cœsalpinia Sappan.
Phala-vriksha	... See "Panasa."
Phalini	... See "Priyangu."
Phanji	... Clerodendron Siphonanthus
Phenila	... Sapindus Triofoliotus.
Phanijjhaka	... See "Arjaka."
Pilu	... Salvdora persica.
Pindálu	... Dioscorea globosa.
Pinda-kharjura	... Phoenix Dactylifera.
Pinditaka	... Randia Dumeterum.
Pippali	... Piper longum.
Pita-Sála	... Pterocarpus Marsupium.
Piyála	... Buchanania Latifolia.
Plaksha	... Ficus Infectoria.
Práchinámalaka	... Flacourtia cataphracta.
Prapaundarika	... Nymphoea Lotus.
Prapunnáda	... Cassia Tora.
Pras'árani	... Pæderea Fœtida.
Prikká	... Trigonella Corinculata.
Prisniparni	... Hemionites Cordifolia.
Priyangu	... Aglaia Roxburghiana.
Puga	... Areca Catacchu.
Punarnavá	... Boerhavia diffusa.
Pundarika	... Nelumbium speciosum.

Punnága	... Culophyllum Inophyllum ; Ochrocarpus Longifolius.
Pushkara	... Sassurea Lappa. Costus Speciosus.
Putaná	... Mentha Arvensis.
Putika	... Guilandina Bonducella ; Cæsalpinia Bonducella.
Putiká	... Besella Rubra.
Puturájiva	... Putranjiva Roxburghii.
Puti-karanja	... Caesalpinia Bonducella.

R

Rájádana	... Mimusops Indica.
Raja-druma	... See "Aragvadha"
Rája-koshátaki	... Luffa Cylindrica.
Raja-másha	... Vigna Sinensis.
Rajani	... See "Haridrá."
Rája-Sarshapa	... Brassica Juncea.
Raja-Vriksha	... See A'ragvadha.
Ra'jiká / **Ráji**	... See "Sarshapa."
Rakta-Chandana ...	... Pterocarpus Santalinus.
Rakta-Chitraka	... Plumbago Rosea.
Rakta-Eranda	... Ricinus Communis.
Rakta-Kánchana ...	... Bauhimia Variegata.
Rakta-kuruntaka ...	... Barlaria Cristola.
Rakta-Sáli	... Oriza Sativa.
Raktotpala...	... Nymphoea Rubra.
Rála	... Mimosa Rubicanlis.
Ra'sná	... Vanda Roxburghii.
Rasona	... Allium Sativum. Garlic.
Rasála	... Mangifera Indica. Mango.
Rasánjana	... Extract of Berberis Asiatica.
Renuká / **Reunka**	... Piper Anantiacum.
Rohisha	... Andropogon Schaenanthus.
Rohitaka	... Amoora Rohitaka.
Rodhra	... See "Lodhra."

S

Sahachara	... Barlaria Cristata.
Sahadevá	... See "Balá."
Śailaja	... A species of Lichen.

S'alvála ... ... Blyxa Octandra.
Sáka... ... ... Sectona grandis.
Sakra ... ... See "Kutaja."
Sákhotaka ... ... Streblus asper.
Sála ... ... Shorea robusta.
Sálmali ... ... Bomba malabaricum.
Sála-parni ... ... Desmodiumgan Geticum.
Sáli ... . Oryza Sativa.
Sálincha ... ... Alternanthera Sessilis
Sallaki ... ... Boswellia Serrata.
Sáluka ... ... Bulbs of different species of Nymphoea.
Sami ... ... Accacia Suma.
Samkha-pushpi ... ... Andropogon Aciculatum. Causcorc Decassata.
Samkhini ... ... Andropogon Ocicularis.
Sana ... ... Crotalaria Juncea.
Sankhálu ... . Pachyrizno Angulius.
Saptalá ... ... Accaia Concinna.
Sapta-chchháda, Saptaparna ... ... Alstonia Scholaris.
Sara ... ... Saccharum Sara.
Sarala ... ... Pinus Longifolia.
Sarala' ... ... See "Trivoit."
Sara-pumkha ... ... Tephrosia purpurea.
Sáriva' ... ... Hemidesmus Indicus.
Sarjikshára ... ... Carbonate of Soda.
Sarja ... ... Shorea Robusta.
Sarpagandhá ... ... Ophioxylon Serpentinum.
Sarpa'kshi ... ... Ophiorrhiza Mungos.
Sarshapa ... ... Brassica Campestris. Sinapis Jungca.
Satáhvá ... ... Pencedanum Sawa. P. Graveolens.
Satamuli, Sata'vari ... ... Asparagus Racemosus.
Sataparva' ... ... Bamboo.
Satapushpi ... ... See Satáhvá.
Sathi ... ... Curcuma Zerumbet.
Satina ... ... Pisum Sativum.
Sebunda, Sehundi ... ... Euphorbia Neriifolia.
Selu ... ... Cordia Myxa.
Sepha'lika' ... ... Nyctanthus Arbortristis.

Śigru	... Moringa Pterygospermum.
Śikhari	... Boswellia Serrata.
Śila'jatu	... Bitumenous substance.
Śimbi	... Dolichos gladíatus.
Śimśapa'	... Dalbergia Sissoo.
Sindhuva'ra	... Vitex Negundo.
Śirisha	... Albizzia Lebbek.
Śita-śiva	... Cinnamomum Camphora.
Śleshma'taka	... See "S'elu."
Śobhánjana	... Moringa Pterygospermum.
Souvira'njana	... Antimony.
Śra'vani	... Sphaeranthus Indicus.
Śriga'la-Kantaka ...	... Argemone Mexicana.
Śriga'la-Koli	... Zizyplus Oenoplia.
Śrikhanda	... Yellow variety of Sandal-wood.
Śringa'taka	... Trapa Bispinosa.
Śringavera	... Gingiber officinal.
Śringi	... See "Karkata-S'ringi."
Śriparni	... Gmelina arborea.
Śriphala	... Aegle Marmellos.
Śriva'sa	... Resin of Pinus longifolia.
Śriveshtaka	... Gum of Boswellia Thuripera.
Śuka-s'imbi	... Mucuna pruriens.
Śuka-na'sa'	... Orxylum Indicum.
Śukla-dugdha'	... See "S'ringátaka"
Śukla-Mudga	... Phaseolus Subloleatus.
Śunthi	... Gingiber officinal.
Śurana	... Amorphophallus Compomulatus.
Śweta-chandana	... Santalum Album.
Śya'ma'	... See "Sárivá and Trivrit." See also "Dhánya."
Śya'ma'ka	... Panicum Frumentaceum.
Śya'ma'latá, Sáriva'	... Ichnocarpus Frutescens.
Śyona'ka	... Colosanthes Indica. Oroxylum Indicum.
Singhi, Singhika'	... See "Vrihati."
Sirdha'rtha, Sirdha'rthaka	... See "Sarshapa."
Soma, Soma-lata'	... Sarcostemna Brevistigma.

Soma-ra'ji	Vernonia Anthelmintica.
Snnbi	Euphorbia Neriifolia.
Srotonjana	Antimony.
Sthala-padma	Hibiscus Mutabilis.
Sthulaila'	Amomum Subulatum.
Sudha'	See "Snuhi."
Sukshmaila'	Elettaria Cardamomum.
Sunnishannaka	Marsiba quadrifolia.
Sura-da'ru	
Sura-druma	See "Devadáru."
Surja'-varta	Cleome Viscosa.
Sushavi	Momordica Charantia.
Suvarchika'	Carbonate of Soda.
Suvarna-kshiri	Cleome felina.
Swarna-ma'kshika	Iron Pyrites.

T

Tagara	Tabernaemontana Coronaria.
Tál	Borassus Flabellisormis.
Ta'la	Yellow orpiment. See "Haritála."
Ta'la-muli	Circuligo orchioides.
Ta'lisa	
Ta'lisa'-patra	Abies Webbiana.
Tama'la	Zanthochymus Pictorius.
Ta'mbula	Peper Bettle.
Tandula	Oryza Sativa, rice.
Tandula	
Tanduliyaka	Amoranthus spinosus.
Tangana	Borax.
Ta'ra	Silver.
Teja-patra	Leaf of Lauruscassia.
Tejovati	Cardiosdermum Halicacabum.
Tila	Sesamum Indicum.
Tilvaka	See Lodhra.
Tinduka	Dyospyros Glutinosa. Eubyopteris.
Tinisa'	Dalbergia Oujeinensis.
Tintida	Tamarindus Indica.
Trapusha	Cucumis Sativus.
Tra'yanti	
Tra'yama'na'	Ficus Heterophylla.

Tvak-kshiri ... ... Curcuma Anguslifolia.
Tri-kantaka ... . See "Gokshura."
Triputi ... ... Lathyrus Sativus.
Trivrit ... ... Ipomea Turpethum.
Tuda ... ... Morus Indica.
Tulasi ... ... Ocimum Sanctum.
Tumburu ... ... Zanthoxylum Alatum.
Tuttha ... ... Sulphate of Copper.
Tuvari }
Tuvarika' } ... . Cajanus Indica.
Tvak ... ... Cinnamon bark. See "Guda-tvak."

U

Udumbara ... ... Ficus Glomerata.
Upodika' ... ... Bsella Alba, Rubra Cordifolia.
Uśira ... ... Andropogon Neuricatum.
Utpala ... ... Nymphœa Stellata.

V

Vacha }
Vacha' } ... ... Acorus Calamus.
Vadara ... ... Ziziphus Jujuba.
Va'g'uji ... ... See "Somarάji"
Vajri ... ... Euphorbia Antiquorum.
Vakula ... ... Mimusops Elengi.
Vamśa ... ... Bambusa Arundinacae. Bamboo.
Vandhujiva .. .. Pentapetes Phœnica.
Vamśaka ... ... Saccharum Afficonarum.
Vams'a-lochana ... ... Bamboo Mama.
Vana-ka'rpa'sa ... ... Hibiscus Vitiolius.
Vana-yama'ni ... ... Seseli Sambae.
Vanjula ... ... Calamus Rotong.
Va'ra'hi ... ... Randla Dumetorum.
Va'ra'hi-kanda ... ... Dioscorea Globosa.
Va'rta'ku ... ... Bringal.
Varuna ... ... Crataeva Nurvala ; C. Religiosa.
Va'sa' }
Va'saka } ... ... Adhatoda Vasika.
Va'stuka ... ... Chenopodium Album.
Vata ... ... Ficus Bengalensis.
Vata-patri ... ... Coleus Amboinicus.

Vetasa	... Calamus Rotong.
Vida'ri / **Vidári-kanda**	... Batatas paniculata
Vidanga	... Embelia Ribes ; E. Robusta.
Vijaya'	... Canabis Sativa.
Vimbi	... Ciphalandra Indica.
Vit-Kharkdira	... Accacia Fernisiana.
Vibhitaka	... Terminalia Bebrica.
Vrihati	... Solanum Indicum.
Vrihi...	... Oryza Sativa. See "Dhánya."
Vrischika'li / **Vrischira**	... A variety of Punarnavá.
Vrisha	... See "Vásá."
Visha	... Aconitum Ferox.
Visa	... Lotus-root.
Vya'ghri	... See "Kantakári."

Y

Yajnodumvura	... Ficus Glomerata.
Yama'ni / **Yama'nika'**	... Lingusticum Ajwan; Carum Copticum
Yashti-madhu	... Glycyrrhiza Glabra. Liqucorice.
Yava	... Hordeum Hexastichum. Barley.
Yavaksha'ra	... Carbonate of Potash.
Yava'saka (Yása)... ...	... Alhgi Maurorum.
Yuthika'	... Jasminum Auriculatum.

N. B. In the preparation of Appendices we have gratefully laid under contribution "Vaidyaka-Sabdasindhu," "Wilson's Sanskrit and English Dictionary," "Indian Plants and Drugs", "Kavirāji S'ikshá," etc.

PRINTED BY HARI CHURN RAKSHIT AT THE BHARAT MIHIR PRESS,
25, ROY BAGAN STREET, CALCUTTA.

Spotted something that isn't quite right?

Let us know and we'll fix it for future reprints. And as a thank you for your diligence, we'll send you a free Sothis book of your choice.

publisher@sothis.press

This page intentionally left blank

Made in United States
Orlando, FL
05 November 2026

90229677R00308